COMPUTED TOMOGRAPHY IN RADIATION THERAPY

Computed Tomography in Radiation Therapy

Editors

C. Clifton Ling, Ph.D.

Professor and Head
Physics Section
Division of Radiation Oncology
and Biophysics
The George Washington University
Medical Center
Washington, D.C.

Charles C. Rogers, M.D.

Professor and Director
Division of Radiation Oncology
and Biophysics
The George Washington University
Medical Center
Washington, D.C.

Robert J. Morton, M.Sc.

Chief
Radiation Therapy Branch
Division of Training
and Medical Applications
Bureau of Radiological Health
Rockville, Maryland

Raven Press ■ New York

Raven Press, 1140 Avenue of the Americas, New York, New York 10036

Made in the United States of America

Library of Congress Cataloging in Publication Data
Main entry under title:

Computed tomography in radiation therapy.

Based on material presented at the symposium held Sept. 18–19, 1981, Arlington, Va., sponsored by the American Association of Physicists in Medicine.
Includes bibliographies and index.
1. Cancer—Radiotherapy—Congresses.   2. Tomography—Congresses.   I. Ling, C. Clifton.   II. Rogers, Charles C.   III. Morton, Robert J.   IV. American Association of Physicists in Medicine. [DNLM: 1. Neoplasms—Radiotherapy.   2. Tomography, X-ray computed. QZ 269 C738]
RC271.R3C65   1982   616.99′40642   81–48496
ISBN 0–89004–831–2

Preface

Computed tomography (CT) plays an increasingly important role in furthering the success of the treatment of human oncological diseases by radiation therapy. With its use, traditional problems such as uncertainties in tumor delineation, errors in critical normal tissue localization, and dose computation inaccuracies owing to tissue inhomogeneity can be avoided or significantly reduced. Many studies have yielded convincing evidence on the potential impact of CT in improving the prognosis of cancer patients treated by radiotherapy. Further research and studies are necessary on a broad front, however, to optimize the usefulness of CT in radiotherapy planning. In the present context, the term radiotherapy planning is used in the broad sense, encompassing the processes of tumor diagnosis, delineation of tumor extent, localization of critical normal tissue, selection of radiation modality and beam energy, simulation of therapy treatment, and clinical dosimetry calculation. Thus a team effort is required by radiation oncologists, diagnosticians, clinical physicists, computer scientists, and others.

The present volume was organized to provide a multidisciplinary exchange of the various important aspects of applying CT to radiation therapy. The first section of this book addresses the application of CT data to clinical radiotherapy as viewed from the perspectives of radiation oncologists and diagnosticians; the usefulness of CT data in therapy planning for lesions of various sites and types is considered. The second section deals with the technical aspects of and current developments in the use of CT data in radiotherapy. The third group of chapters considers the implication of CT data relative to clinical dosimetry calculation, particularly regarding inhomogeneity correction for different types of radiation. The fourth and final section contains a summary viewed from the clinical and the physics and engineering perspective. Radiotherapists, radiation oncologists, and radiologists will find this material helpful in the utilization of computed tomography in radiotherapy planning.

C. Clifton Ling, Ph. D.

Acknowledgments

This volume is based on material presented at the symposium "Computed Tomography in Radiotherapy" (September 18–19, 1981, Arlington, Virginia) sponsored by the American Association of Physicists in Medicine and supported in part by Grant CA/FD 31160-01 from the National Cancer Institute and the Bureau of Radiological Health.

Contents

Technical Aspects of the Utilization of CT
in Radiotherapy Planning

Computed Tomography in Clinical Dosimetry

Review and Projection

Contributors

Mark Abrams
Division of Radiation Biophysics
Department of Radiation Medicine
Massachusetts General Hospital and
*   Harvard Medical School*
Boston, Massachusetts 02114

Sucha O. Asbell
Department of Radiation Therapy
Albert Einstein Medical Center
Philadelphia, Pennsylvania 19141

A. M. Bedford
Departments of Oncology and Physics as
*   Applied to Medicine*
Middlesex Hospital Medical School
London, United Kingdom

R. J. Berry
Departments of Oncology and Physics as
*   Applied to Medicine*
Middlesex Hospital Medical School
London, United Kingdom

George T. Y. Chen
Division of Biology and Medicine
Lawrence Berkeley Laboratory
Berkeley, California 94720

Prakairut Cook
Department of Diagnostic Radiology
University of Kansas Medical Center
Kansas City, Kansas 66103

J. R. Cunningham
Physics Division
The Ontario Cancer Institute
Toronto, Ontario, Canada M4X 1K9

Samuel Dwyer
Department of Diagnostic Radiology
University of Kansas Medical Center
Kansas City, Kansas 66103

Robert S. Fields
Department of Radiotherapy
The University of Texas System Cancer
*   Center and M. D. Anderson Hospital*
*   and Tumor Institute*
Houston, Texas 77030

Benedick A. Fraass
Radiation Oncology Branch
Division of Cancer Treatment
National Cancer Institute
National Institutes of Health
Bethesda, Maryland 20205

Hal A. Fredrickson
Computer Systems Laboratory
Division of Computer Research and
*   Technology*
National Institutes of Health
Bethesda, Maryland 20205

Eli Glatstein
Radiation Oncology Branch
Division of Cancer Treatment
National Cancer Institute
National Institutes of Health
Bethesda, Maryland 20205

A.S. Glicksman
Department of Radiation Oncology
Rhode Island Hospital
Section on Radiation Medicine
Brown University
Providence, Rhode Island 02912

Michael Goitein
Division of Radiation Biophysics
Department of Radiation Medicine
Massachusetts General Hospital and
*   Harvard Medical School*
Boston, Massachusetts 02114

David J. Goodenough
Division of Radiation Physics
The George Washington University
*   Medical Center*
Washington, D.C. 20037

Mahroo Haghbin
Departments of Radiation Oncology and
*   Diagnostic Radiology*
Wayne State University
Detroit, Michigan 48201

R. Mark Henkelman
*Ontario Cancer Institute and Department
of Medical Biophysics
University of Toronto
Toronto, Ontario, Canada M4X 1K9*

Kenneth R. Hogstrom
*Department of Physics
The University of Texas System Cancer
Center and M. D. Anderson Hospital
and Tumor Institute
Houston, Texas 77030*

R. E. Land
*Section on Radiation Medicine
Brown University
Department of Radiology
St. Joseph Hospital
Providence, Rhode Island 02907*

John S. Laughlin
*Department of Medical Physics
Memorial Hospital
New York, New York 10021*

Kyo Rak Lee
*Department of Diagnostic Radiology
University of Kansas Medical Center
Kansas City, Kansas 66103*

Allen S. Lichter
*Radiation Oncology Branch
Division of Cancer Treatment
National Cancer Institute
National Institutes of Health
Bethesda, Maryland 20205*

L. Loverock
*Departments of Oncology and Physics as
Applied to Medicine
Middlesex Hospital Medical School
London, United Kingdom*

Carl M. Mansfield
*Department of Radiation Therapy
University of Kansas Medical Center
Kansas City, Kansas 66103*

James E. Marks
*Washington University School of
Medicine
The Edward Mallinckrodt Institute of
Radiology
Division of Radiation Oncology
St. Louis, Missouri 63110*

Edwin C. McCullough
*Division of Radiation Therapy
Department of Oncology
Mayo Clinic/Foundation
Rochester, Minnesota 55901*

D. L. McShan
*Department of Radiation Oncology
Rhode Island Hospital
Section on Radiation Medicine
Brown University
Providence, Rhode Island 02912*

Jack E. Meyer
*Department of Radiology
Massachusetts General Hospital and
Harvard Medical School
Boston, Massachusetts 02114*

Radhe Mohan
*Department of Medical Physics
Memorial Hospital
New York, New York 10021*

Peter Mondalek
*Departments of Radiation Oncology and
Diagnostic Radiology
Wayne State University
Detroit, Michigan 48201*

John E. Munzenrider
*Department of Radiation Medicine
Massachusetts General Hospital
Boston, Massachusetts 02114*

Beate Planskoy
*Departments of Oncology and Physics as
Applied to Medicine
Middlesex Hospital Medical School
London, United Kingdon*

Helen Pollari
*Department of Mechanical Engineering
Massachusetts Institute of Technology
Cambridge, Massachusetts 02138*

Satish C. Prasad
*Physics Section
Mallinckrodt Institute of Radiology
Washington University School of
Medicine
St. Louis, Missouri 63110*

James A. Purdy
Physics Section
Mallinckrodt Institute of Radiology
Washington University School of
   Medicine
St. Louis, Missouri 63110

L. E. Reinstein
Department of Radiation Oncology
Rhode Island Hospital
Section on Radiation Medicine
Brown University
Providence, Rhode Island 02912

Richard Riley
Department of Medical Physics
Memorial Hospital
New York, New York 10021

Peter L. Roberson
Battelle Pacific Northwest Laboratories
Richland, Washington 99352

Derek Rowell
Department of Mechanical Engineering
Massachusetts Institute of Technology
Cambridge, Massachusetts 02138

Mary Anne Seago
Department of Radiation Therapy
Albert Einstein Medical Center
Philadelphia, Pennsylvania 19141

H. Gunter Seydel
Department of Radiation Oncology and
   Diagnostic Radiology
Wayne State University
Detroit, Michigan 48201

Robert Smereka
Departments of Radiation Oncology and
   Diagnostic Radiology
Wayne State University
Detroit, Michigan 48201

N. Suntharalingam
Thomas Jefferson University
Philadelphia, Pennsylvania 19107

Jan van de Geijn
Radiation Oncology Branch
Division of Cancer Treatment
National Cancer Institute
National Institutes of Health
Bethesda, Maryland 20205

Kenneth E. Weaver
Division of Radiation Physics
The George Washington University
   Medical Center
Washington, D.C. 20037

Judy Wiles
Department of Mechanical Engineering
Massachusetts Institute of Technology
Cambridge, Massachusetts 02138

John W. Wong
Ontario Cancer Institute and Department
   of Medical Biophysics
University of Toronto
Toronto, Ontario, Canada M4X 1K9

Darwin Zellmer
Department of Radiation Therapy
University of Kansas Medical Center
Kansas City, Kansas 66103

Alkis Zingas
Departments of Radiation Oncology and
   Diagnostic Radiology
Wayne State University
Detroit, Michigan 48201

COMPUTED TOMOGRAPHY IN RADIATION THERAPY

Computed Tomography in Radiation Therapy,
edited by C. C. Ling, C. C. Rogers, and
R. J. Morton. Raven Press, New York © 1983

An Overview of Clinical Requirements and Clinical Utility of Computed Tomography Based Radiotherapy Treatment Planning

Allen S. Lichter, Benedick A. Fraass, Jan van de Geijn,
*Hal A. Fredrickson, and Eli Glatstein

*Radiation Oncology Branch, Division of Cancer Treatment, National Cancer Institute, National Institutes of Health, Bethesda, Maryland 20205; and *Computer Systems Laboratory, Division of Computer Research and Technology, National Institutes of Health, Bethesda, Maryland 20205*

Radiation therapy treatment planning depends heavily on the physician's and physicist's abilities to accurately reconstruct cross-sectional anatomy. For this reconstruction, body contour outlines have been typically obtained with wire, plaster, or other devices. Outlines representing tumors and normal structures were then drawn into the contours with information obtained from orthogonal radiographs and conventional x-ray and isotope studies. At best, these cross-sectional reconstructions were crude approximations, but until quite recently they were the best available data, and treatment planning was based entirely on them.

During the second half of the 1970s a new diagnostic technique, computed tomography (CT), has seen increasing use, and the information obtained from CT scans has literally revolutionized treatment planning. With CT, a true, accurate reproduction of cross-sectional anatomy is readily available on multiple levels. Studies in the literature indicate that this single test results in a major modification of treatment volume or treatment technique in 30 to 60% of cases even after all other conventional information is taken into account (6). Diagnostic radiologists have been quick to explore the applications of this new technology, to the point where keeping current in the CT literature is by itself a formidable task. The 1980 *Index Medicus* lists more than 1,300 articles pertaining to CT. Radiotherapists have also been investigating how this new information can be used to improve dose delivery to patients. The Radiation Oncology Branch at the National Cancer Institute (NCI) has been fortunate to have a dedicated whole-body scanner (EMI5005), and the machine has seen increasing use during the last 2 years as our interface between the CT scanner and treatment planning system has been improved. The purpose of this chapter is to present an overview of the use of CT scanning in clinical radiotherapy based on both personal experience and reports in the literature.

1

IMAGING REQUIREMENTS IN RADIOTHERAPY

It is little wonder that cervical cancer and head and neck cancer were among the first noncutaneous tumors approached with radiotherapy at the beginning of this century. These tumors are, for the most part, visible and palpable to the clinician, and thus localization can be done by clinical examination. Tumor response can be monitored daily if necessary.

The majority of cancers at other sites are neither visible or palpable. Yet the radiotherapist must be able to accurately localize these tumors and target areas, as well as relate the targets quantitatively to their anatomic surroundings. This localization must be performed, for the most part, "on instruments," and the radiotherapist relies heavily on imaging techniques transposed from diagnostic radiology. Once located, the tumor area must be treated, not once but reproducibly 20 to 30 times over a period of many weeks. To make matters more complicated, the localization, planning, and treatment are done with different instruments, at different times, and often by different personnel.

Most imaging equipment is designed and built for the major user of such machines—diagnostic radiologists. There are, however, fundamental differences between the needs of diagnostic imaging and radiotherapeutic imaging. For the most part, diagnostic radiology is called on to answer a *qualitative* question: "Is there pathology on this particular study?" Certainly this job is complex, as secondary questions such as, "Is the pathologic process better or worse?" or "What might be causing this pathology?" come into play. However, the fundamental question of normal versus abnormal is of overriding concern. In contrast, radiotherapy patients usually arrive with pathology slides in hand, so the question is no longer, "Is there disease?" We know there is. The questions become: "Where is the tumor? How big is it? What lies nearby? Where has it spread? Where is it likely to spread?" Thus radiotherapy imaging techniques must be *quantitative* in nature. Furthermore, as the typical radiotherapy treatment machine is large and has limited maneuverability, the proper treatment position is often a major factor in producing a proper therapeutic plan. Thus any quantitative imaging techniques used by radiotherapists should allow for optimal patient positioning. In other words, imaging equipment must be compatible with treatment machinery. Yet another difference between diagnostic and radiotherapy imaging is the concern for three-dimensional information by radiotherapy. Whereas diagnostic radiologists view information mostly with two-dimensional planar images, radiotherapists deal with three-dimensional (3-D) volumes, and our imaging techniques must be able to yield such 3-D information as a basis for radiotherapy treatment planning.

CT AS A SOLUTION TO IMAGING NEEDS IN RADIOTHERAPY

There is little doubt that CT scanners represent a major advance toward satisfying the complex imaging requirements of radiotherapy. Fundamentally, multislice CT scanning produces a three-dimensional matrix of information elements from which two-dimensional images in any plane can be reconstructed, as well as quasi-three-dimensional images. If done carefully, the information is quantitatively accurate, readily interpretable, storable, retrievable, and easily displayed on film, paper, or video screen. The technique of CT scanning is virtually tailor-made for radiotherapy treatment planning. When exploring this technology, several important questions arise:

1. The CT scanner is a device basically in the domain of the diagnostic radiologist. Can scans taken for diagnostic purposes be used for radiotherapy treatment planning? If not, why?
2. What specifications are required in a CT scanner used for radiotherapy treatment planning?
3. How is this new technology used in radiotherapy treatment planning?
4. What improvements, if any, have resulted from CT treatment planning?

DIAGNOSTIC CT SCAN VERSUS RADIOTHERAPY TREATMENT PLANNING SCAN

Over the short time that CT scans have been used for radiotherapy planning, a number of important differences have emerged between the diagnostic and the therapy planning scans (Table 1); we believe that a current diagnostic CT scan is in general not adequate for sophisticated therapy planning. The most obvious difference is the patient couch, rounded in the diagnostic setting but necessarily flat for the therapy scan. A simple insert for the rounded couch can be fabricated from wood or plastic to remedy this problem.

The treatment planning scan requires that the patient be placed in the scanner in such a way as to duplicate the treatment position as closely as possible. Not only must the patient be level, but the extremities should be in the same position they will be in for treatment. Failure to duplicate the treatment position greatly reduces or cancels the usefulness of the study. Obviously, with small scanning apertures this positioning requirement cannot be met in all cases. Fortunately, many of the newer scanners are available with a large aperture that eliminates these "physical" problems.

Most diagnostic scans are done with bolus bags filling the empty spaces between the patient and the scanner aperture. These bolus bags can easily distort the patient contour and should not be used in a scan designated for planning purposes.

TABLE 1. *Differences between diagnostic and therapy planning CT scanning*

Diagnostic scanning	Therapy scanning
Rounded couch	Flat couch
Positioning not critical	Reproducibility of treatment position critical
Bolus acceptable	No bolus
Accurate reproducibility of patient geometry not necessary	Faithful one-to-one geometric reconstruction a must
	Quiet respiration allowed
No motion for best image	External markings define a coordinant system for planning
External markings not necessary	

Many diagnostic scanners are not adjusted to provide a faithful one-to-one reproduction of structure size. For example, the lateral dimension may be slightly enlarged whereas the anterior-posterior dimension is slightly reduced compared with true life-size measurements. This distortion is of little consequence to the diagnostician, who is more concerned with identifying abnormal structures and relationships. However, it is inadequate for the radiotherapist, who requires precision in treatment planning scans. Even if the scanner is accurately calibrated, the appearance of the scan on the video screen and on the hard-copy x-ray film may be distorted (Fig. 1). This discrepancy stems from the difficulty of producing an undistorted picture from a gently curved video screen; a distortion of up to 10% can result (11). In order to guard against these errors, any CT unit used for treatment planning must be monitored to ensure fidelity of film images before these films are used in the treatment planning process. Phantoms containing geometric objects of known size should be scanned and the resulting film images measured. Preferably, the scan data is transferred directly to the treatment planning computer, bypassing completely the film interface.

An additional problem when scanning for treatment planning results from the diagnostician's need for an image as free from motion artifact as possible. Hence scans performed in diagnostic departments are usually done with the patient holding his breath, often in deep inspiration. As patients receiving radiotherapy are treated during quiet respiration, this technique of deep breath holding can dramatically distort the anatomy seen in thoracic and abdominal scans (1). We first noted this problem when comparing CT contours to those obtained on the simulator. The CT contour invariably had a larger anteroposterior (AP) thickness, and several centimeters of difference was not rare. We finally traced this problem to the conventional instructions to patients to "take a deep breath and hold it" for the 20-sec scan time. We then verified this phenomenon by scanning patients in deep inspiration and

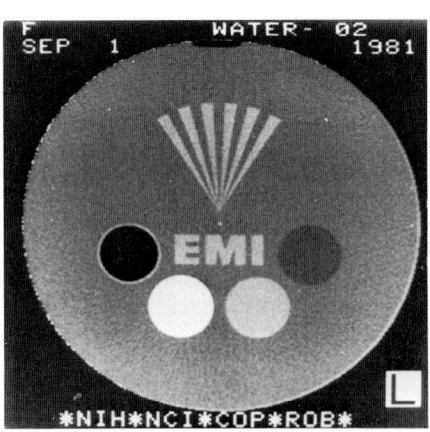 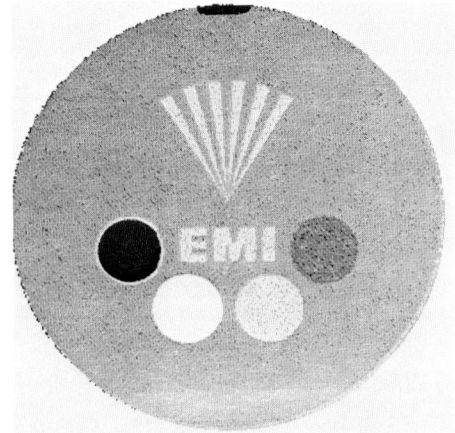

FIG. 1. Left: X-ray of the round water phantom. The resultant image is oblong. **Right:** Same scan from the line printer directly interfaced to the planning computer. The shape is round.

again with quiet respiration (Fig. 2). Not only is the anatomy altered by deep breath holding, but the density of the lung parenchyma changes, a phenomenon that can be of concern if CT-based lung density corrections are used in treatment planning (1). We and others now scan our patients in quiet respiration, accepting a minor motion artifact in our films (8). Diagnostic departments must be instructed to perform the scans in this fashion if they are to be used for radiotherapy treatment planning.

Finally, scans performed for treatment planning purposes should have external markers placed on the patient's skin, either to mark the portals of a previous localization or to form a set of isocentric coordinates for later use in simulation and treatment. Diagnostic scans are rarely done with such external markers.

We caution radiotherapists not to allow a therapy-directed CT scan to be used for diagnostic interpretation. A scan taken with skin markings, in a therapy position on a flat couch, without bolus, with breathing continuing during the scan, and over the limited volume of the treatment portal may not be suitable for diagnostic interpretation and should not substitute for a high-quality diagnostic scan. CT scans for initial diagnosis and follow-up should be performed in a standard manner that is optimal for the diagnostic radiologist. Such scans can then be compared over a period of time. The single therapy-directed scan has a unique purpose and should be used for therapy planning only.

In summary, there are major differences between diagnostic and radiotherapy CT scans, and the radiation oncologist and physicist should be aware that simply photographically enlarging a diagnostic CT scan and planning treatment based on the resultant image is less desirable than repeating the scan with the proper technique compatable with the treatment planning process.

"OPTIMAL" SCANNER FOR CT TREATMENT PLANNING

Several authors have addressed the topic of the optimal scanner for CT treatment planning (4,13,22), and we draw from them as well as from our own experience

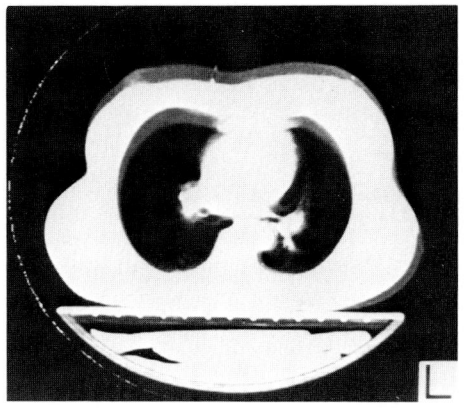

FIG. 2. Influence of deep inspiration on thoracic anatomy. Two scans are superimposed, one taken in quiet respiration and one in deep inspiration. The darkest lung density and whitest soft tissue density is the size of the patient in quiet breathing. The gray areas represent the additional patient thickness and lung volume during deep inspiration.

when making a list of desired features (Table 2). First, the scan time should be relatively short, 5 sec or less. This minimizes motion artifact during respiration and results in higher-quality images. We do not believe, as some authors do (24), that a slow scan time that allows considerable respiration is better, based on the rationale that the patient breathes during treatment. With that reasoning extended, port films or simulator films should also have a 20- to 30-sec exposure, obviously an impossibility except for treatment machine "image" films that are exposed for the entire treatment and are quite poor at displaying detail. The time to check for the effects of respiration is under fluoroscopy on the simulator table. CT scans should be done rapidly to obtain the highest image quality possible. Interestingly, the rapid scan time does not seem to be associated with the ability to scan appreciably more patients per day. In one diagnostic survey, time per patient was reduced only 10% from scanners with a scan time of 5 to 10 sec versus scanners with a scan time of 10 to 60 sec (10).

The scanner should have a thin slice capacity—5 mm is probably adequate— enabling closely spaced scans to be obtained to ensure accuracy of tumor volume determination. Thick slices taken at wider spacing can miss small extensions of tumor and can give a false indication of tumor size. Closely spaced thin slices also provide the data necessary for detailed reconstruction in sagittal or coronal planes.

If one is going to take many rapid, thin slices, then the scanner should be able to accumulate data for many scans without having to take lengthy pauses to reprocess scans. Goitein suggests a 60-scan memory (4).

The ideal scanner should have "scout film" capability, i.e., the ability to take or reconstruct conventional-appearing AP and lateral radiographs with the CT cuts indexed to these "films." This feature is of considerable help when it comes to comparing CT data with conventional x-ray and simulator films. Expansion of this plain film capability coupled with reconstructions in arbitrary planes may replace many of the functions of the simulator in the near future.

The scanner should have a large aperture so that the patient may be simulated in the treatment position; a diameter of 60 cm is the minimum. An effect of the inability to duplicate treatment position is indicated in Figs. 3 and 4. The purpose of CT scanning is not only to reveal occult extensions of the tumor in question but also to verify that a previous simulation was adequate. A patient with Hodgkin's disease is simulated in Fig. 3, and the projection of the mantle blocks is outlined on the skin in radiopaque material. Because the small scanner opening cannot

TABLE 2. *"Optimal" CT scanner for radiotherapy treatment planning*

Rapid scan time
Thin slices (5 mm)
Ability to accumulate 40 to 60 scans without pause
"Scout" film—at least AP and lateral—indexed to scans
Large aperture ($\geqslant$60 cm)
Scan without bolus material
Reconstruction in any plane

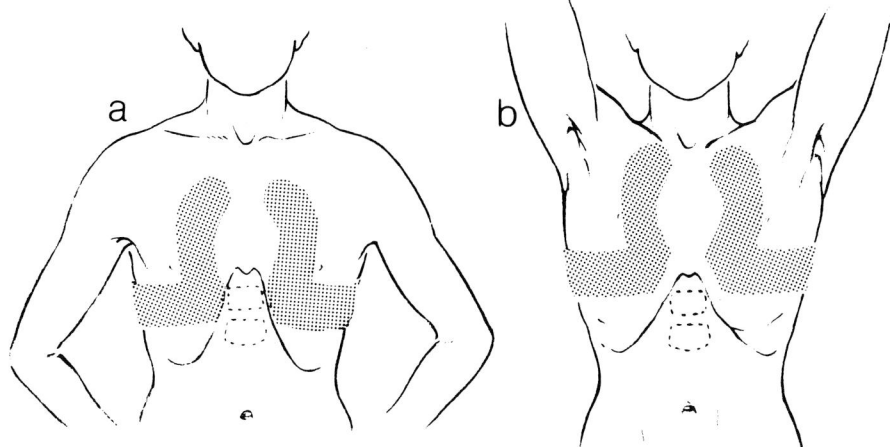

FIG. 3. **a:** Mantle blocks outlined on patient's skin with arms-on-hips position. **b:** With arms-over-head position, required to fit into scanner, the skin marks move appreciably.

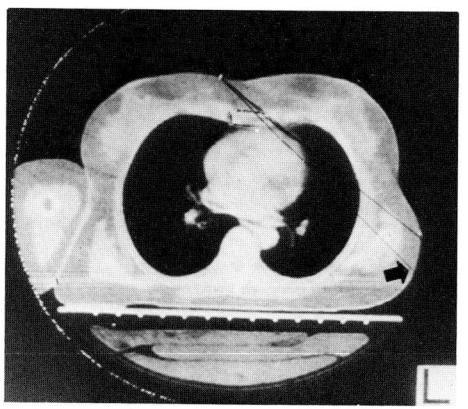

FIG. 4. Influence of arm position during scanning for breast treatment planning. The medial and lateral entrance points for the breast fields are marked on the skin and connected with solid lines. With arm at right angles (actual treatment position), the lateral entrance point is lower *(at arrow)* than it is with the arm raised overhead (scan position). The scan can give a misleading impression of the true treatment volume.

accommodate the patient with hands on hips or even arms at sides, the patient is scanned in an "arms over head" position. This moves the skin marks considerably, making the scan difficult to interpret, as the projection of the mantle blocks is no longer in the simulated position.

A similar situation occurs in patients with breast cancer (Fig. 4). Here the entrance and exit points for the tangential breast fields are marked on the patient's skin. A line between the two points would define the high dose volume. During treatment the patient's arm on the treated side is out at almost a right angle, but for the scan it must be raised overhead. The skin marks again move, creating the false impression that the fields are more shallow in the lung than they really are during treatment. Thus a large scanner aperture is required to reduce positioning errors that are inherent in scanners with small apertures.

It should again be noted that quality scans should be obtainable without the need for bolus material. Finally, the room that houses a CT scanner used for radiotherapy treatment planning should be equipped with side and ceiling lasers to allow rotation-free positioning of patients.

USE OF A CT SCANNER IN RADIOTHERAPY TREATMENT PLANNING

The first step in treatment planning in our opinion remains the standard isocentric simulation (Fig. 5). This localization technique establishes the treatment position for both the body and the extremities, and yields some general ideas as to the margins of the treatment volume. An approximate isocenter is selected, and the lateral and anterior centers are marked. In addition, one can view the treatment region with different gantry angles to gain some insight as to possible field configurations. Standard contours at multiple levels are taken for use as a reference using either a mechanical device or ultrasound. The need for an immobilization device is determined (Fig. 6).

The patient is then CT scanned on a flat couch as close to the treatment position as possible. The anterior and lateral isocentric lines as well as the simulated port dimensions are marked on the skin with opaque angiography catheters which show

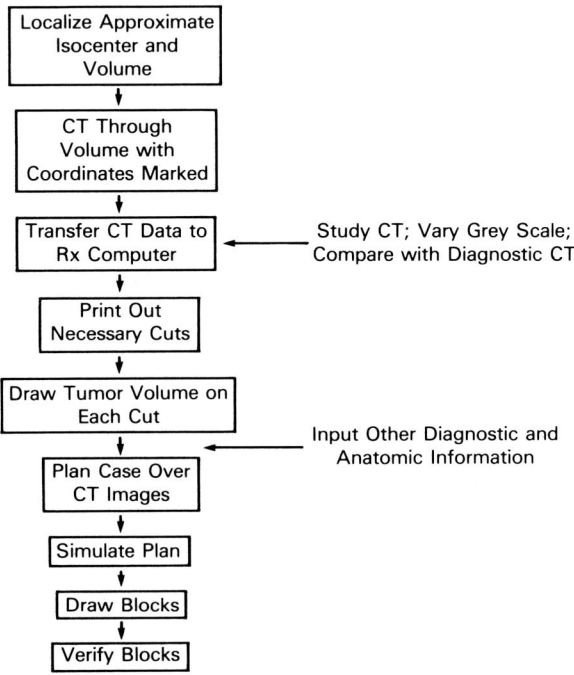

FIG. 5.   Treatment planning sequence when CT is utilized.

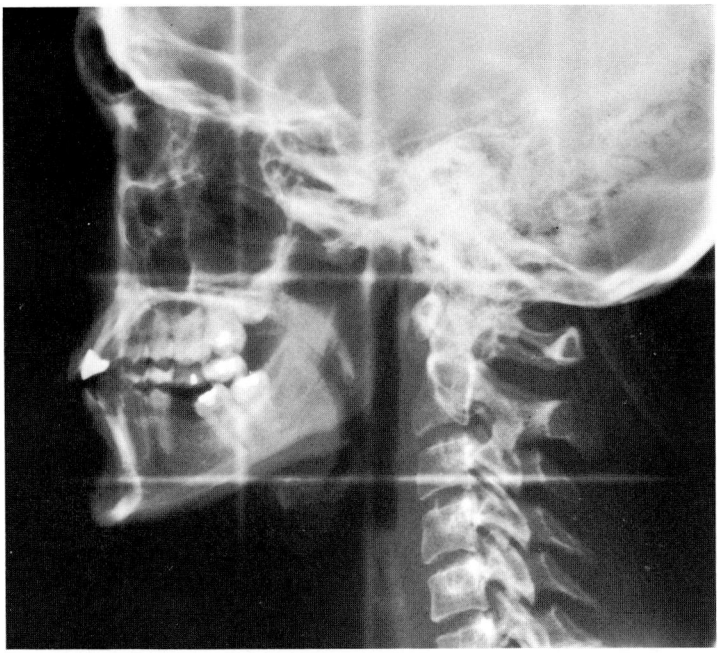

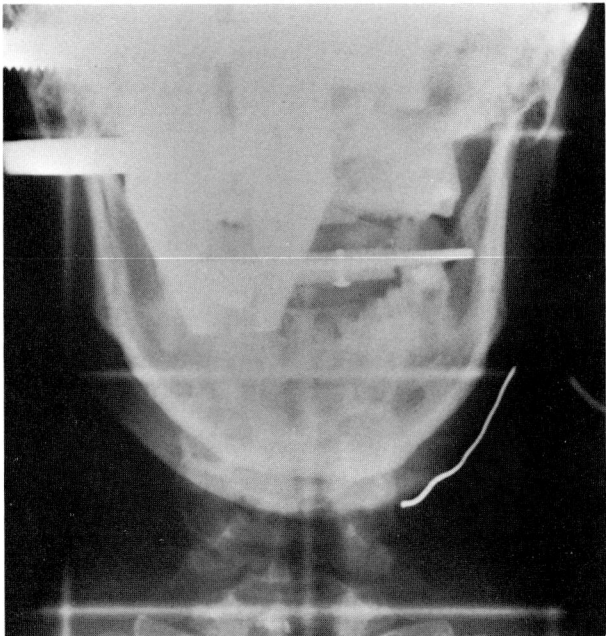

FIG. 6. Top: Lateral localization film in a patient with a submandibular salivary gland tumor. **Bottom:** Anterior localization film.

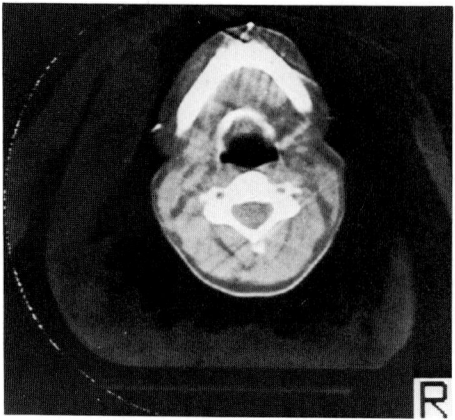

FIG. 7. CT scan through center of volume. Isocentric points are marked with catheters on skin.

up nicely on the scan and do not distort the scan image (Fig. 7). Scans are taken at 1.5 cm spacing on our scanner but can be taken at closer intervals with scanners that have thinner slice capabilities. We always try to scan one cut above and below the marked boundaries of the field to ensure coverage superiorly and inferiorly.

The scan is then viewed, the appropriate window setting is selected, and the scan is transferred to x-ray film for study. The cuts that are to be used for treatment planning are selected and transferred from the scanner tape to the disc pack of our treatment planning computer. It is at this point that comparison with the diagnostic scan and consultation with the diagnostic radiologist is most important. These selected scans are enlarged to life size on a matrix printer (Fig. 8), and the consistency of the CT contour with the previously acquired external contour is confirmed. The treatment volume is carefully outlined on these life-sized printouts, or the scans can be displayed on the television monitor of the computer and the tumor

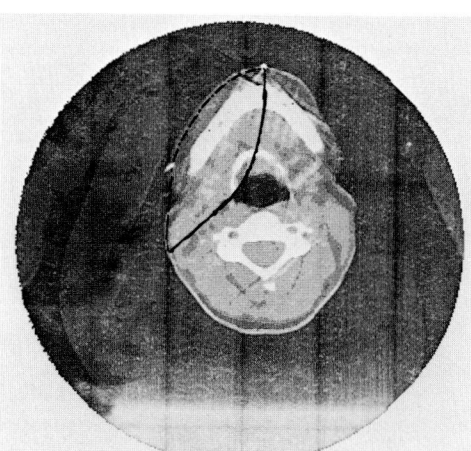

FIG. 8. Scan in Fig. 7 enlarged to life size on the line printer. Target volume is outlined.

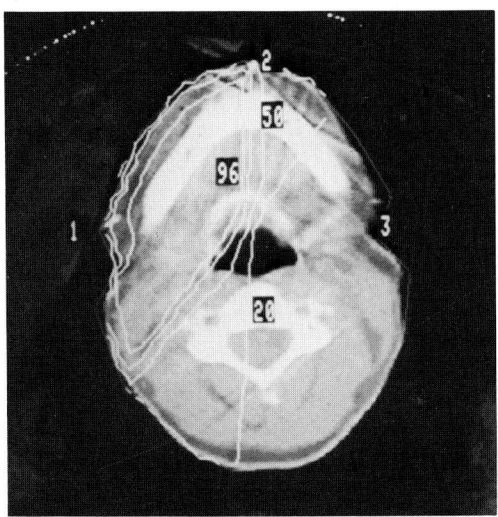

FIG. 9. The beams are selected and the case planned directly on the CT scan.

volumes entered with the "joy stick." The final planning is done directly on the CT scan (Fig. 9). Tissue inhomogeneity factors can be used if desired.

The isocenter of the localization films is taken as the origin of the treatment planning computer coordinate system. Once the treatment plan is completed, the new isocenter, if different, is measured from this origin. The patient is then taken back to the simulator, the new isocenter is located, and the plan is verified with anterior and lateral films as well as films of each treatment portal. These x-rays are inspected to ensure that the intended volume is indeed enclosed within the portals as a check on the entire process. When individualized protection for specific organs is desired, blocks are then drawn and fabricated to shield those normal structures. The location of these blocks is entered into the computer, and the treatment plan is run again so that the influence of the blocks on the dose distribution can be fully appreciated. The anterior and lateral films serve as isocentric reference films for comparison to portal films taken on the treatment machine.

Altogether, the planning process employing CT scans is actually more time-consuming than planning straight from simulator films and external body contours. There must be a tangible payoff for this extra effort, and therapists and physicists have tried for the last few years to quantitate the "improvement" in treatment planning that can be derived from the use of CT scans. These studies are summarized below.

VALUE OF CT-DIRECTED TREATMENT PLANNING

The types of change necessitated by CT planning as compared to conventional planning are summarized in Table 3. Overall, about 40% of plans are altered, with the greatest percentage, roughly 30%, being due to an inadequate target volume that needed to be enlarged after CT planning was performed. The usefulness of CT

TABLE 3. *Changes in treatment plans as a result of CT (all sites)*

Study[a]	No. of patients	Inadequate or marginal tumor volume (No.)	Volume made smaller (No.)	Any change[b] (No.)
Brizel (2)	72	29 (40%)	4 (6%)	44 (61%)
Emami (3)	32	10 (31%)	2 (7%)	17 (53%)
Goitein (7)	77	32 (42%)		40 (52%)
Hobday (8)	123	29 (26%)	5 (4%)	47 (38%)
Lee (15)	22	3 (14%)		3 (14%)
Munzenrider (16)	75	35 (47%)	18 (24%)	41 (55%)
Pilepich (17)	97	21 (22%)		21 (22%)
Prasad (18)	50	11 (22%)	2 (4%)	13 (26%)
Schlager (20)	21	6 (29%)		6 (29%)
Seydel (21)	23	4 (17%)	2 (9%)	6 (26%)
Van Dyk (24)	60			36 (60%)
Totals	652	180 (28%)	33 (5%)	274 (42%)

[a]By first author.
[b]Volume larger or smaller, change modality, change intent, etc.

planning by site of tumor is examined in Table 4. The greatest impact appears to be on abdominal tumors, where conventional radiographic techniques are the weakest. However, it is clear that many other tumor sites show considerable benefit from CT information.

A small note of caution must be sounded concerning the literature (Table 5). One must wonder if the amount of effort that went into conventional planning was similar to that which went into CT planning. If not, could the conventional plan have been improved with a more thoughtful and concentrated approach? Precisely what conventional studies were used to perform the plans that CT later improved on? Were these simple conventional radiographs, or were standard tomography, ultrasound, or contrast studies used? If *all* appropriate conventional studies were used, would CT planning still show the same level of improvement? It must also be pointed out that not all studies published in the literature used consecutive cases.

TABLE 4. *Any change due to CT by tumor site*

Study[a]	Thorax	Abdomen	Pelvis
Brizel (2)			61% (44/72)
Emami (3)	53% (17/32)		
Goitein (7)	44% (7/16)	86% (12/14)	44% (18/41)
Hobday (8)	30% (9/30)	79% (15/19)	31% (20/65)
Lee (15)			14% (3/14)
Munzenrider (16)	67% (14/21)	64% (16/25)	41% (7/17)
Pilepich (17)			22% (21/97)
Prasad (18)	26% (13/50)		
Schlager (20)			29% (6/21)
Seydel (21)	26% (6/23)		
Totals	38% (66/172)	74% (43/58)	36% (119/327)

[a]By first author.

TABLE 5. *Benefits of CT treatment planning: caution when interpreting the literature*

Was a similar amount of effort put forth for conventional and CT planning?
What conventional studies were used—standard radiographs, contrast material, ultrasound?
If consecutive cases were not studied, what factors influenced case selection?
If CT planning suggests a change in treatment planning, is it always assumed to be correct?

Many patients were apparently selected to receive CT scans and then CT planning. If they were selected because their tumor location might have made a CT plan a likely improvement, the study could have been biased and the outcome of superiority for CT planning would have been predetermined. Finally, when CT shows a previously undetected structure adjacent to a tumor region, can anyone be certain that the structure is tumor and not collapsed lung, adjacent bowel, etc.? When CT and conventional planning disagree, is CT always to be assumed correct? Obviously CT scans cannot see microscopic tumor extension or detect internal architectural patterns of small anatomic structures. There is still no substitute for a skilled clinician's understanding of the natural history and spread patterns of tumor; this expertise cannot be superseded by CT.

Additional concerns surface when one attempts to quantify the value of CT treatment planning. Does every "geographic miss" spell disaster for the patient? Clearly not. Some patients have recurrences despite perfect tumor coverage. Others show dissemination of disease. Others will be on a combined treatment with chemotherapy, and the drugs may be able to control the extension of tumor outside the portal. In still other situations the tumor will be missed by only one of several portals; with shrinkage that occurs during therapy, all the responding tumor may eventually be treated in the high dose volume.

One may try to estimate the number of additional "cures" (5-year disease-free survivors) that can be expected as a result of CT scanning. Goitein has elaborated on this point (5), and an adaptation of his calculations appears in Table 6. Briefly, only patients whose tumor coverage was inadequate or marginal would benefit from an increased chance of cure; those whose tumor volume actually was reduced because of CT scanning are most likely to benefit by a smaller chance of normal tissue complications. From the literature, approximately 40% of cases studied have poor tumor coverage that can be improved by CT. If one assumes that local tumor control is likely in 60% of these cases (higher in some cases, e.g., cervical cancer,

TABLE 6. *Increased number of disease-free survivors resulting from CT planning*

Of 100 patients seen	No. benefited
40% with improved coverage of tumor	100 × 40% = 40 patients
60% of these may achieve local control	40 × 60% = 24 patients
50% of these would have had local control despite poor coverage (chemotherapy, implant, etc.)	24 × 50% = 12 patients
50% of these will succumb to metastases	12 × 50% = 6 patients

After Goitein (5).

and lower in other cases, e.g., lung or pancreatic cancer), then the chance of CT-enhanced local cure is 40% × 0.60 = 24%. Of this 24%, some might achieve local control by combined modality therapy (Ewing's sarcoma, small cell lung cancer), and some could be controlled by boost techniques, e.g., cone-down fields or interstitial implantation. In some cases the "marginal" miss was so marginal that with tumor regression after a few treatments the edge of the tumor would have been encompassed within all fields. If one then estimates that one-half of the patients would have achieved local control despite an inadequate initial tumor volume, one can potentially benefit 24% × 0.5 = 12%. Of this 12%, many tumors are destined to disseminate outside the treatment volume. If one estimates that one-half of the cases would disseminate, then the final benefit of CT scanning on ultimate long-term cures would be 12% × 0.5 = 6%.

The purpose of the foregoing discussion is not to suggest that CT treatment planning will cure 6% more patients. Rather, it is presented to suggest a methodology that can be used in individual tumor sites to predict outcome. In most instances the changes will be a few percent at best, and such small differences could never be demonstrated in a prospective trial and probably would get lost in a sea of confounding variables in any retrospective or even prospective analysis. Nonetheless, it is reassuring to be able to calculate that CT scanning probably contributes to the cure of some patients. Increasing the cure rate from radiotherapy by just 1% represents an additional 1,500 to 2,000 lives nationwide. [Approximately 300,000 patients receive radiotherapy per year, about half with curative intent (14).]

The preceding discussion about potential benefits of CT mentioned nothing about decreased complications. Clearly some patients have the size of their treatment portals reduced through CT scanning. Some have a better recognition of the relationship of normal tissue to the tumor volume, so that better shaping of a high dose volume results in a lower dose to normal tissues. These changes result in fewer long-term complications, but the magnitude of such a decrease is virtually impossible to measure or estimate.

CT-directed treatment planning most likely adds a small increment to the overall cure rate stemming from radiotherapy treatment and reduces the number of serious complications. Rarely does a procedure come along that yields this dual benefit.

SITES WHERE CT TREATMENT PLANNING IS LIKELY TO BE OF VALUE

In our experience, treatment planning for almost any tumor site can benefit from CT-based planning. However, the plans are likely to improve the treatment of some sites more than others, as outlined in Table 7. The central nervous system (CNS) is the region where CT scanning had its first applications, and it remains the most frequently scanned area diagnostically. From a therapy standpoint, most CNS malignancies require whole-brain irradiation, and CT-based planning is therefore not crucial. However, coning-down of fields can be greatly facilitated by CT-based planning, and tumors of the pituitary region are most often planned with CT guidance.

TABLE 7. *Probable impact of CT on radiotherapy planning by primary site*

Site	Better coverage of tumor volume	Avoidance of normal tissue
CNS	+/−	+ (cone down)
Head and neck	−	+ (cone down)
Thorax	+ +	+ +
Abdomen	+ +	+ +
Pelvis	+ +	+ +

− = seldom important (<10%). + = occasionally important (10 to 30%). + + = frequently important (>30%).

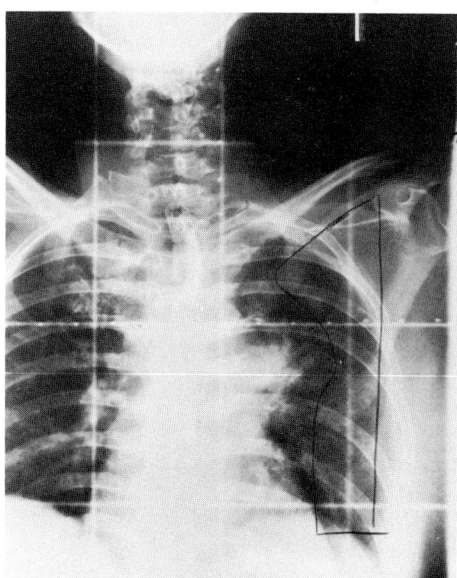
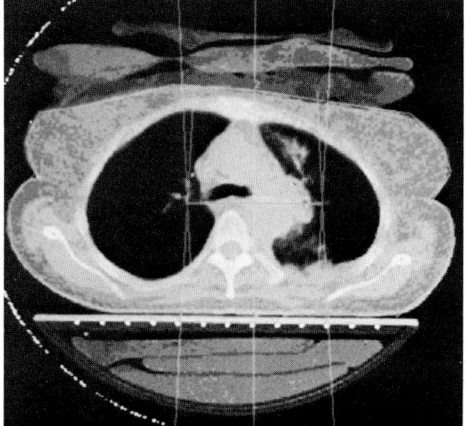
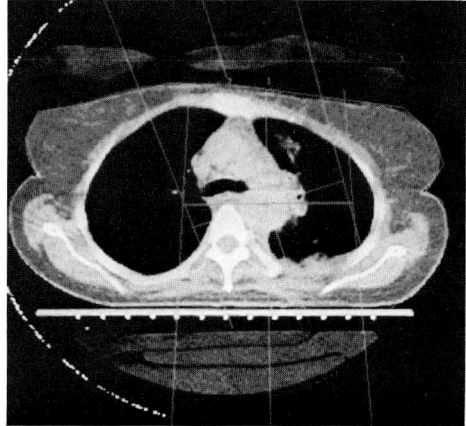

FIG. 10. **Left:** Simulator film of a patient with a small-cell lung cancer in the left hilum. Shielding block to protect normal lung is drawn. **Top right:** Fields superimposed on the CT scan through the hilar mass. Posterior pleural-based tumor is being missed. **Bottom right:** Treatment fields are enlarged and angled to encompass all of the tumor.

The head and neck area is a region where CT is very useful for quantitating tumor extent and thus accurately staging disease. This appears to be especially true in regions that cannot be palpated or directly visualized, e.g., the paranasal sinuses (9). However, it is unlikely that CT scanning will significantly change the treatment volume, as most head and neck tumors are treated with large fields that encompass all known regions at risk. Thus tumor volumes are rather standardized based on site. CT is valuable in designing field arrangements that spare normal tissue in head and neck cancer, e.g., coned-down wedged oblique fields to avoid the spinal cord. CT is also useful for determining tissue inhomogeneity factors in areas such as the paranasal sinuses.

It is in the thorax, abdomen, and pelvis where CT treatment planning has made its biggest impact. Examples in each region where CT proved invaluable are presented in Figs. 10, 11, and 12.

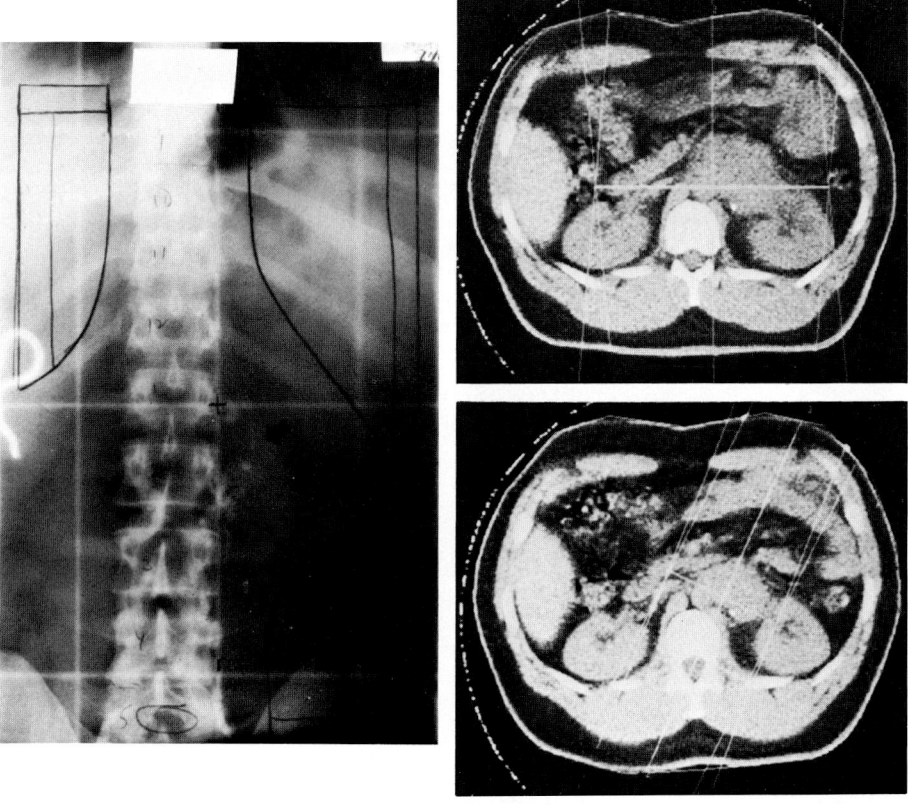

FIG. 11. Left: Simulator film of a patient with a seminoma. Lymphangiography (unilateral) suggests possible nodal involvement *(arrow)*. **Top right:** Huge nodal mass in the renal hilus is easily seen on CT. Large fields are used to begin the therapy. **Bottom right:** As the tumor mass shrinks, CT shows that oblique fields will treat the tumor while sparing the kidneys.

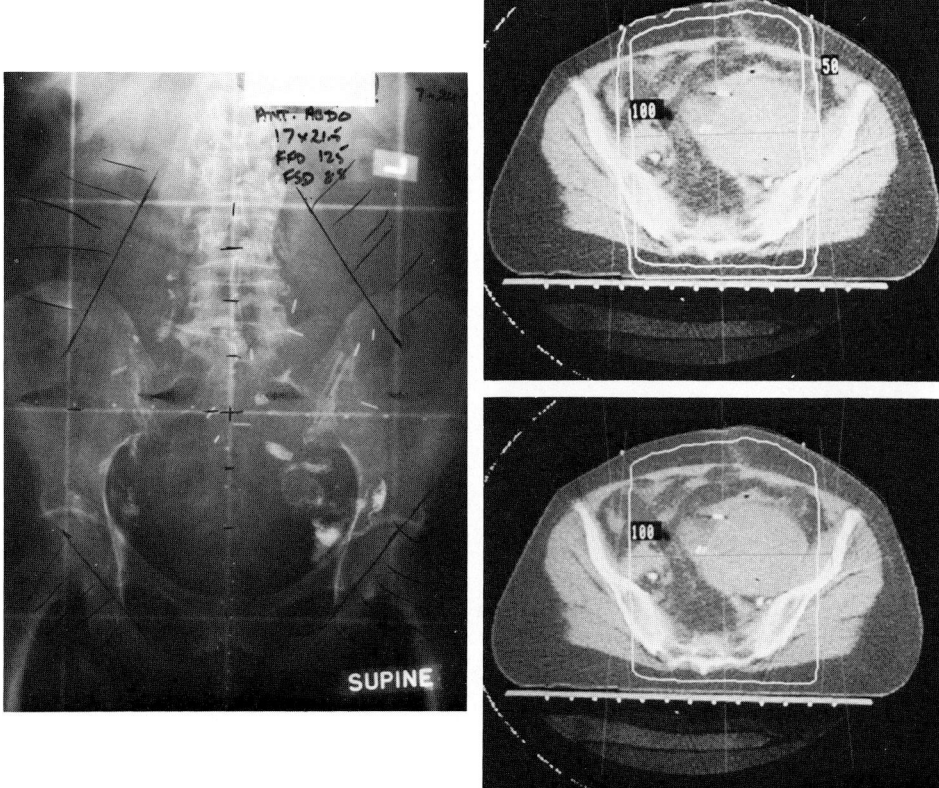

FIG. 12. **Left:** Simulator film of a patient with cervical cancer. Abnormal nodes are within the field. **Top right:** Scan through the central axis. The tumor mass extends outside the 100% isodose line. **Bottom right:** Fields are enlarged on the involved side to encompass the tumor.

ADDITIONAL USES OF CT SCANNING IN RADIOTHERAPY

More than simply providing better information to design tumor volume, CT scanning has additional uses in radiotherapy (Table 8). First, CT scanning provides accurate anatomic information that can improve the quality of daily radiotherapy

TABLE 8. *Additional uses of CT in radiotherapy planning*

Documentation of basic anatomic information
Determination of tissue inhomogeneity factors
Display of brachytherapy dosimetry—interstitial, intracavitary

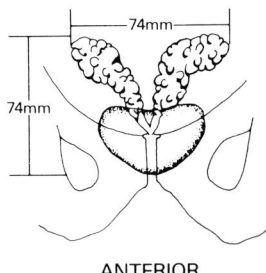

ANTERIOR

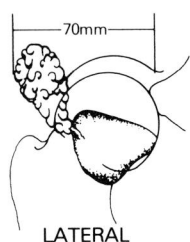

LATERAL

FIG. 13. Anatomy of the prostate and seminal vesicles: Average size in 100 patients. If the seminal vesicles are involved, a standard 8 × 8 cm portal does not allow an adequate margin in most cases. (From Pilepich et al., ref. 17, with permission.)

practice. Figure 13 illustrates this type of study. The authors (17) quantitated the size of the prostate and seminal vesicles in 100 patients with prostate cancer; appropriate portal sizes for prostate irradiation can be determined from these data. It is clear that the standard 8 × 8 cm prostate boost field inadequately covers the area at risk if the seminal vesicles are involved. In radiotherapy departments where CT scanning is not easily available, such anatomic data, unavailable prior to CT, are critical to improving practice. A similar anatomic study in breast cancer therapy was performed in our department (19). Dose to lung during primary breast irradiation was determined based on CT scans of 15 breast cancer patients. The study showed a surprising similarity of lung dose irrespective of technique, illustrating the point that plain radiographs of tangential breast fields can be misleading when estimating the amount of lung treated by a particular field configuration. CT data is far more qualitative.

Another use of CT is to quantitate tissue inhomogeneities so that appropriate correction factors can be applied. These inhomogeneity factors are crucial for charged-particle radiotherapy, as charged particles traverse a finite tissue equivalent path length. Interposition of a material of increased density may result in attenuation that causes the particles to stop before they have traversed the entire target volume. Interposition of a material of low density may allow the particles to continue well beyond the target volume and into a critical normal tissue that should have been spared.

The utility of inhomogeneity corrections for photons is less clear-cut. How big an effect on dose is seen by using inhomogeneity corrections, and how is the clinician to interpret such information? To answer the first question, we performed some sample calculations. In healthy lung, density (relative to water) has been found to vary from 0.25 to 1.0 (12). The dose distribution from a three-field esophagus plan was calculated using lung density corrections of 1.0, 0.2, and 0.5 (Fig. 14), with the equivalent path length density correction method (23). The doses to the tumor volume are seen to differ by 6%. The size of this difference implies that for lung, a pixel-by-pixel multiplane density correction is probably unnecessary, and a lung density of 0.35 would not produce greater than a 3% error even at the extremes of true lung density.

A final use applies to brachytherapy dosimetry, both interstitial and intracavitary. The ability to printout the dose distribution in such cases superimposed on the CT

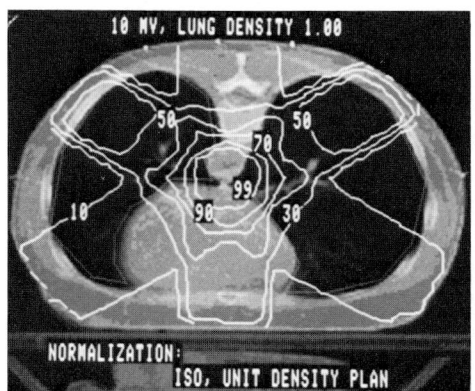
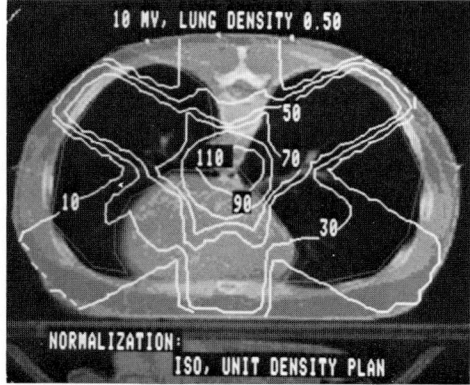
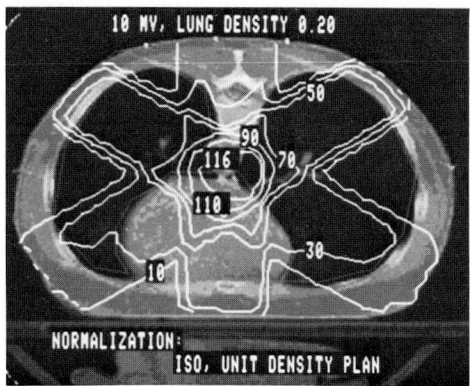

FIG. 14. Influence of lung densities on dose distribution in a patient with esophageal cancer. Lung densities of 1.0 **(left)**, 0.5 **(right)**, and 0.2 **(bottom)** are presented. Isodose plots are normalized to isocenter of the uncorrected plan. Correcting for lung density changes the high dose volume and increases the maximum dose. The differences between the plans is no more than ± 3%, suggesting that an average lung correction of 0.35 may suffice in clinical practice.

scan can help make the important transition from considering dose to points (e.g., point "A" in cervical cancer) to considering dose to volumes of tissue. In gynecologic brachytherapy, dose to a single rectal or bladder point has had a poor correlation with complications. This may be due in large measure to our inability to visualize the volume of these organs that receive a particular dose. CT scanning displays that volumetric information. Brachytherapy dosimetry is discussed further in the chapter by Mansfield et al.

FUTURE OF CT SCANNING IN RADIOTHERAPY PRACTICE

Developments in the use of CT scanning in radiotherapy treatment planning will be of two main types: (a) new technologic developments, and (b) development and extension of currently available techniques. New hardware which allows for larger apertures, faster scan times, and better resolution will clearly improve the utility of CT scanning, especially for diagnostic purposes. However, it is in the development of currently available technology where we see the greatest progress. Genuine three-dimensional imaging of anatomic structures with the possibility of viewing from any vantage point could greatly add to the planning process. Expansion of the "scout film" direction of newer scanners in conjunction with the ability to reconstruct in any arbitrary plane may obviate the need for a separate simulator. The "scout film" function could be rotated and would serve as the simulated gantry angle. Outlines of field sizes could be projected onto the scout film and the scan, including beam divergence. This type of system need not be fluoroscopically controlled, as fast scan times with video presentation of the image make such a system highly interactive. The field dimensions would have to project onto the skin using a light field or laser points so that clinical appreciation of portal location could continue and technologists could mark the skin for transfer of the patient to the treatment machine. The CT table and aperture will need modification so that patient positioning and the use of immobilization devices would not be limited by the scanner. We anticipate that progress along these lines will make the CT scanner a fundamental tool of every major radiotherapy department in the coming years.

REFERENCES

1. Battista, J. J., Rider, W. D., and Van Dyk, J. (1980): Computed tomography for radiotherapy planning. *Int. J. Radiat. Oncol. Biol. Phys.*, 6:99–107.
2. Brizel, H. E., Livingston, P. A., and Grayson, E. V. (1974): Radiotherapeutic applications of pelvic computed tomography. *J. Comput. Assist. Tomogr.*, 4:453–466.
3. Emami, B., Melo, A., Carter, B. L., Munzenrider, J. E., and Piro, A. J. (1978): Value of computed tomography in radiotherapy of lung cancer. *Am. J. Roentgenol.*, 131:63–67.
4. Goitein, M. (1979): Computed tomography in planning radiation therapy. *Int. J. Radiat. Oncol. Biol. Phys.*, 5:445–447.
5. Goitein, M. (1979): The utility of computed tomography in radiation therapy: an estimate of outcome. *Int. J. Radiat. Oncol. Biol. Phys.*, 5:1799–1807.
6. Goitein, M. (1980): Benefits and cost of computerized tomography in radiation therapy. *JAMA*, 244:1347–1350.
7. Goitein, M., Wittenberg, J., Mendiondo, M., Doucette, J., Friedberg, C., Ferrucci, J., Gunderson, L., Linggood, R., Shipley, W. V., and Fineberg, H. V. (1979): The value of CT scanning in

radiation therapy treatment planning: a prospective study. *Int. J. Radiat. Oncol. Biol. Phys.*, 5:1787–1793.

8. Hobday, P., Hodson, N. J., Husband, J., and Macdonald, J. S. (1979): Computed tomography applied to radiotherapy treatment planning: techniques and results. *Radiology*, 133:477–482.

9. Hodson, N. J., Parsons, C. A., and Hobday, P. A. (1981): The role of CT in the management and therapy planning of tumours of the paranasal sinuses. *Br. J. Radiol. [Suppl.]*, 15:29–31.

10. Hughes, G. M. K. (1980): National survey of computed tomography unit capacity. *Radiology*, 135:699–703.

11. Ibbott, G. S. (1980): Radiation treatment planning and the distortion of CT images. *Med. Phys.*, 7:261.

12. International Committee on Radiation Units (1976): Report No. 24, p. 16.

13. Kelsey, C. A., Berardo, P. A., Smith, A. R., and Kligerman, M. M. (1980): CT scanner selection and specification for radiation therapy. *Med. Phys.*, 7:555–558.

14. Kramer, S. (1981): An overview of process and outcome data in the patterns of care study. *Int. J. Radiat. Oncol. Biol. Phys.*, 7:795–800.

15. Lee, D. J., Leibel, S., Shiels, R., Sanders, R., Siegelman, S., and Order, S. (1980): The value of ultrasonic imaging and CT scanning in planning radiotherapy for prostatic carcinoma. *Cancer*, 45:724–727.

16. Munzenrider, J. E., Pilepich, M., Rene-Ferrero, J. B., Tchakarova, I., and Carter, B. L. (1977): Use of body scanner in radiotherapy treatment planning. *Cancer*, 40:170–179.

17. Pilepich, M. V., Prasad, S. C., and Perez, C. A. (1982): Computed tomography in definitive radiotherapy of prostatic carcinoma. II. Definition of target volume. *Int. J. Radiat. Oncol. Biol. Phys. (in press).*

18. Prasad, S. C., Pilepich, M. V., and Perez, C. A. (1981): Contribution of CT to quantitative radiation therapy planning *Am. J. Roentgenol.*, 136:123–128.

19. Roberson, P. L., Bodner, A., Lichter, A. S., Frederickson, H. A., Padikal, T. N., Kelly, B. A., and van de Geijn, J. (1980): Treatment planning in primary breast irradiation: the influence of technique on lung dose and dose to opposite breast. *Int. J. Radiat. Oncol. Biol. Phys.*, 6:1416 (abstract).

20. Schlager, B., Asbell, S. O., Baker, A. S., Sklaroff, D. M., Seydel, H. G., and Ostrum, B. J. (1979): The use of computerized tomography scanning in treatment planning for bladder carcinoma. *Int. J. Radiat. Oncol. Biol. Phys.*, 5:99–103.

21. Seydel, H. G., Kutcher, G. J., Steiner, R. M., Mohiuddin, M., and Goldberg, B. (1980): Computed tomography in planning radiation therapy for bronchogenic carcinoma. *Int. J. Radiat. Oncol. Biol. Phys.*, 6:601–606.

22. Stewart, J. R., Hicks, J. A., Boone, M. L. M., and Simpson, L. D. (1978): Computed tomography in radiation therapy. *Int. J. Radiat. Oncol. Biol. Phys.*, 4:313–324.

23. Van de Geijn, J. (1972): EXTDOS 71; revised and expanded version of EXTDOS, a program for treatment planning in external beam therapy. *Comp. Prog. Biomed.*, 2:169–177.

24. Van Dyk, J., Battista, J. J., Cunningham, J. R., Rider, W. D., and Sontag, M. R. (1980): On the impact of CT scanning on radiation planning. *Comp. Tomogr.*, 4:55–65.

Computed Tomography in Radiation Therapy,
edited by C. C. Ling, C. C. Rogers, and
R. J. Morton. Raven Press, New York © 1983

Computed Tomography in Radiation Therapy Treatment Planning: The Diagnostician

Jack E. Meyer

Department of Radiology, Massachusetts General Hospital and Harvard Medical School, Boston, Massachusetts 02114

A major impact of computed tomography (CT) has been in the area of diagnosis, staging, treatment, and follow-up of malignant disease. The heretofore unobtainable cross-sectional information outlining tumor volumes and relationships with adjacent normal anatomic structures has resulted in the design and implementation of potentially more accurate and complex radiation treatment plans. This should result in a higher percentage of local tumor control and a lower incidence of complications.

As few radiation therapy departments at present have the luxury of a dedicated CT unit or radiologist, an open dialogue and understanding between these specialities is necessary to utilize all the potential information available from this modality.

DISCUSSION

The diagnostic radiologist's role in the pretreatment evaluation of a patient with a malignancy is to help outline the tumor boundaries and identify regional or distant metastatic deposits. The selection of the most appropriate treatment strategy is predicated on accurate clinical staging.

A CT examination alone or in conjunction with other diagnostic studies is usually the most accurate means of detecting the extent of tumor involvement. This information is nearly indispensible for treatment planning in many organ systems prior to the initiation of radiation therapy, as well as being an aid for designing smaller boost fields when indicated.

Several studies have documented the positive impact of CT on the process of developing a radiation treatment plan in the cancer patient (5,6,10). Marginal or inadequate tumor coverage was documented in 47% (10), 41% (5), and 24% (6) of patients when CT data were compared to those derived from conventional imaging techniques. The CT information was deemed essential in 55% of patients (10), of major significance in 36% (5), and prompted a change in plan in 38% (6). These studies included combinations of thoracic, abdominal, pelvic, extremity, and head and neck tumors. Speculation based on this type of data suggests that CT scanning might improve local tumor control by an average of 6% and the 5-year survival by 3.5% (4).

Considerable new information has been accumulated on the site-specific impact of CT on the staging and treatment of malignant neoplasms (1,3,8,9,11). CT plays an important yet undocumented role in boost field design and follow-up of patients treated with irradiation. CT can accurately monitor tumor regression, so tailored radiation boost fields may be constructed or consideration given to surgery or chemotherapy when appropriate. With the increasing availability of CT equipment, previously treated patients with tumors located in anatomic areas not easily evaluated on routine radiographic studies should have access to shorter-interval CT follow-up in hopes of identifying a recurrence at the earliest stage so treatment may be more effectively administered.

The diagnostic radiologist should have a firm understanding of the basic principles and techniques of radiation therapy when monitoring a CT scan performed for treatment planning. The need for scanning in the treatment position, placement of radiopaque catheters on proposed radiation portals, and inclusion of the entire anatomy without bolus or restricting clothing seems simple enough but may be overlooked. Problems related to respiration and peristalsis have been obviated with faster scanners.

Localized tumor evaluation should be supplemented with a survey of common sites of metastatic spread. As intraabdominal and pelvic tumors manifest a wide spectrum of metastatic potential, an abdominal study should be part of the work-up of these malignancies. In a recent study of 54 patients with carcinoma of the rectum and sigmoid colon, CT delineated metastasis in the liver in 20%, the para-aortic nodes in 15%, and the adrenal glands in 7% (7). This wealth of information on bone and other organ detail must be studied at the CT monitor by the diagnostic radiologist to document all available information.

Injections of contrast material are given if deemed necessary by the radiologist. In pelvic tumors of genitourinary and gastrointestinal origin, the urine-filled bladder, nonopacified with intravenous contrast material, is easily distinguishable from surrounding structures, and subtle changes in bladder wall thickness and infiltration into the adjacent fat are well delineated. The vagina is easily identified after insertion of a small tampon. Although oral contrast material is given prior to abdominal or pelvic CT examinations, transit through the small intestine and colon varies with each patient. Nonopacified loops of small bowel may mimic tumor masses, but delayed scans and positional changes should obviate this potential diagnostic error. Some malignancies of the head, neck, and spine need separate examinations using intrathecal and intravenous contrast to best outline the complex relationships that may exist between tumor and normal tissue.

When an abnormality is discovered on CT evaluation of a patient with a known malignancy, it may be appropriate to perform a biopsy for histologic confirmation. CT-guided percutaneous aspiration biopsies are safe and accurate, and can be performed on an outpatient basis by the diagnostic radiologist in approximately 1 hr (2). This addition to the diagnostic armamentarium should result in more accurate treatment planning, as decisions would be based on histologically confirmed abnormalities rather than on speculation.

We have allocated a number of CT appointments each week to radiation therapy which are used only for treatment planning. A diagnostic radiologist with a special interest in oncology monitors these examinations after consultation with the therapeutic radiologist. Whether the cooperative effort develops in this manner or on a less formal basis, the patient is the recipient of the potential benefits.

REFERENCES

1. Brizel, H. E., Livingston, P. A., and Grayson, E. V. (1979): Radiotherapeutic applications of pelvic computed tomography. *J. Comput. Assist. Tomogr.*, 3:453–466.
2. Ferrucci, J. T., Wittenberg, J., Mueller, P., Simeone, J., Harbin, W., Kirkpatrick, R., and Taft, D. (1980): Diagnosis of abdominal malignancy by radiologic fine-needle aspiration biopsy. *Am. J. Roentgenol.*, 134:323–330.
3. Ginaldi, S., Wallace, S., Jing, B. S., and Bernadino, M. (1981): Carcinoma of the cervix: lymphangiography and computed tomography. *Am. J. Roentgenol.*, 136:1067–1091.
4. Goitein, M. (1979): The utility of computed tomography in radiation therapy: an estimate of outcome. *Int. J. Radiat. Oncol. Biol. Phys.*, 5:1799–1807.
5. Goitein, M., Wittenberg, J., Mendiondo, M., Doucette, C., Friedberg, C., Gunderson, L., Lingood, R., Shipley, W. U., and Fineberg, M. V. (1979): The value of CT scanning in radiation therapy treatment planning: a prospective study. *Int. J. Radiat. Oncol. Biol. Phys.*, 5:1787–1798.
6. Hobday, P., Hodson, N. J., Husband, J., Parker, R. P., and MacDonald, J. S. (1979): Computed tomography applied to radiotherapy treatment planning: techniques and results. *Radiology*, 133:477–482.
7. Mayes, G. B., and Zornoza, J. (1980): Computed tomography of colon carcinoma. *Am. J. Roentgenol.*, 135:43–46.
8. Meyer, J. E., and Munzenrider, J. E. (1981): Computed tomographic demonstration of internal mammary lymph node metastasis in patients with locally recurrent breast carcinoma. *Radiology*, 139:661–663.
9. Moss, A., Schnyder, P., Thoeni, R., and Margulis, A. (1981): Esophageal carcinoma: pretherapy staging by computed tomography. *Am. J. Roentgenol.*, 136:1051–1056.
10. Munzenrider, J. E., Pilepich, M., Rene-Ferrero, J. B., Tchakarova, I., and Carter, B. L. (1979): Use of body scanner in radiotherapy treatment planning. *Cancer*, 40:170–179.
11. Prasad, S., Pilepich, M., and Perez, C. (1981): Contribution of CT to quantitate radiation therapy planning. *Am. J. Roentgenol.*, 136:123–128.

Computed Tomography in Radiation Therapy,
edited by C. C. Ling, C. C. Rogers, and
R. J. Morton. Raven Press, New York © 1983

Computed Tomography in Radiation Therapy Planning: Thoracic Region

H. Gunter Seydel, Alkis Zingas, Mahroo Haghbin, Peter Mondalek, and Robert Smereka

Departments of Radiation Oncology and Diagnostic Radiology, Wayne State University, Detroit, Michigan 48201

With the explosive spread of computed tomographic (CT) scanning throughout the United States, one of the main applications has been in patients who are treated for cancer by surgery, radiation therapy, or chemotherapy. For the radiation oncologist, the desire to provide local tumor control and avoid geographic misses to achieve an expected prolongation of survival has led to the use of large radiation fields in the treatment of intrathoracic cancer, including bronchogenic carcinoma, cancer of the esophagus, and other malignant tumors. The optimal radiation therapy plan is a balance between local tumor control and the necessity to preserve normal structures by the use of directed and limited fields for bulk disease. CT scanning has been employed to accurately demonstrate the extent of tumor as well as to determine the isodose distribution of radiation, including the spatial distribution of radiation portals in single planar and three-dimensional aspects as well as consideration of tissue inhomogeneities. The accurate planning of the distribution of therapeutic irradiation includes both the tumor-bearing target volume and the critical normal tissues.

This chapter provides information regarding these aspects of the application of CT scanning to radiation therapy for bronchogenic carcinoma and carcinoma of the esophagus. The more technical aspects of CT scanning, e.g., three-dimensional scanning and the use of CT scanning to correct for tissue inhomogeneities, are left to others to discuss.

CT FOR STAGING BRONCHOGENIC CARCINOMA

Among the technical aspects of CT of the thorax, the use of the injection of contrast material is generally accepted to be of great value for distinguishing vascular normal structures and abnormal masses (e.g., aneurysms) from solid masses. The injection of contrast material is recommended when scanning for the staging of lung cancer if only one CT scan is to be performed (Fig. 1).

Another technical detail, the shape of the CT couch, is very important because it alters body contours and normal anatomy; for optimum duplication of a treatment

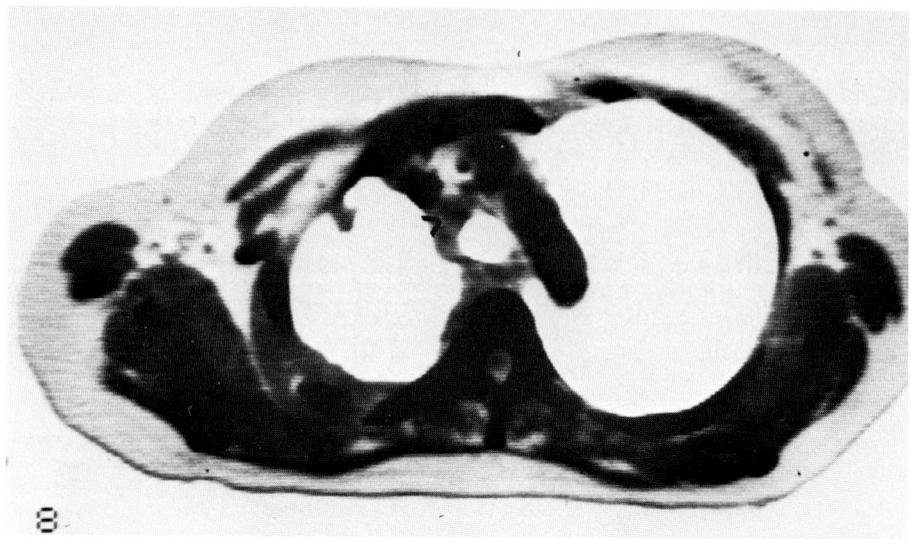

FIG. 1. Squamous cell carcinoma of the right upper lobe of the lung with enlarged mediastinal lymph nodes and pleural involvement. The use of contrast material permits the separation of blood vessels from lymph nodes *(arrowhead).*

setup, the CT scanner should have a flat-topped couch. For many patients CT scans are performed prior to consultation with the radiation oncologist, usually with suspended respiration. This creates an artificial condition because of the need to have patients treated under respiration. Hobday et al. (11) showed that any change in body contour of 1 cm or more may alter the dose delivered to the tumor if the change results in inadequate positioning of the center of the radiation field. However, when they evaluated the effect of respiration on the use of CT scans for radiation therapy planning according to their technique, they described no significant effect on the dose distribution when changes in body contour over 1 cm occurred in 6 of 30 patients. This factor deserves further investigation.

Identification of the position of CT sections for reproduction on the radiation therapy simulator has been greatly aided by the development of the survey film for late generation CT scanners (Fig. 2). Other methods include the use of prescanning radiographs with marking devices to identify the level of CT cross sections, although these techniques have not been as satisfactory.

CT has become an important method for evaluating small nodular lung masses of any origin because it allows lesions as small as 3 mm in diameter to be identified. The majority of pulmonary metastatic lesions are in the periphery of the lung parenchyma, and many of these tumors are subpleural and visualized free of the densities of the chest wall in CT scans. In a study of 54 resected nodules over 3 mm in diameter, Schaner et al. (23) reported that 78% were detected by CT scanning, compared to 59% by conventional tomography. Chang et al. (4) reported on the use of CT in 25 patients who underwent subsequent thoracotomy. CT identified

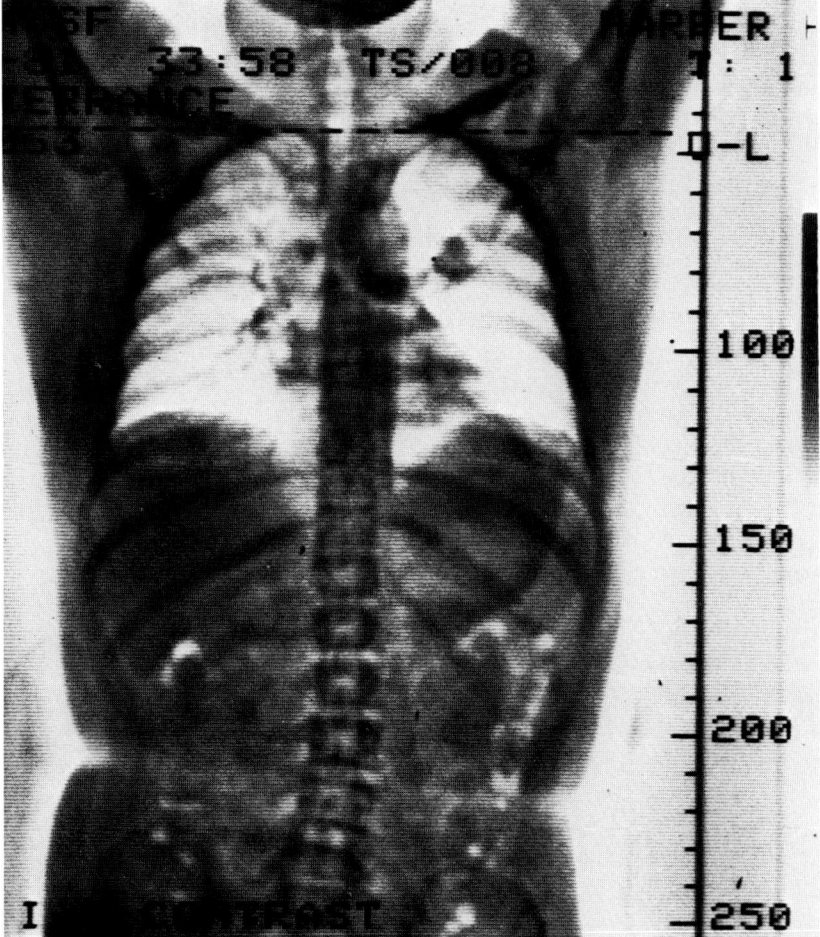

FIG. 2. Survey film of metastatic osteosarcoma.

more nodules than did conventional tomography in 13 of these cases, but a distinction between benign and malignant pulmonary masses was not always possible; of the total number of metastatic nodules present, CT identified 11% more than conventional tomography.

When evaluating malignant pulmonary masses, CT may prove to have considerable value in distinguishing tumor masses from surrounding abnormal lung tissue. However, in a study by Seydel et al. (24), the determination of CT numbers with and without contrast enhancement did not give a definitive distinction between solid tumor and nontumor infiltrates (Table 1), and further research in this area is necessary. On the other hand, the involvement of soft tissues and bony structures of the chest wall can be demonstrated more accurately by CT scans than by other radiographic methods. McLoud et al. (13) described mediastinal and pleural ex-

TABLE 1. *CT numbers based on 12 patients*

Tissue	Hounsfield number ± 1 SD	
	Without contrast medium	With contrast medium
Tumor (primary or node)[a]	49 ± 14	64 ± 6
Tumor and/or infiltrate[a]	29 ± 11[c]	51 ± 27
Muscle	65 ± 12	71 ± 10
Blood vessels	57 ± 20	110 ± 23
Pulmonary fibrosis[b]	25 ± 18[c]	35 ± 11[c]

[a]Before radiotherapy.
[b]After radiotherapy.
[c]Maximum deviation (small population).
From Seydel (24), with permission.

tensions of bronchogenic carcinoma in 9 of 15 patients for whom no such extensions were seen on conventional radiographic examinations.

It is generally agreed that hilar lymph node enlargement is better diagnosed by conventional tomography with 55% angulation than by CT. Mintzer et al. (15) reported on a group of patients with proven hilar metastatic disease, where CT revealed 13 of 20 involved lymph nodes, whereas false-negative results were reported in 2 of these 20 cases. Oblique linear tomography, on the other hand, was accurate in 15 cases, and additional information regarding hilar lymph adenopathy resulted from the examination of the remaining 5 patients.

We demonstrated 75% of proved cases of mediastinal metastasis by CT scanning, whereas conventional tomograms diagnosed only 37%. There was a false-negative CT scan in 10% of the patients.

A correlation of the findings on CT with other means of diagnosis (e.g., thoracotomy and radiographic follow-up) of suspected primary lesions revealed that lung tumors were accurately diagnosed in 90% of the patients (19,24). These authors showed that the accuracy of CT scanning exceeded that of other radiographic methods. CT diagnosed unsuspected malignant lesions in 43 to 65% of patients with bronchogenic carcinoma in studies by Munzenrider et al. (19) and Emani et al. (7), and multiple pulmonary metastases were diagnosed in 34% more patients by Muhm et al. (18). The authors believed that at least 10% of these diagnoses of unsuspected areas of involvement were significant in the management of the patients.

Two recent studies evaluated the accuracy of the CT diagnosis of lymph node involvement in the preoperative staging of bronchogenic carcinoma (6,29). These authors reported on 36 patients with enlarged mediastinal nodes of which only 11 were biopsy-proven to contain metastatic tumor. In one of the series (29), there were 5 additional patients with negative CT scans and positive mediastinoscopy.

The importance of staging lung cancer rests on its impact on treatment policies as well as prognosis. The extent of local tumor affects the decisions of the surgeon as well as those of the radiation therapists. CT scanning has been shown to change the stage of bronchogenic carcinoma in up to 40% of patients (7,10,24). These changes in the stage of the primary tumor rest on the ability of CT to demonstrate direct extraparenchymal extension of primary tumors (T stage), e.g., rib destruction or extrathoracic soft tissue masses, as well as the evaluation of metastatic disease in the mediastinum (N stage) and lung (M stage). The findings in patients with superior vena caval obstruction may be misleading, however, because occasionally lymph node involvement is difficult to demonstrate on CT scans even in the presence of gross clinical symptoms.

CT AND BRONCHOGENIC CARCINOMA

CT has had a significant impact on radiation therapy planning for the treatment of lung cancer. The radiation therapist benefits from improvement in the localization and definition of malignant tumors and normal structures, and, in cooperation with the radiologic physicists and dosimetrists, uses CT information to develop treatment plans. The use of CT absorption coefficients in the treated volume for dose calculations remains in the area of radiologic physics, and the major impact of CT scanning on the radiation therapy of lung cancer requires acceptable systems for use in inhomogeneity calculations and three-dimensional CT reconstructions in addition to the current use of CT for tumor localization.

We consider CT so important that all patients who are treated definitively for lung cancer at our institution undergo scanning of the thorax. Future systems will allow us an integration of the CT scanner, the treatment planning system, and the simulator, but at present we employ a technique which consists of photographic enlargement of the CT scan to conform to the patient contour. We then superimpose clear Xerox copies of the isodoses with beam modification, compensation, or the use of special techniques, e.g., electron beam (Fig. 3).

At the present time, the impact of this use of CT scanning on the treatment of lung cancer can be evaluated only by an analysis of the changes in treatment policy or treatment plan. Outcome studies require follow-up of more patients. The critical effect on tumor control and survival remains to be shown, but it is reasonable to assume such an effect from more adequate coverage of the primary tumor and node metastasis as well as by the modification of the target volume with higher doses to gross tumor masses. Because of the better definition of tumor extension and normal tissues in CT scans, a change in the irradiated volume has been reported in 27 to 66% of patients (7,11,19,22,24). Goitein et al. (10) also examined in detail the type of changes that took place and identified that in 42% of cases there was inadequate or marginal tumor coverage and in 5% a change of normal tissue coverage, compared to plans based on conventional radiographs.

Van Houtte et al. (30) compared the maximum dose in the irradiated tumor volume obtained by the use of conventional radiographs in treatment planning to that used when CT scans were employed. They calculated a factor of 0.97 to 1.09, and for the spinal cord dose this factor was 0.95 to 1.19.

Although CT localization of some normal tissues (e.g., spinal cord) is related to a well-understood mechanism of radiation damage, based on our past experience,

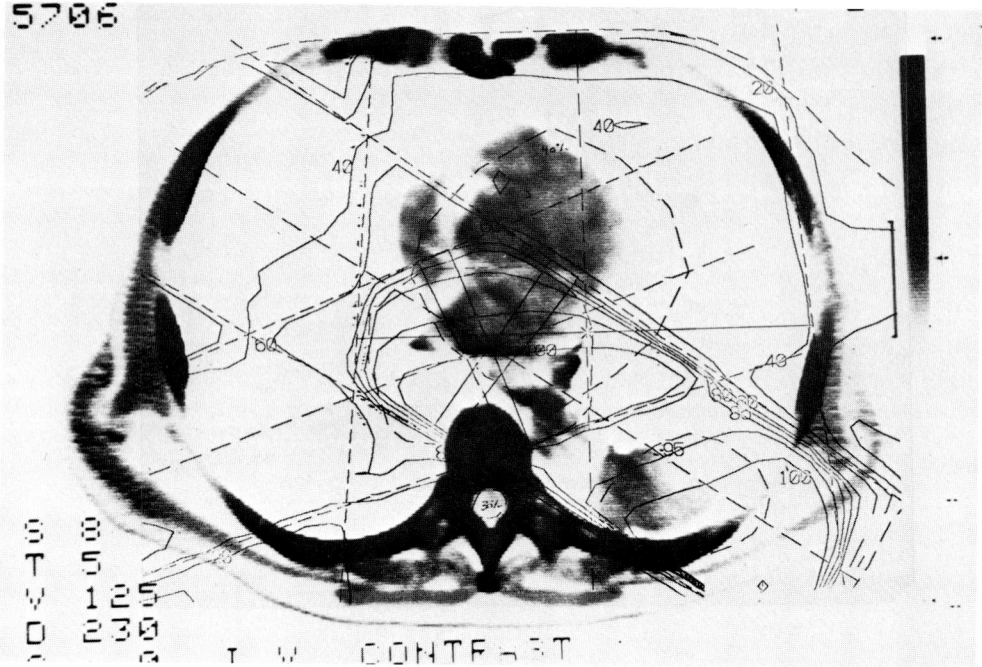

FIG. 3. Composite isodose for large-cell undifferentiated carcinoma of the left lower lobe of the lung using one anterior and two posterior oblique fields (10 MeV photons).

the evaluation of irradiated lung by CT scanning offers prospects of a better understanding of the time-dose-volume effect. Van Houtte et al. (30) studied the development of radiation fibrosis in patients treated postoperatively for lung cancer and found the expected dense fibrosis with compensatory hyperinflation in adjacent lung and often with retraction of mediastinum and the trachea. As expected, the severity of the fibrosis increased with higher doses of radiation. An analysis of their CT data indicated that there was a cumulative incidence of fibrosis in less than 5% of patients who were treated with a dose of approximately 3,000 rads and an approximately 90% incidence at 6,000 rads. Significant work remains in this area, especially with reference to risk factors, e.g., coexisting lung disease.

The dose to the heart can be minimized by appropriate treatment planning using CT scans. There remains, however, a wide field of investigation concerning the unresolved problem of the time-dose-volume relationships of the radiation effect on the heart and pericardium.

The diagnosis of recurrent or persistent carcinoma of the lung becomes even more difficult following radiation therapy because of the superimposition of irradiated lung. Although we have been able to make use of CT scans for this purpose (Fig. 4), the use of tissue-specific CT numbers remains unresolved.

The value of CT scanning for the optimization of radiation therapy is reflected in the reports of Munzenrider et al. (19), Emani et al. (7), and Ragan and Perez (22). These authors indicate that essential information in CT scans was obtained

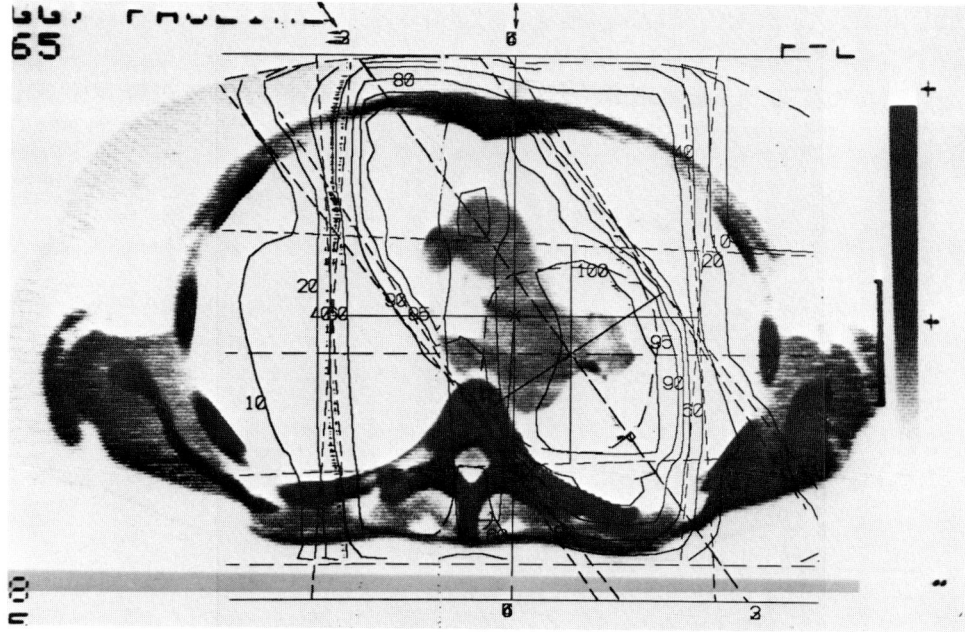

FIG. 4. Recurrent squamous cell carcinoma of the left upper lobe of the lung following lobectomy. Isodose for parallel opposing anteroposterior portals with a posterior cord block and a pair of oblique small fields (10 MeV photons).

for this purpose in 44 to 58% of their selected cases. It is important to realize that CT aids staging, and individualized treatment of non-oat-cell carcinoma of the lung significantly influences the outcome of surgery (17,25,26) as well as the results of radiation therapy (20). Tumor regression after radiotherapy has been shown to be a prerequisite for survival, and there is evidence that higher doses given to involved areas may lead to increased complete tumor response and an increase in survival for localized inoperable non-oat-cell carcinoma of the lung.

Goitein (9) has used a mathematical method to quantify outcome of treatment. He assumed that prolonged survival was clearly a desirable outcome but that other factors are also important: local control of disease, minimization of complications, maintenance of function, and high quality of life. When analyzing his cases, Goitein identified that although there was partial miss of the tumor volume in 42% of the cases, the tumor was out of the field for the entire course of treatment in only 9% because of changes in portal arrangements during the course of therapy. The model suggests an improvement of 3.5% in 5-year survival if CT information is fully utilized.

CT SCANNING IN ESOPHAGEAL CARCINOMA AND OTHER INTRATHORACIC TUMORS

Although preoperative diagnosis of carcinoma of the esophagus usually rests on the use of esophagrams, with or without fluoroscopy, the staging can be significantly aided by CT scanning. Daffner et al. (5) reported that CT accurately showed the extent of mediastinal spread in each of 27 patients with carcinoma of the esophagus. Similarly, Moss et al. (16) described the CT characteristics of carcinoma of the esophagus in 49 patients with surgical data in whom focal thickening of the esophageal wall was present in all cases (Fig. 5). The CT scan accurately identified the mean tumor lengths. Local extension and regional metastases were shown in 60% of the patients with this operative finding, and there were distant metastases in 21%. The value of CT scans in radiation therapy planning is similar to that suggested for bronchogenic carcinoma.

The use of CT scanning in the management of mesothelioma (1,3), lymphoma (12,21), thymoma (14,28), and other intrathoracic cancers remains to be explored, but current reports suggest an excellent potential for improvements in the treatment techniques and survival of patients.

FUTURE PROSPECTS OF CT IN RADIOTHERAPY PLANNING

Integrated systems in which CT scanning, simulation, and computed treatment planning are combined are currently under development. A system already in use combines computerized dose calculations from a modified commercial system with patient specific tissue information obtained from a CT scanner (27); results of the clinical evaluation have been published (2). The currently available systems must be used with caution, as the improved accuracy of dose calculations on the basis

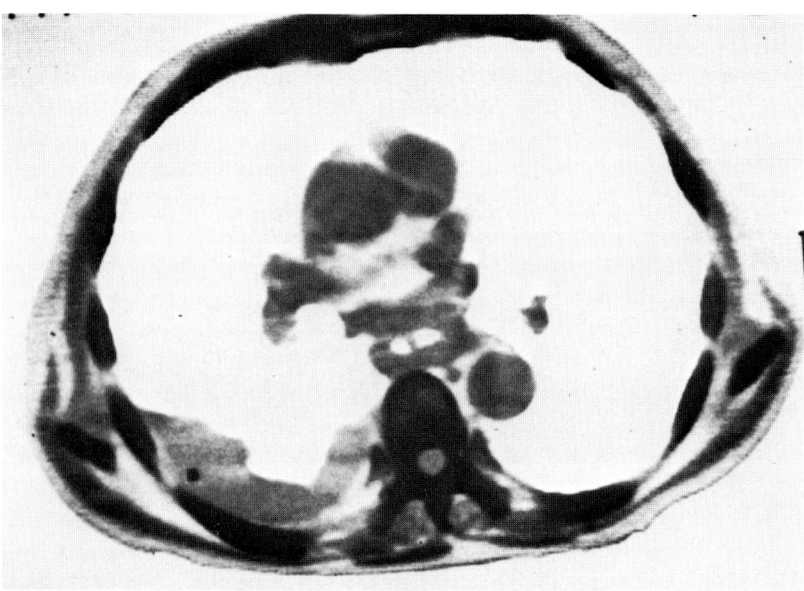

FIG. 5. Squamous cell carcinoma of the thoracic esophagus with local extension and pleural involvement.

of the CT information depends on the accuracy of the inhomogeneity corrections. Battista et al. (2) found good agreement between computed doses and the doses measured *in vivo*, with a maximum difference of 4.3% of the calculated dose.

There are major problems which must still be resolved; Geise and McCullough (8) have shown that present photon beam corrections for inhomogeneity can tolerate uncertainties in electron densities of 10% and still achieve clinically acceptable (± 2%) dose distributions. We may be approaching a degree of potential accuracy in calculation that exceeds the needs of the radiotherapy planning process. On the other hand, the early CT scanners did not satisfy the diagnostic needs of the radiation oncologist, although they may well have been satisfactory for obtaining the necessary physical information.

Furthermore, immobilization and repositioning techniques in radiation therapy must conform to the accuracy possible with a treatment planning system which is based on CT scans, and further effort in this regard is necessary on the part of clinicians. The patient's condition during CT scanning must duplicate that during treatment, especially with regard to positioning and respiration. Corrections for tissue inhomogeneity must be tested for accuracy for each new system. Clinical evaluation remains a task to be pursued by clinicians. Through the systematic investigation of all of these factors and the increased availability of integrated treatment planning systems, there should be further significant improvement in the success of radiotherapy for intrathoracic cancer.

REFERENCES

1. Alexander, E., Clark, R., Colley, D., and Mitchell, S. (1981): CT of malignant pleural mesothelioma. *Am. J. Roentgenol.*, 137:287–291.
2. Battista, J., Rider, W., and Van Dyke, M. (1980): Computed tomography for radiotherapy planning. *Int. J. Radiat. Oncol. Biol. Phys.*, 6:99–107.
3. Bricout, P., and Engler, M. (1981): Computerized tomography scanning and the planning of high-dose radiotherapy for pleural mesothelioma: a report of five patients. *Int. J. Radiat. Oncol. Biol. Phys.*, 7:821–826.
4. Chang, A., Everett, G., Schaner, E., Conkle, D., Flye, W., Doppman, J., and Rosenberg, S. (1979): Evaluation of computed tomography in the detection of pulmonary metastases. *Cancer*, 43:913–916.
5. Daffner, R., Halber, M., Postlethwait, R., Korobin, M., and Thompson, W. (1979): CT of the esophagus. II. Carcinoma. *Am. J. Roentgenol.*, 133:1051–1055.
6. Ekholm, S., Albrechtsson, U., Kegelberg, J., and Tylen, U. (1980): Computed tomography in preoperative staging of bronchogenic carcinoma. *J. Comput. Assist. Tomogr.*, 4:763–765.
7. Emani, B., Belo, A., Carter, B., Munzenrider, J., and Piro, A. (1978): Value of computed tomography in radiotherapy of lung cancer. *Am. J. Roentgenol.*, 131:63–67.
8. Geise, R., and McCullough, E. (1977): The use of CT scanners in megavoltage photon-beam therapy planning. *Radiology*, 124:133–141.
9. Goitein, M. (1981): Computed tomography in radiation therapy. *Br. J. Radiol. [Suppl.]*, 15:173–177.
10. Goitein, M., Wittenberg, J., Mendiondo, M., Doucette, J., Friedberg, C., Ferrucci, J., Gunderson, L., Lingood, R., Shipley, W., and Fineberg, H. (1981): The value of CT scanning in radiation therapy treatment planning: a prospective study. *Int. J. Radiat. Oncol. Biol. Phys.*, 5:1787–1798.
11. Hobday, P., Hodson, N., Husband, J., Parker, R., and MacDonald, J. (1979): Computed tomography applied to radiotherapy treatment planning: techniques and results. *Radiology*, 133:477–482.
12. Jones, S., Tobias, D., and Waldman, R. (1978): Computed tomographic scanning in patients with lymphoma. *Cancer*, 41:480–486.

13. McLoud, T., Wittenberg, J., and Ferrucci, J. (1979): Computed tomography of the thorax and standard radiographic evaluation of the chest: a comparative study. *J. Comput. Assist. Tomogr.*, 3:170–180.

14. Mink, J., Bein, M., Sukov, R., Herrmann, C., Jr., Winter, J., Sample, W., and Mulder, D. (1978): Computed tomography of the anterior mediastinum of patients with myasthenia gravis and suspected thymoma. *Am. J. Roentgenol.*, 130:239–246.

15. Mintzer, R., Malave, S., Neiman, H., Michaelis, L., Vanecko, R., and Sanders, J. (1979): Computed vs. conventional tomography in evaluation of primary and secondary pulmonary neoplasms. *Radiology*, 132:653–659.

16. Moss, A., Schnyder, P., Thoeni, R., and Margulis, A. (1981): Esophageal carcinoma: pretherapy staging by computed tomography. *Am. J. Roentgenol.*, 136:1051–1056.

17. Mountain, C., McMurtrey, M., and Frazier, O. (1980): Regional extension of lung cancer. *Int. J. Radiat. Oncol. Biol. Phys.*, 6:1013–1020.

18. Muhm, R., Brown, L., and Crowe, J. (1977): Use of computed tomography in the detection of pulmonary nodules. *Mayo Clin. Proc.*, 52:345–348.

19. Munzenrider, J., Pilepich, M., Rene-Ferrero, J., Tchakarova, I., and Carter, B. (1977): Use of body scanner in radiotherapy treatment planning. *Cancer*, 40:170–179.

20. Perez, C., Stanley, K., Rubin, P., Kramer, S., Brady, L., Perez-Tamayo, R., Brown, G., Concannon, J., Oatman, M., and Seydel, H. (1980): A prospective randomized study of various irradiation doses and fractionation schedules in the treatment of inoperable non-oat cell carcinoma of the lung. *Cancer*, 45:2744–2753.

21. Pilepich, M., Rene, J., Munzenrider, J., and Carter, B. (1978): Contribution of computed tomography to the treatment of lymphomas. *Am. J. Roentgenol.*, 131:69–73.

22. Ragan, D., and Perez, C. (1978): Efficacy of CT-assisted two-dimensional treatment planning: analysis of 45 patients. *Am. J. Roentgenol.*, 131:75–79.

23. Schaner, E., Chang, A., Doppman, J., Conkle, D., Flye, M., and Rosenberg, S. (1978): Comparison of computed and conventional whole lung tomography in detecting pulmonary nodules: a prospective radiologic-pathologic study. *Am. J. Roentgenol.*, 131:51–54.

24. Seydel, H., Kutcher, G., Steiner, R., Modiuddin, M., and Goldberg, B. (1980): Computed tomography in planning radiation therapy for bronchogenic carcinoma. *Int. J. Radiat. Oncol. Biol. Phys.*, 6:601–606.

25. Shevland, J., Chiu, L., Schapiro, R., Young, J., and Rossi, N. (1978): The role of conventional tomography and computed tomography in assessing the resectability of primary lung cancer: a preliminary report. *J. Comput. Tomogr.*, 2:1–19.

26. Shields, T. (1980): Classification and prognosis of surgically treated patients with bronchial carcinoma: analysis of V.A.S.O.G. studies. *Int. J. Radiat. Oncol. Biol. Phys.*, 6:1021–1027.

27. Sontag, M., and Cunningham, J. (1978): Clinical application of a CT-based treatment planning system. *Comput. Tomogr.*, 2:117–130.

28. Steiger, R. (1980): Personal communication.

29. Underwood, G., Hooper, R., Acelbaum, S., and Goodwin, D. (1979): Computed tomographic scanning of the thorax in the staging of bronchogenic carcinoma. *N. Engl. J. Med.*, 300:777–778.

30. Van Houtte, P., Piron, A., Lustman-Marechal, J., Osteaux, M., and Henry, J. (1980): Computed axial tomography (CAT) contribution of dosimetry and treatment evaluation in lung cancer. *Int. J. Radiat. Oncol. Biol. Phys.*, 6:995–1000.

Computed Tomography in Radiation Therapy,
edited by C. C. Ling, C. C. Rogers, and
R. J. Morton. Raven Press, New York © 1983

Computed Tomography in Therapy Planning: Abdominal Region

John E. Munzenrider

Department of Radiation Medicine, Massachusetts General Hospital, Boston, Massachusetts 02114

Radical radiotherapy of nonlymphomatous malignancies arising in or adjacent to the abdominal cavity is among the more challenging problems encountered by the radiotherapist. The radiation doses required for controlling adenocarcinomas that arise in the gastrointestinal tract, pancreas, biliary system, and kidney, and sarcomas that arise in the abdominal wall and retroperitoneum, are well above the tolerance levels of dose-limiting abdominal organs, e.g., the liver, kidneys, gut, and spinal cord. In addition, the extent of such tumors and their relationship to these dose-limiting structures cannot routinely be determined from the physical examination, and it has been difficult to determine these parameters with traditional radiographic techniques.

The revolutionary nature of computed tomography (CT) was universally and justifiably recognized by the awarding of the 1979 Nobel Prize in Medicine jointly to Hounsfield and Cormack for their independent contributions to the development of that technique. Physicians in general and radiotherapists in particular were called on to respond to the challenge of appreciating the potential and limitations of the new technique, and to define criteria for its application in clinical practice. Early experience with body scanners demonstrated that the technique could identify abdominal lymph node masses, retroperitoneal tumors, and pancreatic disease, frequently more completely than other methods or where other methods had failed to delineate such lesions. Wittenberg and Ferrucci (42) reviewed experience gained with first-generation body scanners in abdominal imaging and concluded that the morphologic representation of abdominal solid tumors provided by computed body tomography (CBT) was superior to all other imaging techniques; moreover, it was noninvasive and was associated with relatively low radiation exposure.

The use of CBT-guided fine needle aspiration of abdominal and pelvic tumors has been reviewed by Ferrucci and Wittenberg (10), and the utility of CBT in the clinical follow-up of abdominal malignancy has been discussed by Kreel (22), Munzenrider et al. (31), and Pilepich et al. (33). Lee and associates (26) demonstrated that CBT is quite useful in following progression or regression of abdominal tumor masses after treatment, with serial scans being helpful in assessing tumor status in 96% of lymphoma patients, 90% of pancreatic cases, and 72% of patients with retroperitoneal disease.

CBT has therefore proved to be of major significance in imaging abdominal tumors, identifying their histological type by guiding percutaneous aspiration biopsy, and following patients with abdominal tumors after treatment.

CT IN RADIATION TREATMENT PLANNING

Early clinical efforts with CBT were directed toward defining its utility as an imaging technique and determining which categories of patients might benefit from its application. It soon became apparent that the technique had great potential for radiotherapy treatment planning, as the scan provided a transverse body contour containing an exact image of the tumor and the relationship of the tumor volume to dose-limiting normal tissues. Munzenrider et al. (32) have critically appraised the value of abdominal CBT to the radiotherapist.

Tufts-New England Medical Center Study

Recognizing that radiotherapy depends heavily on imaging techniques for tumor diagnosis, determination of tumor extent, and localizing tumors for treatment planning, Munzenrider et al. (31) retrospectively analyzed CBT scans of 98 radiotherapy patients to determine the contribution of the scan to the management of those patients. Scans were available for treatment planning in 25 abdominal patients and in 50 with nonabdominal tumors. Availability of CBT data impacted relatively more significantly on the total volume treated, the volume of normal tissue irradiated, and the degree of adequacy of tumor coverage in the abdominal patients. The scan was judged essential for treatment planning in almost two-thirds of abdominal patients and in only 50% of patients with nonabdominal tumors. The contributions of the scan to evaluation of and treatment planning in the patients studied are summarized in Table 1.

Massachusetts General Hospital Study

In a prospective study, Goitein et al. (15) assessed the value of CBT in treatment planning for 77 patients, including 14 with abdominal tumors. Treatment was planned with all available data before CBT scan was performed, then replanned

TABLE 1. *Contribution of scan to treatment planning:*
Tufts-New England Medical Center Study

Contribution of scan	Abdomen 25 pts. (%)	Other sites 50 pts. (%)
Tumor coverage not adequate	60	40
Unsuspected involvement seen	59	33
Normal tissue volume reduced	44	16
Treatment volume changed	56	40
Essential for planning	64	50

with the scan. The scan was of major significance for treatment planning in 64% of patients with abdominal tumors but in only 30% of those with nonabdominal tumors. The scan was also valuable in selecting patient position for treatment, with important changes in normal tissue coverage being produced by treating in a particular position as suggested by the scan. The reproducibility of anatomic relationships defined by CBT was verified with repeat scans in situations where critical normal tissue tolerances were involved or where postsurgical changes were suspected to have occurred. Contributions of the scan to treatment planning in these patients are summarized in Table 2.

Royal Marsden Hospital Study

The application of CBT to radiotherapy treatment planning has also been described by Hobday and associates (19), who studied 123 patients scheduled for radical treatment. Nineteen had abdominal tumors. CBT data was transferred directly from the scanner to the treatment planning computer, and quantitative CBT data were employed directly for inhomogeneity corrections. Respiration degraded the diagnostic image more significantly in the abdomen, relative to the pelvis and thorax, with respiratory motion contributing to poor scan quality in 37% of abdominal scans but in only 12% of pelvic and thoracic scans. Changes in body contour due to respiration were observed in 32% of patients with abdominal tumors and in only 6% of those with nonabdominal lesions. In two cases the treatment volume moved on and off the tumor with the movement of the anterior abdominal wall during respiration. The kidney position for blocking purposes was incorrect in 56% of 9 patients when renal position from the scan was compared with that from other studies. The spinal cord position from conventional studies was incorrect in 3 of 30 patients with thoracic lesions; these data are relevant to abdominal treatment planning, as a significant constraint in irradiating upper abdominal tumors, including those of the pancreas and stomach, as well as para-aortic nodes, is to avoid exceeding spinal cord tolerance. Neither internal anatomy nor tumor was observed to move transversely with respiration. It was concluded that CBT scanning had played a significant role, especially in patients with abdominal tumors. Advantages of direct transfer of CBT data from scanner to treatment planning computer were discussed. Contributions of the scan to treatment planning in the patients studied are summarized in Table 3.

TABLE 2. *Contribution of scan to treatment planning: Massachusetts General Hospital Study*

Contribution of scan	Abdomen 14 pts. (%)	Other sites 63 pts. (%)
Change in plan	86	44
"Miss"		
Large volume	14	13
Boost	43	18
Major significance	64	30

TABLE 3. *Contribution of scan to treatment planning: Royal Marsden Hospital Study*

Contribution of scan	Abdomen 19 pts. (%)	Other sites 104 pts. (%)
Change in body contour with respiration	32	6
Tumor coverage not adequate	58	19
Treatment volume changed	68	22
Total change in treatment	79	31
Kidney position incorrect[a]	56	
Spinal cord position incorrect[b]		10

[a]Nine patients.
[b]Thirty patients with thoracic lesions.

TABLE 4. *Summary: contribution of scan to abdominal treatment planning in three studies*

Contribution of scan	Tufts study 25 pts. (%)	MGH study 14 pts. (%)	Royal Marsden study 19 pts. (%)
Tumor coverage inadequate	60	57[a]	53
Treatment volume changed	56		68
Change in plan		86	79
"Essential"	64		
"Major significance"		64	

[a]Fourteen percent "miss" large field and 43 "miss" boost field.

Three Studies on Abdominal Treatment Planning Compared

These three studies were structured differently and were performed in three separate institutions with varying treatment policies, treatment planning facilities, and computer expertise. Their remarkably similar conclusions are summarized and compared in Table 4. These early studies clearly demonstrated the inherent value of the scan in providing valuable information regarding abdominal tumors and documented the gross inadequacy of conventional techniques in localizing abdominal tumors for radiotherapy treatment planning.

LIMITATIONS AND PITFALLS OF CBT FOR TREATMENT PLANNING

Despite the remarkable improvement in imaging abdominal tumors for radiotherapy treatment planning, documented in the three studies cited above, there are significant limitations to the utilization of CBT in treatment planning. Numerous pitfalls await the unwary treatment planner using this revolutionary new tool. These limitations and pitfalls are discussed in detail below.

Special attention must be paid to *registering* the level of the transverse scan showing the tumor and surrounding normal structures to external or internal landmarks employed for treatment simulation and setup. The patient must be positioned in a reproducible way so that transverse image data will not only accurately localize the tumor and adjacent normal organs in nontransverse planes but will allow external and internal landmarks to be used in relating a specific transverse scan to external and internal landmarks for simulation and treatment. Newer scanners capable of multiplanar reconstructions are most helpful in this regard. Organs and/or tumors may shift significantly with changes in *patient position*, making hazardous or potentially disastrous localization of structures of interest on a scan taken in one position if treatment will be in another position. Patient immobilization, for both scanning and treatment simulation and execution, may be necessary, especially if nonsupine techniques are employed, either to shift normal structures out of the treatment volume or because of constraints of therapy unit beam direction, etc. *Involuntary patient motion*, especially that due to respiration, may alter the location of both the tumor and the adjacent normal structures relative to each other or relative to external or internal landmarks. Allowance must be made for such changes based on knowledge of how such movements affect the contents of the treatment volume during treatment. Each of these problems is discussed below.

Registration of Scan Level to External Skin Marks or Internal Landmarks

Registration of transverse scan level to external skin marks was achieved by placing barium paste (19,31) and radiopaque catheters (15) on skin reference marks during scanning.

The relationship of surface landmarks to vertebral level for determining scan level of cross-sectional images has been discussed by Kuhns et al. (24). External landmarks, including the tip of the xiphoid, the ends of the 11th rib, the umbilicus, and the iliac crests, were studied in relation to corresponding vertebral segments as determined on anterior-posterior (AP) radiographs and abdominal scans in 50 patients undergoing intravenous urography. It was concluded that these landmarks could be used only as a rough guide to approximate abdominal organ level for CBT scanning due to variability in organ level caused by body habitus and respiratory motion. They were, however, relatively constantly related to vertebral segment and hence were more reliable for localization of vertebral body level or retroperitoneal structures which move somewhat less with respiration than abdominal viscera.

Kreel (22) has described a simple yet relatively accurate technique to relate scan level to vertebral level, in which each CT section is related to a radiograph taken with metal markers over fixed bony points. A similar technique has been described by Dossetor et al. (7): A conventional radiograph is taken through a lead grid lattice with pinpoint holes separated by a distance equivalent to the thickness of the CBT cuts, with aluminum markers placed on the skin at 5-cm intervals. The aluminum markers are left in place for the scan, produce little if any artifact, and allow accurate registration of scan level with vertebral level on the radiograph.

Scan artifacts produced by external foreign objects (e.g., barium paste or other radiopaque skin markers) can hinder accurate tissue boundary localization and interfere with quantitative use of CT numbers for tissue heterogeneity corrections in radiotherapy treatment planning. The CT level indicator described by Villafana et al. (41) allows relatively precise correlation between scan level and an AP radiograph, and introduces no artifacts. A rectangular Plexiglas plate with linear grooves of lengths which vary by 1-cm increments, and which are 1 cm apart, is placed under the patient at a previously marked level during scanning. Air filling the grooves is clearly seen on the scan and allows registration of each scan section to the external reference mark. A duplicate plate with copper wires filling the grooves is employed during conventional simulation. When the marking plate is carefully positioned under the patient for scanning and simulation, an overall accuracy of 5 mm is observed.

Current scanners capable of taking a "scanogram," or a scout film, in the scanning position with appropriate markers projected on the film would simplify the task of registering the scan section to the appropriate anatomic level of the patient. Such films can also be readily compared with other studies (e.g., arteriograms) and would also be of significant value in radiotherapy treatment planning for comparison with simulator radiographs. A typical scanogram and a corresponding CBT section are shown in Fig. 1.

Effect of Patient Position on Internal Anatomy

The effect of patient position on organ and tumor location relative to fixed bony landmarks must be considered when using CBT data in treatment planning. This can be of particular significance if either the tumor volume moves out of, or a dose-limiting organ moves into, the treatment volume when the patient's position is other than that during the scan. Haaga et al. (18) described organ shifts on scans performed in the supine and the right decubitus positions. A pancreatic tumor was seen more clearly in the latter position due to anterior and inferior shifts of the stomach, duodenum, and liver away from the tumor; in the supine scan those organs lay directly on the pancreas. In the decubitus scan the left kidney moved anteromedially.

Lee et al. (28) have scanned patients with gastric malignancies in supine, prone, and decubitus positions, and observed that the shift in the stomach and its contents with positional change allowed evaluation of the thickness of the anterior and posterior walls, which were outlined alternately by air and contrast material in the various positions.

Changes in organ and tumor location may occur after surgery; preoperative scans must be used with caution for treatment planning, especially after extensive surgery. Bernardino et al. (3) demonstrated that the postnephrectomy renal fossa normally contains only bowel. Alter et al. (1) stated that the right renal fossa in postnephrectomy patients may be occupied by liver, colon, and the junction of the second and third portions of the duodenum; following left nephrectomy, loops of small bowel may occupy the left renal fossa, and the spleen and descending colon are located more posteromedially than usual. The tail of the pancreas may also occupy the medial left renal bed, whereas after splenectomy and nephrectomy the descending colon was seen there. Figure 2 shows the duodenum occupying the right renal

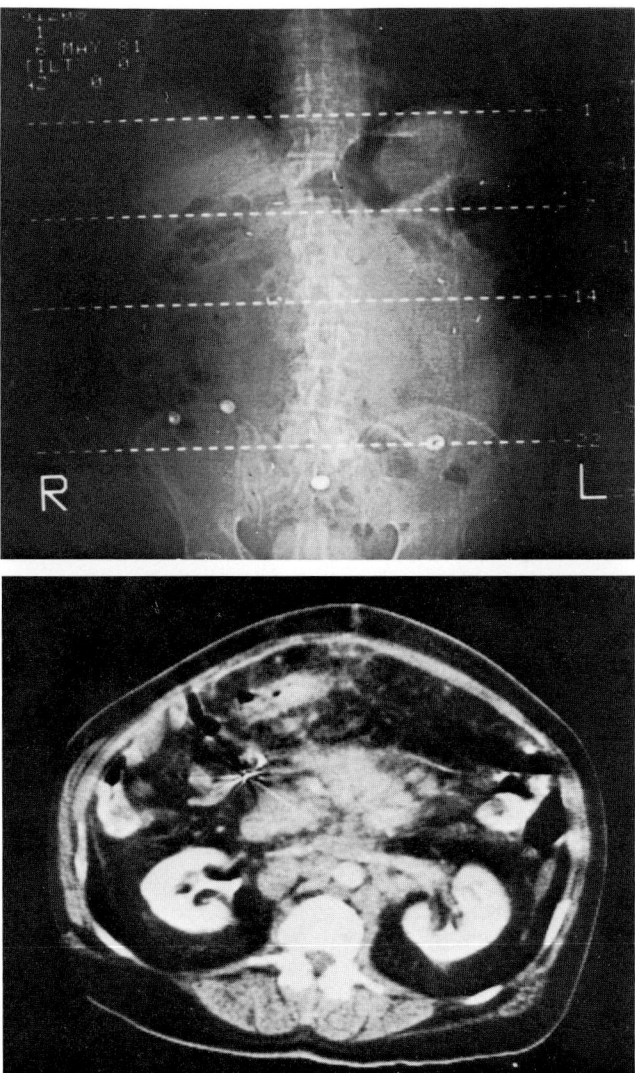

FIG. 1. **Top:** "Scanogram" of patient with pancreatic carcinoma. **Bottom:** Section 13 of patient shown in the scanogram showing large exophytic pancreatic cancer. (Courtesy of Dr. L. L. Gunderson, Mayo Clinic.)

fossa in a patient whose right kidney was removed along with a retroperitoneal sarcoma.

Sagel et al. (37) alluded to the potential utility of the scan for kidney shielding purposes during radiotherapy. Hobday and associates (19) observed that the renal position on the scan differed from that determined by conventional techniques in 5 of 9 patients studied. Neither group, however, specifically mentioned the pos-

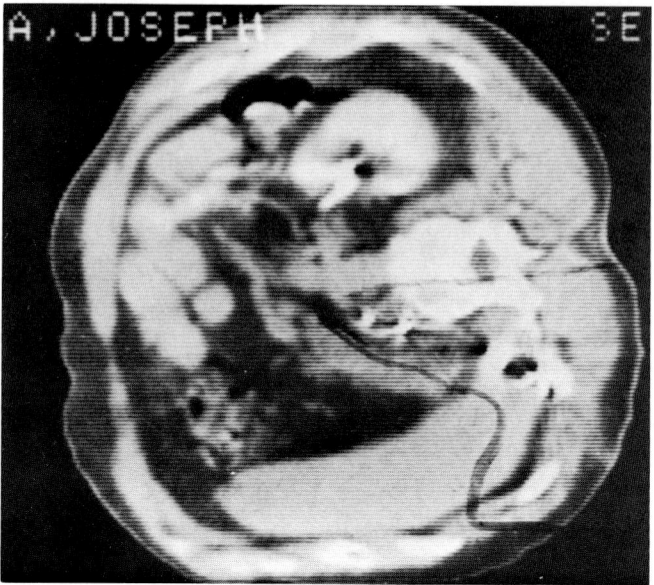

FIG. 2. Scan at level of L2, showing a loop of barium-filled duodenum (ring-shaped structure) filling the right renal fossa after nephrectomy.

sibility of renal position change with patient position change, although Hobday et al. stressed the importance of performing the scan used for treatment planning in the same position as that used for treatment.

The renal position shifts between the supine and the prone positions. Prone scan sections at the levels of the first and second lumbar vertebral bodies are shown in Fig. 3, top, and supine scans are shown in Fig. 3, bottom. The left kidney on both levels and the right kidney on the L2 scan are located more anteromedially on the prone scan (Fig. 3, top) relative to their position on the supine scan (Fig. 3, bottom). The degree of displacement observed is 19, 14, and 16 mm in the AP direction and 9, 3, and 9 mm in the transverse direction for the left kidney at both levels and the right kidney at the lower level, respectively. The AP and transverse diameters of the kidneys at these levels ranged from 5.0 to 6.6 cm. Thus the observed kidney shift from the prone to the supine position approximates one-third (27 to 37%) of the AP renal diameter and 10% (5 to 15%) of the transverse diameter at these levels.

These renal shifts have obvious significance in terms of planning renal shielding based on renal position taken from the scan: with anterior and posterior para-aortic portals, the medial portion of the kidney might be completely excluded from the treatment field in the supine position and included in the prone position. The anterior renal margin might be excluded from lateral portals directed at the pancreatic area in the supine position, and included to a significant degree if treatment were to be given with the patient prone. Lateral portals directed at the para-aortic area would

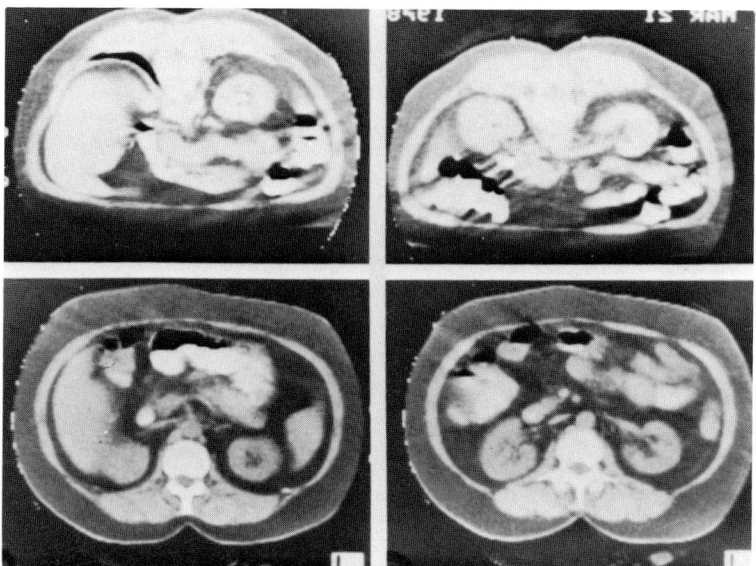

FIG. 3. Top: Prone scans at level of L1 **(left)** and L2 **(right)** of patient with cervical cancer metastatic to the para-aortic nodes. **Bottom:** Supine scans at the same levels. Note the anteromedial displacement of the kidneys in these prone scans, relative to the position of the kidneys in the supine scans. Also note the posterior external air gap.

cover less than half of the kidney area at these levels with the patient supine, and include almost the entire organ if the patient were treated in the prone position. Similar renal shifts occur, as noted above (18) when moving the patient from the supine to the decubitus position, and probably also occur when going from the recumbent to the upright position.

Similar shifts of liver, small bowel, stomach, and the mobile portions of the large intestine, as well as the pancreas, occur with positional change as documented by Gunderson (17). Figure 4, left, shows a prone X-ray film of the small bowel in a patient with cecal carcinoma following right ileocolectomy. The barium-filled bowel is quite evenly distributed over the entire adbomen, with a significant amount of bowel seen lateral to the sacroiliac joint in the tumor bed overlaying the right iliac fossa. However, with the patient in the left lateral decubitus position (Fig. 4, right), almost all the visualized bowel is medial to the sacroiliac joint. Tumor bed irradiation with anterior and posterior portals in that position treats a significantly smaller volume of intestine than would have been treated with the same portals in the prone position. Significant displacement of bowel out of the target volume can be achieved by treating in the decubitus position when the target volume includes the lateral abdominal gutters, the iliac fossa, or the iliac bone itself.

Patients can be positioned for scanning and treatment with a simple decubitus board (17). Retroperitoneal vascular structures and lymph nodes also shift by 1 to 2 cm toward the dependent side in the decubitus position (16).

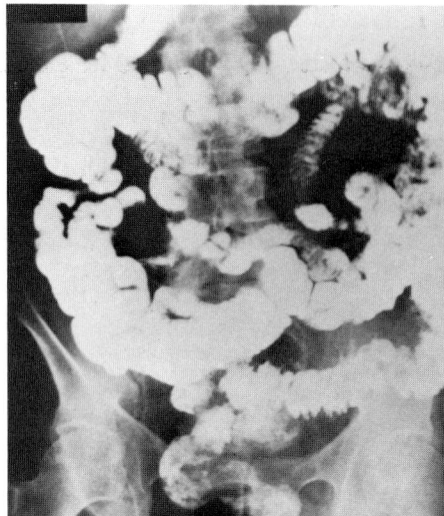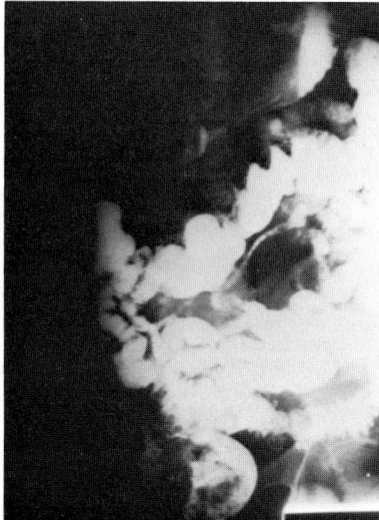

FIG. 4. Small-bowel series in prone **(left)** and left lateral decubitus **(right)** positions, showing bowel displaced to the left in the decubitus position.

Effect of Involuntary Patient Motion on Internal Anatomy

Involuntary patient motion, especially respiration and peristalsis, degraded the diagnostic image obtained with first-generation scanners, which had relatively long scan times. However, these problems have been largely eliminated by giving intravenous glucagon to inhibit peristalsis for use with slow scanners and the development of fast scanners, which can complete a scan section during a single suspended respiration by the patient. Sagel et al. (37) reported that 91% of 131 patients with renal masses were able to suspend respiration for at least the 18 sec required to complete a single scan. However, abdominal organ mobility with respiration must be considered when planning abdominal radiotherapy, as few therapy units can complete treatment in less than 18 sec. For treatment planning purposes, extremes of organ and tumor excursion during normal breathing in the treatment position should be considered when designing treatment portals or shielding blocks.

Kuhns et al. (25) studied the variation in renal and diaphragmatic positions with repeated suspension of respiration in 32 patients undergoing intravenous urography. The position of the superior pole of the kidney on 1-, 2-, and 3-min films in the same patient had mean variations ranging from 4.9 mm to 7.7 mm despite the patient being given the same specific breathing instructions for each film. The apex of the diaphragm was seen on each film in 12 patients: The mean variation in diaphragm position was 8.0 mm. These data were cited to emphasize the difficulty of scanning an identical level on subsequent scans due to internal organ mobility with respiration, and to demonstrate that internal anatomy cannot be voluntarily reproduced even by cooperative patients.

Haaga and associates (18) have noted that increased pressure from the weight of the abdominal viscera in the right lateral decubitus position decreases right diaphragmatic excursion and aids visualization of the pancreas on abdominal scans. Kivisarri et al. (21) observed that the pancreas moved with respiration as much as two vertebral segments, and cited this great mobility as an impediment to rescanning an identical abdominal section. The stomach, duodenum, kidney, and liver probably move as much as the pancreas, although CBT data in this regard are lacking.

The effect of respiration on treatment planning was studied by Hobday and associates (19), who detected contour change in 6 of 19 (32%) abdominal patients. In 2 patients respiration caused anterior displacement of the isocenter, which moved the treatment volume off the tumor during treatment. No transverse motion of tumor or of internal organs was detected during quiet breathing.

The treatment planning implications of abdominal organ motion with respiration are significant. Accurate sagittal and coronal reconstructions would be extremely valuable for treatment planning by allowing three-dimensional appreciation of tumor extent in a format similar to AP and lateral radiographs usually obtained from conventional treatment simulators. However, resolution of sagittal and coronal reconstructions is limited by both scan thickness and anatomic overlap of contiguous scan sections due to patient respiration (11). Errors in multiplanar reconstructions due to changes in internal anatomy with time because of the respiratory motion of abdominal organs might be avoided by obtaining multiple scans at contiguous levels during a single suspension of respiration in order to obtain accurate density data for reconstruction in other planes (25). For routine treatment planning, however, scanning should probably be done during quiet respiration (19).

The therapist must realize that tumors or organs displayed on a given transverse section may not always be there, relative to fixed bony landmarks or skin marks, during any one treatment or during a course of treatment; this is due to motion of mobile abdominal organs with respiration. If a mobile organ (e.g., the pancreas, stomach, or kidney) is involved by tumor, the treatment volume must be large enough to include the tumor in all phases of respiration. Figure 5 shows a simulator radiograph outlining the portal employed when treating a pancreatic carcinoma defined by clips placed at surgery; it illustrates the degree of margins required superiorly and inferiorly to allow for diaphragmatic excursion of the pancreas during quiet respiration.

Treatment could be gated to the respiratory cycle—if a high-dose rate (≈ 500 rads/min) therapy unit is available— with cooperative patients being treated during a particular phase of respiration. However, the variation in diaphragmatic and renal positions in "cooperative patients" (25) suggests that significant margins would still be required for irradiating tumors that involve mobile abdominal organs. Allowance should also be made for kidney mobility with respiration when renal shielding is planned from CBT scans.

Movement of mobile tumors or organs in the AP direction with respiration has not been evaluated, with either CBT or conventional techniques. Such motion could be particularly significant if lateral or oblique portals are employed to reduce the

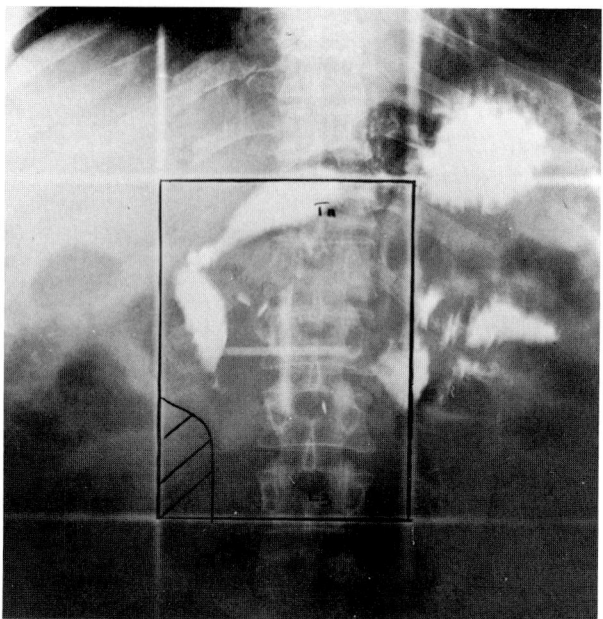

FIG. 5. Simulator radiograph of pancreatic cancer patient. Clips placed at surgery define the gross tumor extent, and barium outlines the duodenum. Solid lines show the radiation portal needed to encompass the mass during all phases of respiration due to mobility of the tumor and organ with breathing. (Courtesy of Dr. L. L. Gunderson, Mayo Clinic.)

volume of normal tissue irradiated. Further studies are urgently needed to confirm that the rate of "significant" change in treatment plans with respiration is no greater than the 10% change found by Hobday et al. (19) due to anterior abdominal wall skin excursion with respiration.

Multiplanar Reconstructions from Transverse Images

Tumors arising in the adrenal gland and the retroperitoneum have been well demonstrated by Foley et al. (12) using reformatted coronal display of upper abdominal transverse CT scans. Exophytic pancreatic cancers were not well demonstrated by that technique because of poorly defined tumor margins, which were attributed to incomplete duodenal opacification in the cases studied. Coronal, off-axis coronal, and off-axis coronal images tilted in the cephalocaudal plane were employed in the study, suggesting the possibility of "simulation" of obliquely angled treatment portals or of portals unconventionally angled relative to the long axis of the patient, i.e., with the central axis of the treatment beam being angled in a craniocaudad orientation. Such unconventional portal arrangements could have important implications in terms of normal tissue coverage when treating abdominal malignancies, as suggested by Goitein et al. (15). Multiplanar reconstructions from transverse scan sections done with the patient in the supine, decubitus, or upright position are routinely employed in proton treatment planning at the Massachusetts General Hospital, using a VAX computer and a raster graphics scan display unit designed by Goitein and Abrams (14). That system can generate a "projection view" which shows what a simulation X-ray or a portal radiograph should look like if taken at the prescribed angle.

Influence of Scan Speed on Image Quality

The influence of scan speed on image quality was studied by Robbins et al. (36) in 75 patients undergoing abdominal scanning. One section in each patient which clearly demonstrated a diagnostic abnormality was rescanned at four scan speeds: 2.25, 4.5, 9.0, and 18.0 sec. The number of motion artifacts per scan increased progressively with longer scanning times, as did the number of unreadable scans. None of the 2.25-sec scans but 10% of the 18-sec scans were unreadable. The diagnosis was apparent in all 2.25- and 4.5-sec scans, whereas it was not made on 1 of 75 and on 12 of 75 (16%, $p < 0.0001$) of the 9- and 18-sec scans, respectively. Five of the 12 scans misdiagnosed with the 18-sec studies were in patients with neoplastic conditions (three pancreatic cancers, one liver mass, and one retroperitoneal nodal mass). Of the 12 misdiagnosed scans, 11 were in patients with upper abdominal pathology, leading the authors to suggest that cardiac and respiratory motion might be responsible for image degradation in upper abdominal scans studied at longer scan times.

Because a 16% error rate occurred in the interpretation of 18-sec abdominal scans (36), it is pertinent to note that the three abdominal treatment planning studies described above were all done with "slow" scanners: Munzenrider et al. (31) used a 2.5-min scanner, Goitein et al. (15) used an 18-sec scanner, and Hobday et al. (19) used a 20-sec scanner. Thus it is possible that the value of CT scanning in abdominal treatment planning was underestimated in these three studies due to a failure to totally appreciate the diagnostic information present in the scans. Although the question of scan speed in abdominal treatment planning has not been studied, it appears prudent to employ scanners with scan times of 9 sec or less in abdominal treatment planning where possible.

Quantification of Tissue Inhomogeneities for Abdominal Treatment Planning

Tissue inhomogeneities may produce significant variations in dose distribution, especially with electrons, heavier charged particles, or neutrons. Inhomogeneities of potential concern in abdominal planning include (a) vertebral bone; (b) subcutaneous, retroperitoneal, and intraperitoneal fat; and (c) air cavities in bowel or external to the patient (Fig. 3). Supervoltage photon beam treatment planning may ignore fat or bone inhomogeneities, as such beams are insignificantly perturbed by their presence in the treatment volume. Neutron treatment planning would have to consider and allow for the presence of fat. Bowel air can produce significant alterations in photon dose distribution, and efforts to compensate for that inhomogeneity should be considered. However, currently available programs which apply pixel by pixel corrections for photon beams should be used with caution in abdominal planning. The planning scan shows what air is present on the day of the scan. However, patients undergoing daily fractionated radiotherapy would probably have varying amounts of air in the bowel, and it would occupy different positions from day to day. Transmission measurements during fractionated abdominal irradiation can quantitate dose variations due to different amounts of air in the bowel during pelvic irradiation (6). However, transmission measurements would not reveal if the air was in the entrance or the exit dose region and would be of limited value for compensation on a day-to-day basis. A worthwhile study would be to scan the same section daily to determine the variation in gut air on a day-to-day basis; the effect of diet, drugs, and other factors could be assessed, and techniques developed to compensate daily for whatever air is shown to be present.

Particle beams are significantly perturbed by air and bone inhomogeneities. Location of such inhomogeneities can be readily determined from the scan for particle therapy planning.

Alterations in external contour which might not be appreciated with a conventionally obtained contour can be detected on the scan (Fig. 3). The posterior air gap between the table top and the midline skin would produce an overdose to the midplane of the illustrated abdomen if treated with uncompensated, equally weighted, anterior and posterior portals directed to the pancreas or para-aortic area of 5%, 3%, and 1.5% with ^{60}Co, and 10 and 25 mV X-rays, respectively.

DIAGNOSTIC CBT STUDIES OF ABDOMINAL MALIGNANCIES

Data relevant to radiotherapy treatment planning contained in primarily diagnostically oriented publications has been presented above. Selected articles relating to diagnostic aspects of abdominal CBT are briefly summarized below.

CBT and Abdominal Lymphoma

CBT has been evaluated in patients with abdominal lymphoma using first-generation scanners by Redman et al. (35), Pilepich et al. (33), Jones et al. (20), Lee et al. (27), and Schaner et al. (38). A more recent study by Ellert and Kreel (8) reviewed the results of CBT scanning in 160 abdominal lymphoma patients studied with 18- and 20-sec scanners. CBT was thought to be superior to bipedal lymphangiography for defining disease extent, especially in patients with nodal involvement in high para-aortic, retrocrural, mesenteric, and hepatic and splenic hilar regions. The techniques provided the same diagnosis on 81% of 97 patients evaluated with both techniques. Forty-nine percent were positive by both techniques; among these, CBT demonstrated more nodal involvement in two-thirds of the cases. After the initial experience with both procedures, CBT became the study of choice, and lymphangiography was thought to be needed for complete assessment in only four cases. Each of these four cases had no fat planes to aid in the delineation of abdominal and retroperitoneal structures. Extranodal abdominal involvement was less well defined than was nodal involvement.

CBT scanning in lymphoma, generally, is of particular value in defining unsuspected disease and has significant implications for staging, altering portal placement, or changing treatment modality. It also furnishes an accurate contour for treatment planning and can assess treatment response, thereby aiding in therapeutic decisions about whether to stop or continue with treatment, etc.

CBT appears to be the procedure of choice for evaluating patients with proved or suspected abdominal lymphoma (4,8), with lymphangiography reserved for patients with no abnormalities on CBT, or for very thin patients without abdominal and retroperitoneal fat.

CBT in Gastric Malignancies

The use of CBT for evaluating patients with stomach cancer has been discussed by Kressell et al. (23) and Lee et al. (28). Balfe and associates (2) recently used CBT to study the stomach in 100 normal and 31 gastric disease patients. Stomach thickness was less than 1 cm in 90% of normal patients and in only 6% of patients with gastric disease; it ranged up to 14 cm in the latter group. Focal thickness in 12 adenocarcinoma patients ranged from 1.2 to 4.0 cm, with 11 of the 12 showing an intraluminal or concentric pattern of tumor growth. Retrogastric spread, indicated by obliteration of the fat plane between the posterior stomach and the pancreas, was correctly diagnosed in 3 patients; recurrence was indicated in 2 cases by a mass at the gastrojejunostomy site. Although 8 of 9 lymphoma patients also had thickened walls, ranging from 1.2 to 3.0 cm, growth patterns alone could not distinguish lymphoma from adenocarcinoma, although secondary signs of lymphoma (splenomegaly in 5 and diffuse retroperitoneal and mesenteric adenopathy in 6) suggested the diagnosis. A large extragastric mass separable from the gastric wall ranging in diameter from 4.5 to 14 cm was present in each of 4 patients with leiomyosarcoma. CBT accurately predicted the presence or absence of metastasis or direct extension in those four cases. One patient with malignant fibrous histiocytoma had a lymphoma-like CBT scan, which also correctly predicted splenic invasion.

Therefore, although scanning is not the primary diagnostic modality for evaluating gastric malignancies, it can provide valuable information regarding tumor extent and adjacent organ involvement. It can also suggest the need for additional diagnostic studies and aid in reaching therapeutic decisions.

CBT and Pancreatic Cancer

CBT in the evaluation of patients with suspected pancreatic cancer has been described by Haaga et al. (18), Sheedy et al. (39), Stanley et al. (40), Cotton et al. (5), Foley et al. (13), and Moss et al. (30). Redman (34) recently reviewed the role of radiologic procedures, including CBT, in the diagnosis of pancreatic cancer. He conceded that small, potentially curable cancers are not routinely diagnosed by CBT but acknowledged that CBT can provide a simple and effective demonstration of pancreatic masses. Particular problems in imaging the organ in emaciated patients who have no peripancreatic fat and in visualizing scirrhous cancers were discussed, as were techniques for scanning. Implications for treatment planning, in addition to mass demonstration [e.g., liver metastasis, exophytic extension (obliteration of peripancreatic fat planes), and portahepatic masses, indicating nodal involvement or direct extension] were discussed. The importance of scan speed when studying the pancreas was stressed, with totally failed examinations said to be rare with fast scanners but to occur with 18-sec or slower instruments.

CBT and Colon Cancer

Mayes and Zornoza (29) reviewed scans on 80 patients with colon cancer studied with an 18-sec scanner; 26 lesions were proximal to the sigmoid colon. Fifteen abnormalities were seen in 11 patients with cecal cancer, and 11 abnormalities were seen in 15 patients with cancers arising in the ascending, transverse, or descending colon. A pelvic mass was seen in 3 of 26 patients with abdominal lesions; other abnormalities included para-aortic nodes in 4, adrenal involvement in 4, liver metastases in 9, and other sites of involvement in 9. Routine use of the technique in all patients with colon cancer was recommended because of the need to assess disease extent so that appropriate treatment decisions can be based on a more complete understanding of tumor extent.

Ellert and Kreel (9) also reviewed their experience with 55 malignant colonic tumor patients studied with CBT, including 14 colon cancers proximal to the sigmoid. The majority of patients were scanned at varying intervals postoperatively to determine what contribution the scan could make to earlier diagnosis of recurrent disease, to define the extent of disease in such patients, and to aid in reaching practical treatment decisions. Among the patients with recurrence, the scan revealed local recurrence only in 44%, distant metastases only in 10%, and both local recurrence and distant metastases in 46%. The technique was particularly helpful for detecting clinically occult recurrence. In patients with clinically apparent disease, it aided in defining disease extent and in making practical decisions regarding patient management. Some patients did achieve pain relief with local irradiation directed to the CBT-defined recurrence.

SUMMARY AND CONCLUSIONS

The radiotherapy community is continuing to appreciate the significant contribution CBT can make to planning abdominal radiotherapy and is also beginning to appreciate the pitfalls and limitations of the technique. Specific attention should continue to focus on patient registration with the scanner and simulator radiographs, patient position during scanning and treatment, and effects of involuntary patient motion, especially breathing, on organ and tumor localization. Effects of patient positional changes and of involuntary motion during treatment on treatment planning and execution should be quantitated, as should effects of inhomogeneities, especially gut air, on abdominal dose distribution.

Radiotherapy planned with CBT data can impact significantly on morbidity and mortality associated with abdominal malignancies. Faster scanners (with a scanning time of 9 sec or less) should be employed where possible to obtain maximum diagnostic information. Multiplanar reconstruction and true three-dimensional treatment planning can enhance significantly the value of CBT in treatment planning. Radiotherapists, radiodiagnosticians, radiation physicists, and oncologists must continue to meet the challenge of realizing the true potential of CBT for the benefit of the cancer patients entrusted to their care.

ACKNOWLEDGMENTS

The assistance of Cynthia Palma and Barbara Weigel in the preparation of the manuscript is gratefully acknowledged. Supported in part by NIH grant C421239.

REFERENCES

1. Alter, A. J., Uehling, D. T., and Zwiebel, W. J. (1979): Computed tomography of the retroperitoneum following nephrectomy. *Radiology*, 133:663–668.
2. Balfe, D. M., Koehler, R. E., Karstaedt, N., Stanley, R. J., and Sagel, S. S. (1981): Computed tomography of gastric neoplasms. *Radiology*, 140:431–436.
3. Bernardino, M. E., deSantos, L. A., Johnson, D. E., and Bracken, R. B. (1979): Computed tomography in the evaluation of post-nephrectomy patients. *Radiology*, 130:183–187.
4. Best. j., and Blackledge, G. (1981): Do we need CT for the management of lymphomas? In: *Computerized Axial Tomography in Oncology*, edited by J. E. Husband and P. Hobday, pp. 59–68. Churchill Livingstone, Edinburgh.
5. Cotton, P. B., Denyer, M. D., Kreel, L., Husband, J., Meire, H. B., and Lees, W. (1978): Comparative clinical impact of endoscopic pancreatography, grey-scale ultrasonography, and computed tomography (EMI scanning) in pancreatic disease: preliminary report. *Gut*, 19:679–684.
6. Dische, S., and Zanelli, J. D. (1976): Bowel gas—a cause of elevated dose in radiotherapy. *Br. J. Radiol.*, 30:543–549.
7. Dossetor, R. S., Veiga-Pires, J. A., and Kaiser, M. (1979): Localization of scanning level in computed tomography of the spine. *J. Comput. Assist. Tomogr.*, 3:284–285.
8. Ellert, J., and Kreel, L. (1980): The role of computed tomography in the initial staging and subsequent management of the lymphomas. *J. Comput. Assist. Tomogr.*, 4:368–391.
9. Ellert, J., and Kreel, L. (1980): The value of CT in malignant colon tumors. *CT*, 4:225–240.
10. Ferrucci, J. T., Jr., and Wittenberg, J. (1978): CT biopsy of abdominal tumors: aids for lesion localization. *Radiology*, 129:739–744.
11. Foley, W. D., Lawson, T. L., and Quiroz, F. (1979): Sagittal and coronal image reconstruction: application in pancreatic computed tomography. *J. Comput. Assist. Tomogr.*, 3:717–721.
12. Foley, W. D., Lawson, T. L., Berland, L. L., Chintapalli, K., Berninger, W. H., and Reddington, R. W. (1981): Reformatted coronal display of upper abdominal computed tomography: comparison with ultrasound. *J. Comput. Assist., Tomogr.*, 5:496–502.
13. Foley, W. D., Stewart, E. T., Lawson, T. L., Greenan, J., Loguidice, J., Maher, J., and Unger, G. F. (1980): Computed tomography, ultrasonography, and endoscopic cholangiopancreatography in the diagnosis of pancreatic disease: a comparative study. *Gastrointest. Radiol.*, 5:29–35.
14. Goitein, M., and Abrams, M. (1981): This volume.
15. Goitein, M., Wittenberg, J., Mendiondo, M., Doucette, J., Freidberg, C., Ferrucci, J., Gunderson, L., Linggood, R., Shipley, W. U., and Fineberg, H. V. (1979): The value of CT scanning in radiation therapy treatment planning: a prospective study. *Int. J. Radiat. Oncol. Biol. Phys.*, 5:1787–1798.
16. Graffman, S., Urie, M., Verhey, L. J., and Munzenrider, J. E. (1981): Potential contribution of modulated proton beam therapy to radical irradiation of para-aortic nodes. *Int. J. Radiat. Oncol. Biol. Phys.*, 9:1214 (abstract).
17. Gunderson, L. (1979): Radiation oncology. In: *Alimentary Tract Radiology. Abdominal Imaging*, Vol. 3, edited by A. R. Margulis and H. J. Burhenne, pp. 600–619. Mosby, St. Louis.

18. Haaga, J. R., Alfidi, R. J., Zelch, M. G., Meany, T. F., Boller, M., Gonzalez, L., and Jelden, G. L. (1976): Computed tomography of the pancreas. *Radiology*, 120:589–595.
19. Hobday, P., Hodson, N. J., Husband, J., Parker, R. P., and McDonald, J. S. (1979): Computed tomography applied to radiotherapy treatment planning: techniques and results. *Radiology*, 133:477–482.
20. Jones, S. E., Tobias, D. A., and Waldman, R. S. (1978): Computed tomographic scanning in patients with lymphoma. *Cancer*, 41:480–486.
21. Kivisaari, L., Kormano, M., and Rantakokko, V. (1979): Contrast enhancement of the pancreas in computed tomography. *J. Comput. Assist. Tomogr.*, 3:722–726.
22. Kreel, L. (1977): Computerized tomography using the EMI general purpose scanner. *Br. J. Radiol.*, 50:2–14.
23. Kressell, H. Y., Callen, P. W., and Montagne, J. P., (1978): Computed tomographic evaluation of disorders affecting the alimentary tract. *Radiology*, 129:451–455.
24. Kuhns, L. R., Borlaza, G. S., Seigel, R., and Thornbury, J. R. (1978): External anatomic landmarks of the abdomen related to vertebral segments: applications in cross-sectional imaging. *Am. J. Roentgenol.*, 131:115–117.
25. Kuhns, L. R., Thornbury, J., and Seigel, R. (1979): Variation of position of the kidneys and diaphragm in patients undergoing repeated suspension of respiration. *J. Comput. Assist. Tomogr.*, 3:620–621.
26. Lee, J. K. T., Levitt, R. G., Stanley, R. J., and Sagel, S. S. (1978): Utility of body computed tomography in the clinical follow-up of abdominal masses. *J. Comput. Assist. Tomogr.*, 2:607–611.
27. Lee, J. K. T., Stanley, R. J., Sagel, S. S., and Levitt, R. G. (1978): Accuracy of computed tomography in detecting intra-abdominal and pelvic adenopathy in lymphoma. *Am. J. Roentgenol.*, 131:311–315.
28. Lee, K. R., Levine, E., Moffat, R. E., Bigongiari, L. R., and Hermreck, A. S. (1979): Computed tomographic staging of malignant gastric neoplasms. *Radiology*, 133:151–155.
29. Mayes, G. B., and Zornoza, J. (1980): Computed tomography of colon carcinoma. *Am. J. Roentgenol.*, 135:43–46.
30. Moss, A. A., Federle, M., Shapior, H. A., Ohto, M., Goldberg, H., Korobkin, M., and Clemett, A. (1980): The combined use of computed tomography and endoscopic retrograde cholangiopancreatography in the assessment of suspected pancreatic neoplasm: a blind clinical study. *Radiology*, 134:159–163.
31. Munzenrider, J. E., Pilepich, M., Rene-Ferrero, J. B., Tchakarova, I., and Carter, B. L. (1977): Use of body scanner in radiotherapy treatment planning. *Cancer*, 40:170–179.
32. Munzenrider, J. E., Verhey, L., and Doucette, J. (1981): A critical appraisal of the value of CT to the radiotherapist—the abdomen. In: *Computerized Axial Tomography in Oncology*, edited by J. E. Husband and P. Hobday. Churchill Livingstone, Edinburgh.
33. Pilepich, M., Rene, J. B., Munzenrider, J. E., and Carter, B. L. (1978): Contribution of computed tomography to the treatment of lymphomas. *Am. J. Roentgenol.*, 131:67–73.
34. Redman, H. C., (1981): Standard radiologic diagnosis and CT scanning in pancreatic cancer. *Cancer*, 47:1656–1661.
35. Redman, H. C., Glatstein, E., Castellino, R. A., and Federal, W. A. (1977): Computed tomography as an adjunct in the staging of Hodgkin's disease and non-Hodgkin's lymphomas. *Radiology*, 124:381–385.
36. Robbins, A. H., Pugatch, R. D., Gerzof, S. G., Spira, R., Rankin, S. C., and Gale, D. R. (1981): An assessment of the role of scan speed in perceived image quality of body computed tomography. *Radiology*, 139:139–146.
37. Sagel, S. S., Stanley, R. J., Levitt, R. G., and Geisse, G. (1977): Computed tomography of the kidney. *Radiology*, 124:359–370.
38. Shaner, E. G., Head, G. L., Doppman, J. L., and Young, R. C. (1977): Computed tomography in the diagnosis, staging, and management of abdominal lymphoma. *J. Comput. Assist. Tomogr.*, 1:176–180.
39. Sheedy, P. F., Stephens, D. H., Hattery, R. R., and MacCarty, R. L. (1977): Computed tomography in the evaluation of patients with suspected carcinoma of the pancreas. *Radiology*, 124:731–737.
40. Stanley, R. J., Sagel, S. S., and Levitt, R. G. (1977): Computed tomographic evaluation of the pancreas. *Radiology*, 124:715–722.
41. Villafana, T., Lee, S. H., Vider, M., and Wu, R. K. (1979): Device for correlating CT and radiation therapy portal images. *Am. J. Roentgenol.*, 133:1191–1193.
42. Wittenberg, J., and Ferrucci, J. T., Jr. (1978): Computed body tomography. *Gastroenterology*, 74:287–293.

Computed Tomography in Radiation Therapy,
edited by C. C. Ling, C. C. Rogers, and
R. J. Morton. Raven Press, New York © 1983

Computed Tomography in Therapy Planning: Pelvic Region

Sucha O. Asbell and Mary Anne Seago

*Department of Radiation Therapy, Albert Einstein Medical Center,
Philadelphia, Pennsylvania 19141*

Since computed tomographic (CT) body scanning became generally available in 1977, it has proved valuable in diagnosing the extent of tumors as well as in the dynamic physiological localizing of certain pelvic organs for radio-oncologic treatment. CT provides a contour at multiple levels of tumor and frequently demonstrates disease not shown on other x-ray studies; it may also define nonpalpable disease. CT scans help to decide if the tumor is so extensive that a palliative pre- or postoperative approach is necessary. It also permits following tumor regression with decreasing portal size. CT is being used to refine tumor dose calculations by providing accurate density and inhomogeneity factors. Several authors have reported improved accuracy of dosimetry with CT data; it is hoped that the 30% alteration in treatment planning from information learned from CT scans will result in improved palliation, decreased injury to normal tissue, and increased survival (5,11,27,30).

This chapter reviews the role of CT scanning in radio-oncologic treatment planning of the pelvis, i.e., bladder carcinoma (CA), prostate CA, recurrent rectal CA, gynecologic malignancy, and lymph nodal involvement in cancer and lymphoma.

GYNECOLOGIC MALIGNANCY

There has been little in the literature (1,4,17,29,36) up to the present time regarding the use of CT scanning in gynecologic oncology. Between January 1977 and June 1981, 119 cases of CA of the uterus, 65 of the cervix, 25 of the ovary, 6 of the vulva, and 1 of the vagina were seen in the radiation therapy department of our institution. Only 39 of these patients were evaluated with abdomen and pelvic CT scans, as we had learned from early evaluations that these scans did not appear to be particularly useful. Only 13 of the 39 scans were interpreted as abnormal, and they were from patients with advanced bulky disease; 26 of the scans were interpreted as normal, although five of these showed some uterine enlargement. Each of the 26 patients whose scans were negative had disease more extensive than 2 cm but mostly centrally located, and in 13 patients CT abnormality failed to reflect bulky clinical parametrial extent of disease. We found that in stage I CA of the cervix and stage II CA of the uterus there were rarely abnormalities or masses in the true pelvis. Because tumor has virtually the same density as normal tissue, one could not expect the CT to differentiate from one pelvic tissue to another unless the anatomy were distorted. Central disease was hidden by the contour of the uterus; and unless contrast was utilized in the bladder, addition of shadows made interpretation of central disease quite difficult. We agree with Bernardino and Dodd (4) that ultrasound has been more or as useful in determining the port borders when there was a need to encompass the entire uterus. Thus little information for treatment planning was gleaned except if there was enlargement of nonpalpable high iliac or low para-aortic nodes in the false pelvic region.

CT scans, however, are quite useful in the more advanced stages of carcinoma of the uterus, cervix, and ovaries in treatment planning. Abnormalities found on CT did not always reflect the full extent of disease noted clinically. This finding is in contrast with that of Ginaldi et al. (10), who found a good correlation between the physical findings and CT; their patient number, however, was small. Frequently tumor margins which could not be identified clinically, in one or several dimensions, were provided in both the primary as well as the cone-down portals. If patients had had previous surgery (e.g., hysterectomy or abdominal-perineal resection), evaluation of the remaining pelvic structures or tumor masses became easier. However,

TABLE 1. *Average bladder area at the level of femoral heads*

Subject	Sex	Bladder area (cm)		Residual area post-void/pre-void
		Pre-void	Post-void	
Bladder CA (av. age 65)	M	56.2	41.5	0.74
	F	50.0	38.9	0.78
Prostate CA (av. age 69)	M	50.7	37.4	0.74
	F	—	—	—
Normal (av. age 45)	M	51.8	20.2	0.39
	F	55.7	33.1	0.59

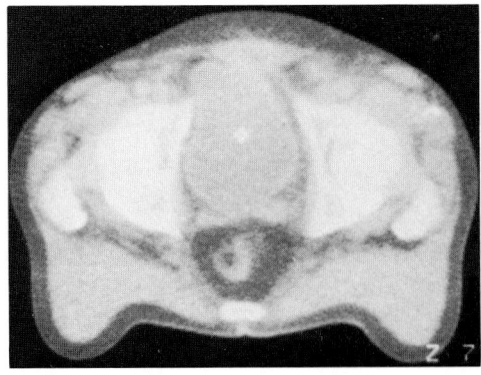 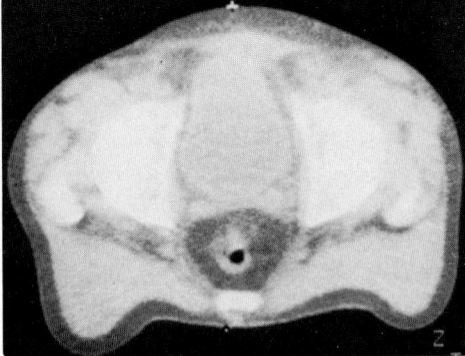

FIG. 1. **Left:** Pre-void scan of bladder at the level of the femoral heads. **Right:** Post-void scan of same patient showing no significant change in the anterior aspect of the bladder.

TABLE 2. *Comparison of methods used in treatment planning for bladder carcinoma*

Area evaluated	IVP	Cystogram	CT scan
Bladder walls (lateral, superior, inferior)	+	+	+
Anterior bladder wall	+/−	+/−	+
Posterior bladder wall	+/−	+/−	+
Extent of tumor mass	−	−	+

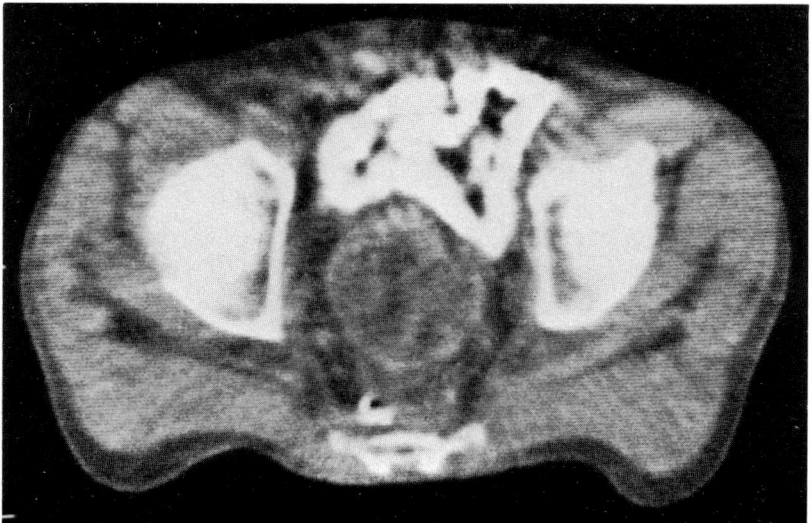

FIG. 2. **A:** CT scan in a male patient showing the posterior shift of the bladder after A-P resection. Note the contrast material in the small bowel anterior to the bladder.

recent literature revealed the failure of CT to identify masses surgically confirmed of less than 2 cm, especially small peritoneal and surface of the liver seedings. Thus CT cannot be totally relied on to determine the extent of disease if it is inadequately staged surgically. CT cannot replace the "second-look operation." Treatment portals which are confined to large abdominal masses seen on CT may be inadequate to treat disease.

BLADDER

The use of CT scanning in the management of carcinoma of the bladder has only begun (11,13–15,18,30,32,33,35). The physiological status of the bladder, both full and empty in its normal and malignant states, differs. We have learned that it is the older population, who frequently present with bladder cancer, who have atony or poor tone. This may be secondary to age or to chronic obstruction in the male but more likely is due to tumor extending into the muscle. Frequently the bladder

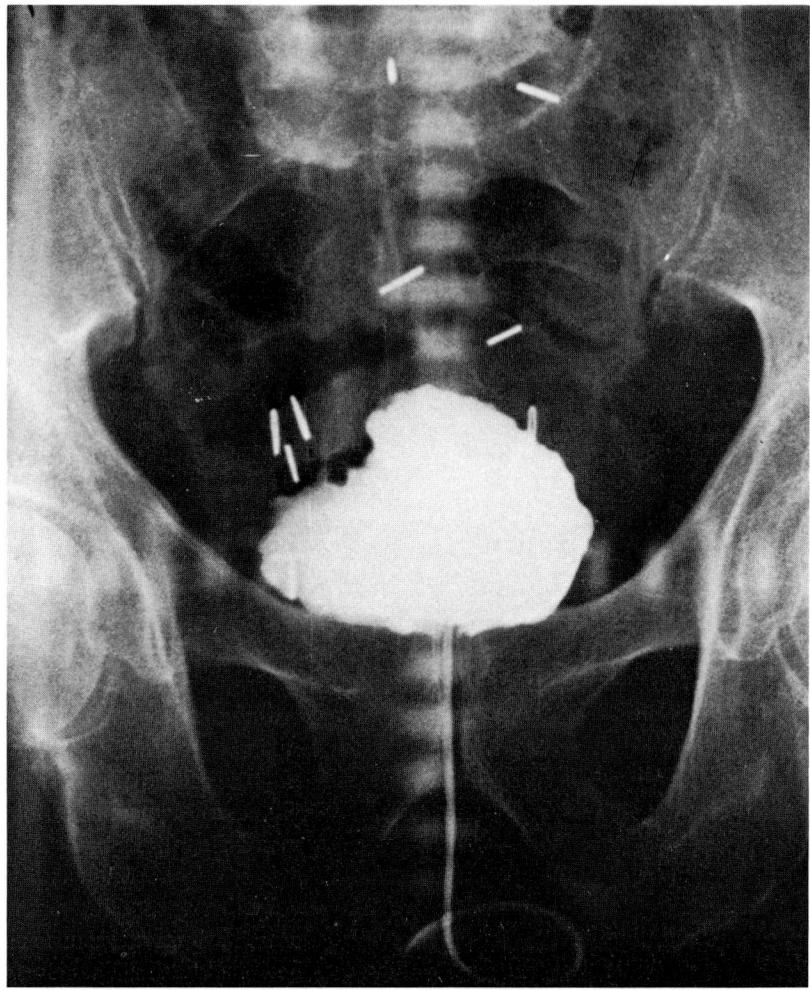

FIG. 2. B: Cystogram, AP view, in the same patient as in **A**.

does not appear to empty as completely in patients with carcinoma as it does in normal individuals (Table 1). The area identified as bladder on CT scans at the level of the femoral heads after voiding, divided by its pre-void area, can be called the residual area. One notes that the residual area is greatest in the elderly and in patients with carcinoma in contrast with the normal or middle-aged patient. Before CT was available at our institution, for radiation therapy treatment, planning consisted of: (a) asking the patient to void completely prior to (b) catheterizing him, (c) introducing 30 cc air and 30 cc contrast material, and (d) taking x-ray simulation portals, anteroposterior (AP) and lateral, in preparation for the four field box technique.

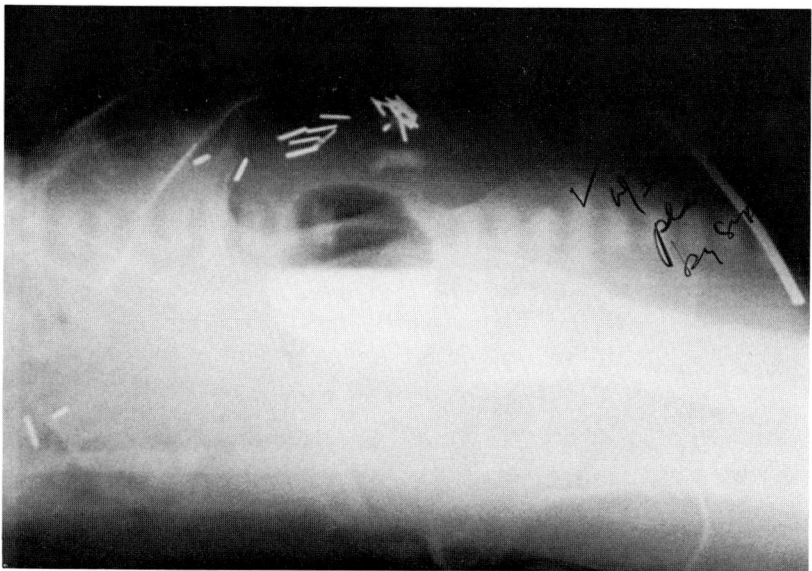

FIG. 2. C: Lateral simulation film in a male after A-P resection, with contrast material.

We noted that many of our patients had post-void residual urine (as much as 250 ml). Frequently their bladders assumed odd shapes, or there were diverticuli. If the condition of the patient is to resemble his status under routine post-void circumstances and if CT scanning is not available to evaluate bladder size and location under routine physiological conditions, then the procedure should consist of: (a) having the patient void; (b) inserting a catheter; (c) calculating the amount of residual urine; (d) placing contrast material equal in volume to that of residual urine in the bladder.

Thus the simulation will approximate the size of the bladder that would normally be present in the post-void state and allow a more accurate confirmation of the treatment volume in all dimensions. If simulation is to be utilized along with CT, a comparison of bladder size and location will be more accurate. However, simulation with invasive techniques probably can be safely eliminated, as reconstruction in many planes is possible. Only CT scans will show extension of extraluminal disease, the way the bladder empties, and how much small bowel falls into its previous position with pre- and post-void scans. We have learned that the anterior extent of the bladder at the level of the femoral heads does not change significantly and does not fall behind the pubic bone after voiding (Fig. 1). The dome and upper portions of the bladder disappear from the CT levels seen on pre-void scans. Even with contrast material in the bladder, lateral films in the obese patient may not demonstrate the anterior wall. CT measures all dimensions of the bladder more accurately than any invasive technique (Table 2).

The effect of previous surgical procedures on the location of the bladder must be taken into account in the treatment planning in the pelvis. This is especially true

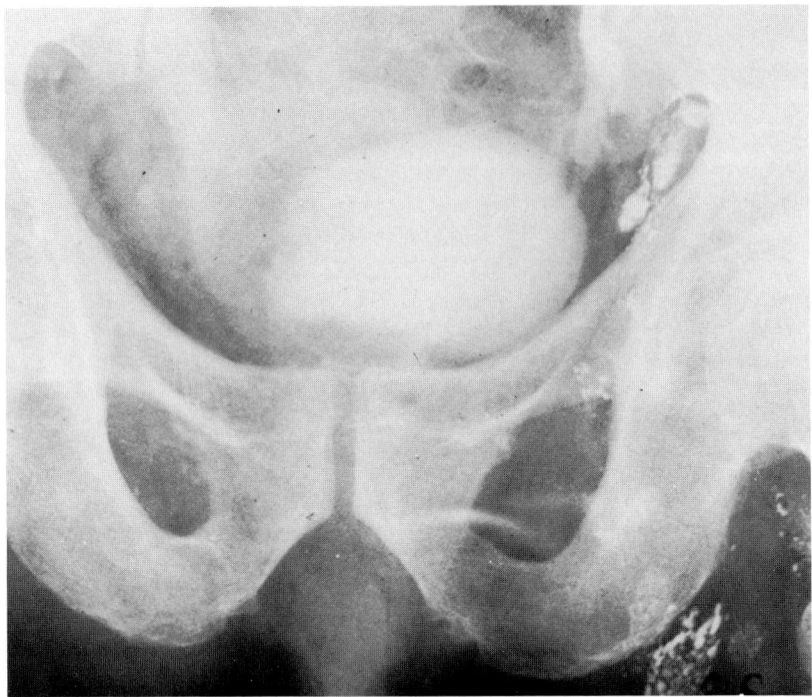

FIG. 3. **A:** An intraluminal defect in the bladder visualized on IVP, demonstrated by the irregular right margin, in a 70-year-old male patient with carcinoma of the bladder.

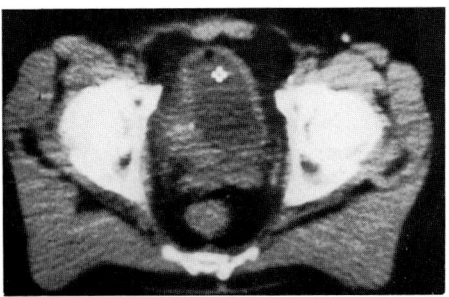

FIG. 3. **B:** CT scan at the level of the femoral heads showing extension of this lesion to the pelvic wall.

for the male urogenital tract when there has been an abdominal-perineal (A-P) resection for carcinoma of the rectum. In a few patients we evaluated several weeks postoperatively, the bladder sometimes shifted posteriorly, falling into the sacral hollow (Fig. 2A). Despite the patient's prone position for prophylactic treatment of stage C carcinoma of the rectum (Asler-Collier modification of Duke's staging classification) after A-P resection, cystitis could not have been anticipated from a cystogram (which is not routinely done in most radiation therapy departments) (Fig. 2B). The posterior shift of the bladder may be confirmed as well by lateral simulation

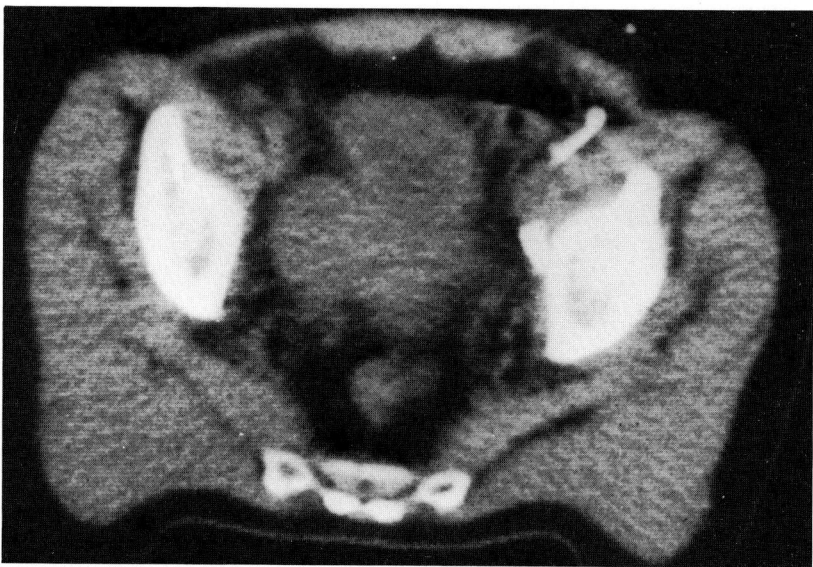

FIG. 3. C: CT scan above the level of the femoral heads showing an extraluminal mass.

(Fig. 2C) as by CT, but placing contrast material in the bladder would not be done routinely for this malignancy.

Kenny et al. (19) demonstrated that 56% of patients with bladder cancers had been inaccurately staged at surgery. These inaccuracies may result from the inability to adequately examine the patient bimanually or because the tumor mass is too small to be noted by the examining finger. The accuracy of staging, especially in the obese patient where bimanual examination is difficult, is improved with CT scanning. Seidelmann et al. (33), Kellet et al. (18), and Yu et al. (41) have demonstrated a greater than 80% accuracy in staging with CT scanning, especially noting disease outside the bladder wall, which is most easily ascertained on CT (15).

Thirty percent of our patients who were prescribed bladder or pelvic and bladder boost irradiation for carcinoma have had their treatment plans changed from information gained on the CT scan, whether due to abnormal location of the bladder, peculiar shape, indefinite margins at simulation, or a mass outside the bladder (30).

In radiation therapy treatment planning and dosimetry, the extent of intravesicular disease in carcinoma of the bladder does not have a major effect on the management, as the entire bladder is treated. Thus the air insufflation technique described by Seidelmann et al. (32) seems to be an unwarranted additional instrumentation for initial pretreatment evaluation. Seidelmann's technique of air insufflation, however, may provide us with insight about the sites and patterns of recurrence in the follow-up evaluation. This remains to be determined.

Although bimanual examination and simulation may reveal no mass extending through or outside the bladder wall, the CT scan may indicate the maximum tumor

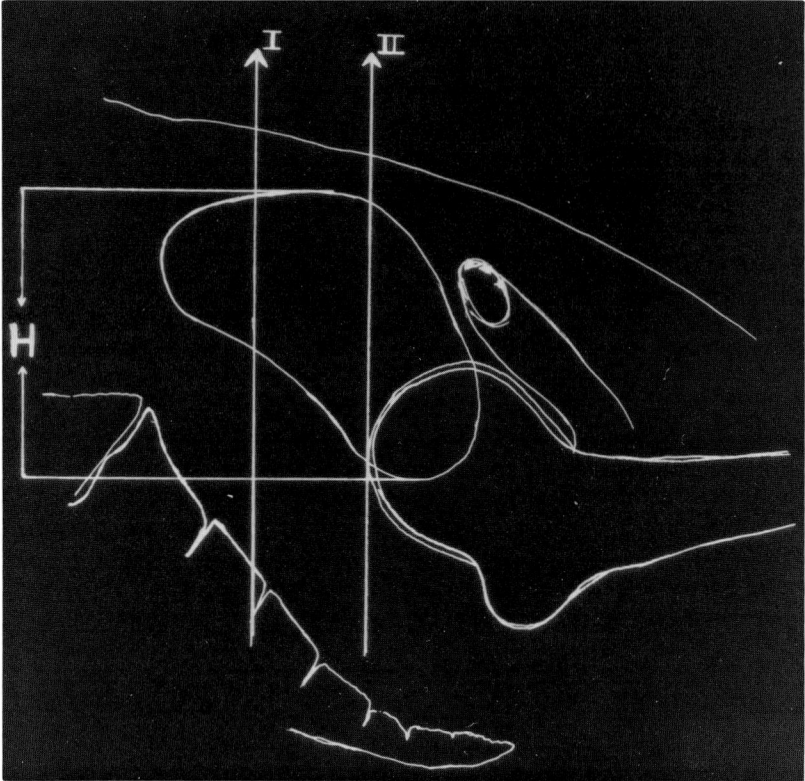

FIG. 3. **D:** Diagram of lateral view of bladder showing it at the level of the femoral heads (II) above (I), corresponding respectively to **B** and **C**.

volume necessary when multiple CT levels are summated (Fig. 3). At times what is clinically palpable has not been visualized on CT; this may be due to a failure to change normal tissue planes. CT is certainly not foolproof, and small lesions may be missed. A question remains: If the disease is not palpable but is seen on CT, is the prognosis still as grave? There may be a critical mass or extent of disease seen on CT which we previously would have incorrectly felt incurable. Only time will resolve these questions.

We have noted that extraluminal masses do not shrink away rapidly during the course of treatment. Repeat scanning was performed during the middle or near the end of a course of 6,000 to 6,500 rads of therapy, and there was no apparent change in the size of the tumor. Thus tumor volume could not be reduced as in ovarian CA or lymphoma. Later regression of tumor masses did occur, however.

For example, a 70-year-old male with carcinoma of the bladder had a CT scan that showed a mass which was palpable at the seminal vesicles. He underwent a CT scan during radiation therapy; no changes were noted. At 6 months, however, there seemed to be tumor regression (Fig. 4). Doubleday and Bernardino (8) described postradiation changes but in only 26 patients with various malignancies.

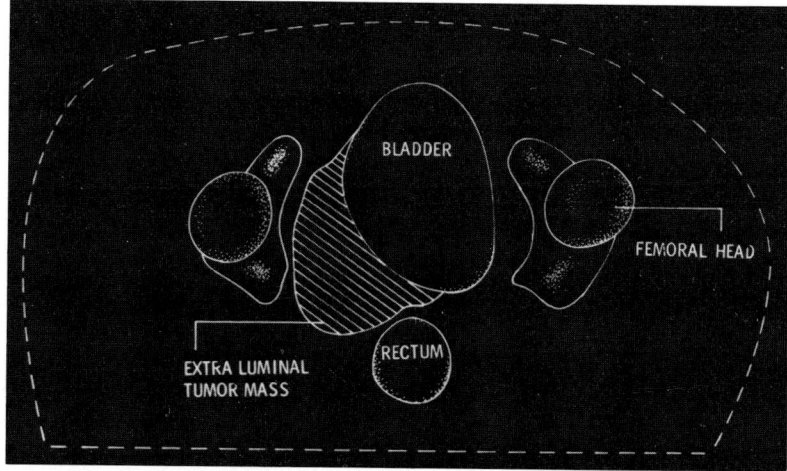

FIG. 3. **E:** Diagram of summated tumor volume reconstructed at the isocenter of the treatment volume from **B** and **C**.

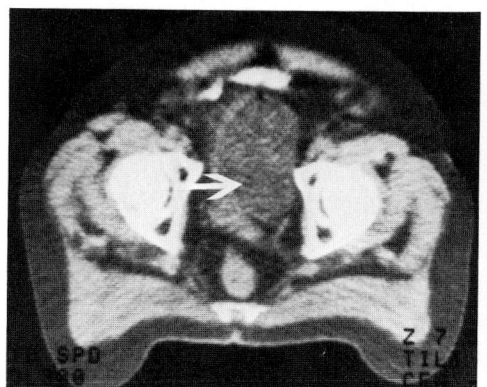 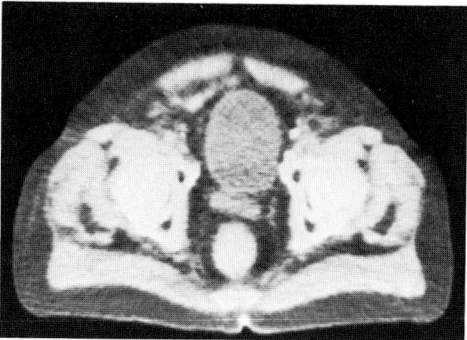

FIG. 4. **Left:** CT scan of a 70-year-old male patient with CA of the bladder who had a clinically palpable mass *(arrow)* at the seminal vesicles. **Right:** CT scan showing tumor regression 6 months after radiation therapy.

However, CT scans were not performed on each patient before and after treatment. Thus the only confirmation of some of these abnormalities are those on diagnostic x-rays, as described by Lipshitz (25), and even he admits that the frequency of these alterations after radiation therapy is not routine, although no frequency testing has been done. After a review of many patients after radiation therapy, we were unable to confirm Doubleday and Bernardino's findings with any regularity.

PROSTATE

The prostate gland is not easily seen on diagnostic x-ray evaluation. CT scans now provide the major source of organ and tumor definition, aside from clinical evaluation and ultrasound (21,26,37). In addition to defining the dimensions of the gland (2,38), CT provides help in staging by defining the extension outside of the gland. Involvement of the seminal vesicles and paraprostatic tissues increases the stage. Extension to these areas was not easily determined on clinical examination or by any x-ray examination other than seminal vesiculography. Fewer than 300 vesiculograms have been reported in the American and English journals during the past 30 years. This is probably because of the aversion of patients and surgeons to have invasive manipulation of the vas (31). Inclusion of the seminal vesicles in treatment planning may be of importance in stage C (American staging system) prostatic carcinoma, as by definition tumor extends outside the prostatic tissue at this stage. This may also be of importance in 17 to 36% of the stage B patients, as the extent of tumor may be greater than is clinically appreciated; this was noted by several authors (Table 3). Vickery and Kerr (39) reported that in 65% of their patients with poorly differentiated carcinoma of the prostate there was invasion of the seminal vesicles at surgery.

The treatment volume in radiation planning must include organs with a high probability of involvement, as well as tumor, if treatment is to be successful. It is not yet known if inclusion of the seminal vesicles will increase the successful treatment of prostatic carcinoma, stages B and C. Treatment planning is done if the seminal vesicles are to be included, as they sit above the prostate (Fig. 5, top). A CT scan must be sufficiently superior to the prostate (Fig. 5, middle) to detect these organs (Fig. 5, bottom). They are usually posterior to the prostate and may hug the rectum. There has been some motion of the seminal vesicles (34). However, we have found insufficient movement of the seminal vesicles in the prone position to allow for a change in treatment planning to accommodate the rectum when including the seminal vesicles in the treatment plan via this manipulation. If one is to simulate a four-field "box" technique (i.e., AP and lateral films), filling the bowel and bladder with contrast material for prostate localization, the treatment volumes will be inadequate. Localization of the prostate and paraprostatic tissues

TABLE 3. *Literature review of seminal vesicle involvement in CA of prostate*

Author	Date	%	No.	Stage or histology
Colby	1953	36.0	20/56	Clinical stage B
Arduino	1962	24.0	17/71	Clinical stage B
Vickery	1963	38.6	32/83	Well differentiated
Vickery	1963	64.9	24/37	Poorly differentiated
Scott	1969	27.0	9/33	—
Jewett	1970	17.0	17/103	Clinical stage B
Byar	1972	16.0	30/178	Stage C
Byar	1972	18.0	37/208	Clinical stage B
Mostofi	1973	17.0	30/175	—
Dahl	1974	0.0	0/18	Clinical stage B
Barzel	1977	31.0	31/100	Stage C
Veenema	1977	10.0	16/159	Clinical stages A & B

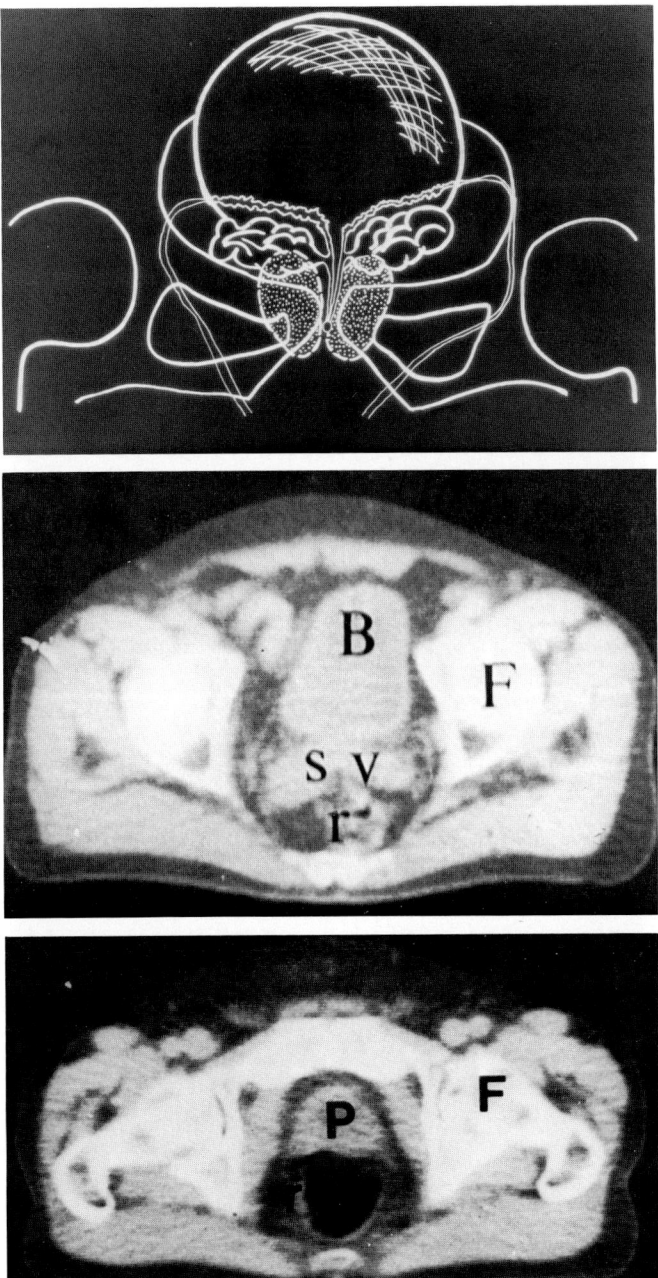

FIG. 5. **Top:** Diagram showing superior location of seminal vesicles to prostate. **Middle:** CT at the level of the seminal vesicle. B = bladder. F = femoral head. r = rectum. sv = seminal vesicles. **Bottom:** CT scan at the level of the prostate. P = prostate. F = femoral head. r = rectum.

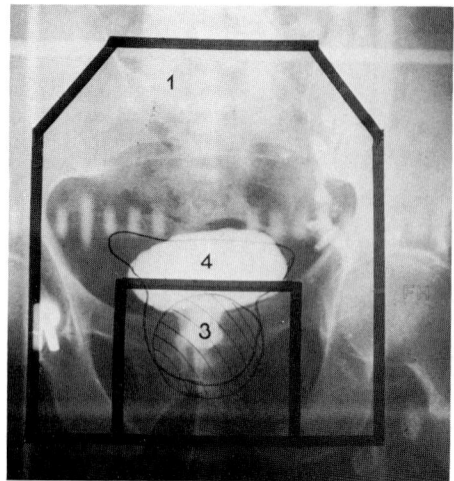
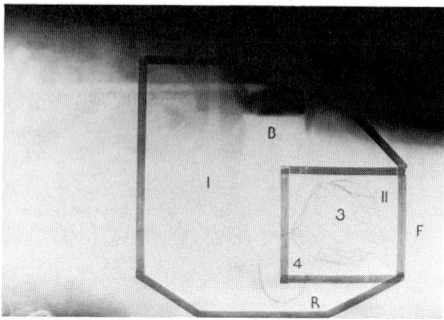

FIG. 6.   Left: AP simulation film with heavy black lines outlining the large (area 1) and reduced (area 2) fields. The cross-hatched area (3) represents the prostate, as determined from the simulation films. Area 4 outlines the region occupied by the seminal vesicles and prostate as defined by the CT scan. **Right:** Lateral simulation film with heavy black lines outlining the large (area 1) and reduced (area 2) treatment portals. Area 3 *(cross-hatched)* represents the prostate as deduced from the simulation film and radiographs. Area 4 represents the composite of the prostate and seminal vesicles as obtained from the CT scan. B = bladder. F = femoral head. R = rectum.

may be inaccurate if the scan is performed in this manner (Fig. 6). The diagrammatic estimation of prostatic size and location from simulation in a typical case is demonstrated in Fig. 7.

The simulations in CT localization for prostatic and seminal vesicular tumor volumes and prostate alone are compared in Tables 4 and 5. It is obvious that on small fields directed to the prostate alone the greatest error is in the posterior and superior directions. When the prostate and seminal vesicular volume are included, inaccuracies are present in all dimensions, and part of the tumor or organ is missed. The following suggestions are offered after review of 24 patients with prostatic CA, stage B or C, diagnosed after transurethral resection (TUR):

1. The size and location of the prostate is not accurately deduced or estimated from x-ray simulation with contrast material in the bladder or rectum.

2. CT scanning demonstrates prostatic size and location within the pelvis.

3. The average size of the prostate measured on CT, post-TUR, was 4.9 ± 0.7 cm (lateral), 4.8 ± 0.8 cm (AP), and 4.4 cm (craniocaudad), with a range of 3.9 to 6.5 cm.

4. Utilizing an 8 × 8 × 8 cm treatment volume for inclusion of the prostate gland alone, without benefit of a CT scan, allows an error in any one of the three dimensions in 18 to 25% of the cases studied.

5. A literature review revealed that prostatic invasion of the seminal vesicles occurred in 65% of the patients with poorly differentiated carcinoma subclinically

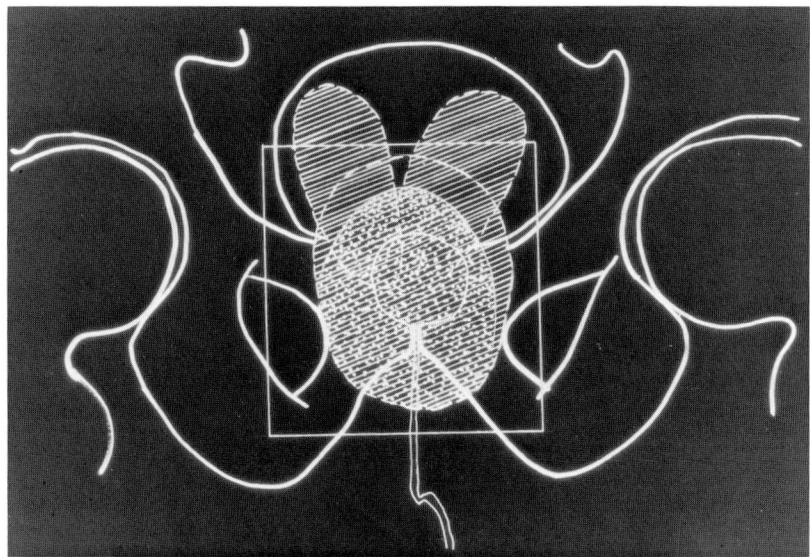

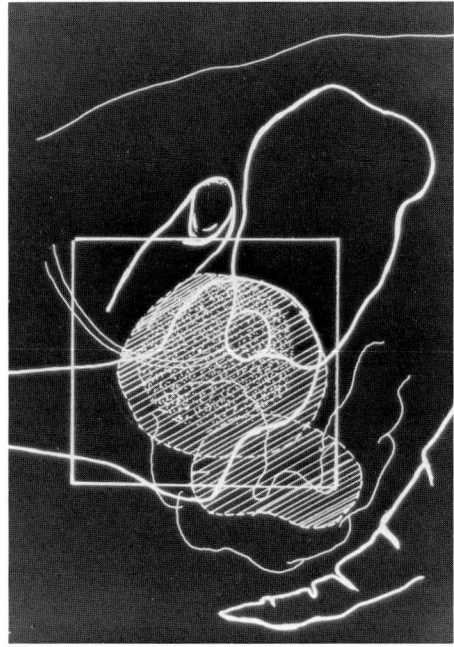

FIG. 7. Top: AP diagram of a simulated estimation of the prostate *(heavy dots)* included within an 8 × 8 cm portal compared to the actual size of the prostate and seminal vesicles *(diagonal lines)* seen by CT. **Left:** Lateral diagram of the same area as top.

TABLE 4. *Comparison of simulation and CT for prostatic tumor volume in 24 patients*

Area	Pelvic field, prostate, & lymph nodes (%)		Field limited to prostate (%)	
Lateral margins	Inadequate	0	Inadequate	18
	Portion missed	0	Portion missed	0
	<1 cm margin	0	<1 cm margin	18
Craniocaudad margins	Inadequate	0	Inadequate	21
	Portion missed	0	Portion missed	0
	<1 cm margin	0	<1 cm margin	21
Anterior-posterior margins	Inadequate	17	Inadequate	25
	Portion missed	0	Portion missed	0
	<1 cm margin	17	<1 cm margin	25

TABLE 5. *Comparison of simulation and CT for prostatic and seminal vesicular tumor volume in 24 patients*

Area	Pelvic field prostate, seminal vesicles, and lymph nodes (%)		Field limited to prostate and seminal vesicles (%)	
Lateral margins	Inadequate	0	Inadequate	43
	Portion missed	0	Portion missed	25
	<1 cm margin	0	<1 cm margin	18
Craniocaudad margins	Inadequate	0	Inadequate	65
	Portion missed	0	Portion missed	50
	<1 cm margin	0	<1 cm margin	15
Anterior-posterior margins	Inadequate	50	Inadequate	75
	Portion missed	10	Portion missed	50
	<1 cm margin	40	<1 cm margin	25

and in 0 to 36% of the patients whose disease was clinically stage B; this was substantiated at prostatovesiculectomy and represents an average of 17%.

6. All stages of prostatic carcinoma equal to or greater than stage C, and all poorly differentiated tumors, should probably include seminal vesicles in the treatment volume at the time of X-ray therapy.

7. Invasion of the seminal vesicles from prostatic carcinoma cannot be substantiated on CT scan from our small series, predominantly stage B, although we substantiate localization of the routinely radiographically silent seminal vesicles.

8. If the seminal vesicles are to be included in the treatment volume, an 8 × 8 × 8 cm field for the prostate would be inadequate. These tissues would be missed in 25 to 50% of patients in any one dimension; in 43 to 75% there would be less than a 1-cm margin.

9. A 9 × 9 × 9 cm treatment volume, if properly placed, provides the smallest volume that would include the prostate and seminal vesicles and eliminate most marginal errors if CT is unavailable.

10. CT scans provide quick, accurate localization of the prostate and seminal vesicles. It allows for individualized treatment planning without any invasive pro-

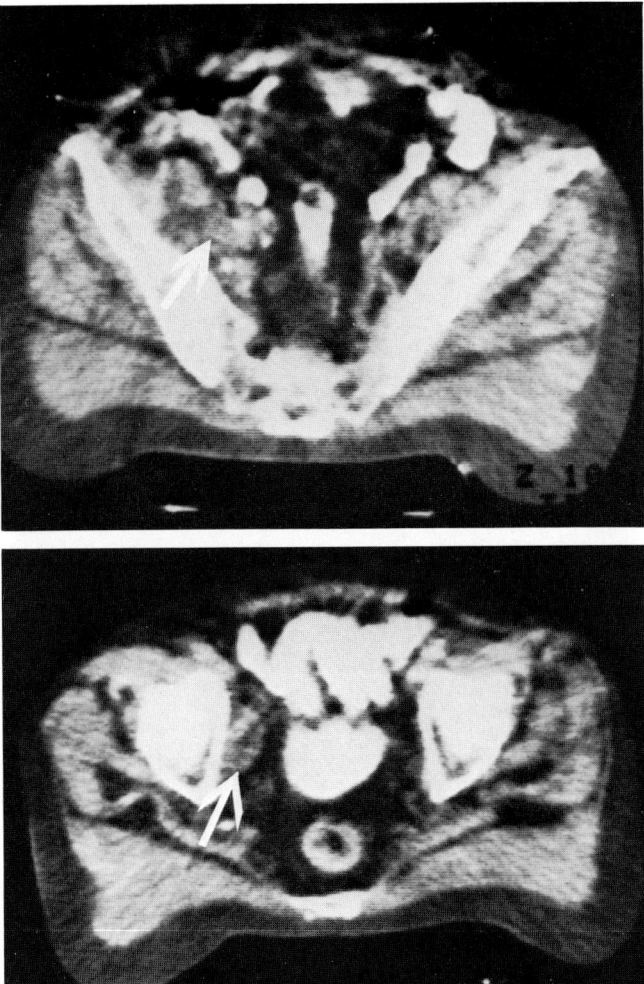

FIG. 8. Top: A 72-year-old male patient with CA of the prostate who presented several years after diagnosis with right leg edema. CT shows obstructing lymphatics at the level of the iliac crest. **Bottom:** CT scan taken slightly above the acetabuli.

cedure and may permit less than a $9 \times 9 \times 9$ cm reduced or small field tumor volume.

Along with diethylstilbestrol, or after its failure, radiation therapy may still be utilized to decompress the ureter. Although some investigators describe a change in seminal vesicle angle as classic for this situation, others do not agree (28). We believe a lack of definition of the seminal vesicles on CT accompanies intravenous pyelogram (IVP) evidence of obstruction. Tumor growing up the posterior aspect of the bladder along the region of the seminal vesicles leads to the obstruction of

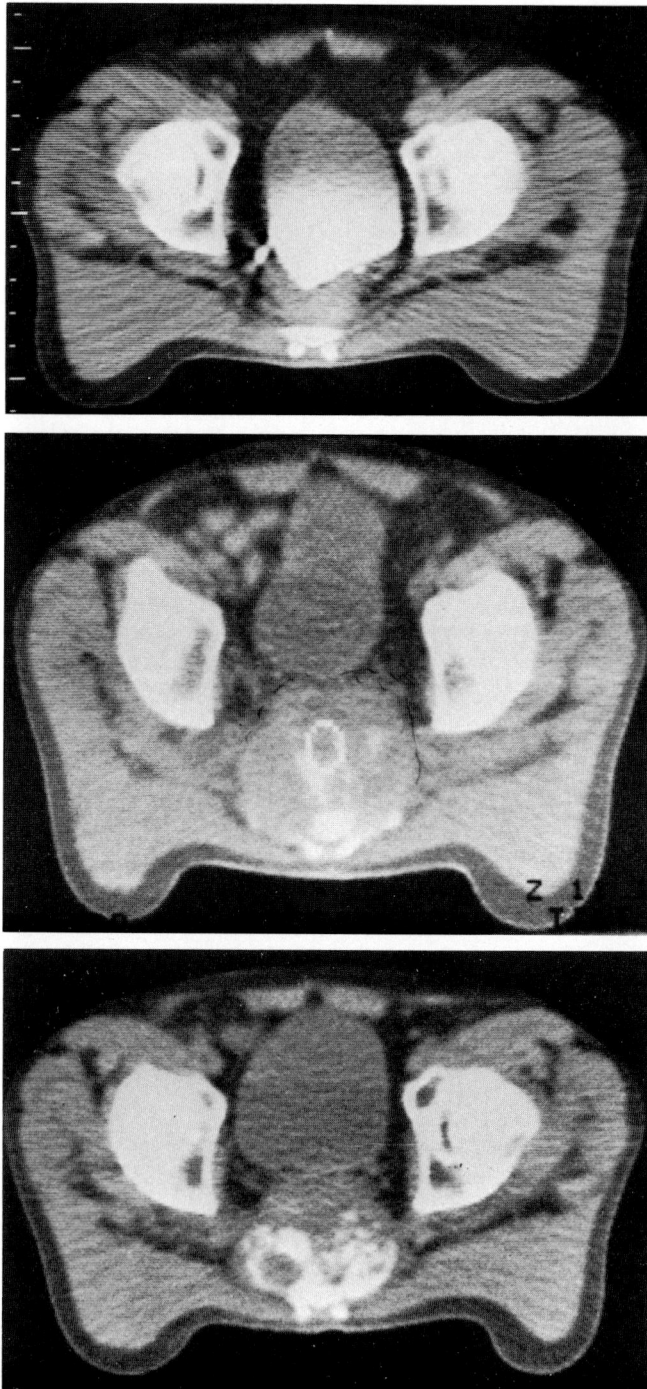

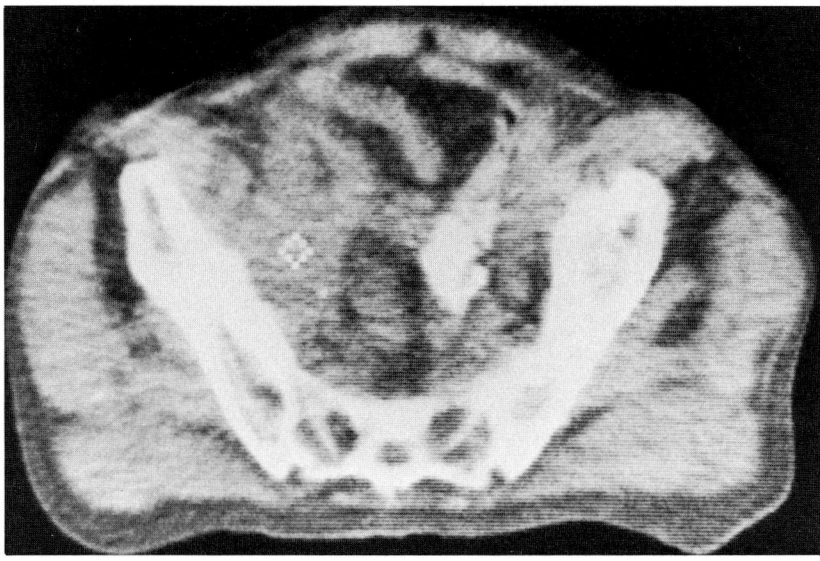

FIG. 10. A 70-year-old patient with carcinoma of the rectum after A-P resection, who tried to commit suicide because of severe right back pain. See metastasis to right iliac nodes *(asterisk)*, undiagnosed on all other x-ray studies.

the ureteral orifices. The tumor density is similar to that of normal tissue. All that is lost is the lack of normal tissue planes in this region of the growth unless there is very bulky disease showing as tumor mass.

LYMPH NODES

Until sufficient data accrue, it will be difficult to assess in which malignancies CT of the pelvis should be accompanied by CT of the abdomen. Certainly in advanced carcinoma of the bladder, prostate, cervix, and uterus, CT scanning of the abdomen as well as of the pelvis should be performed, especially if the tumor is poorly differentiated, longstanding, or recurrent. The risk of disease outside the pelvis as well as para-aortic metastasis is greater under these circumstances. If CT scans show enlargement of the lymph nodes in the pelvis or low para-aortic area, a change in treatment plan might be considered and perhaps a palliative instead of a curative approach followed.

More than 40 of our patients had lymphangiography prior to CT scanning in hopes that a three-dimensional evaluation and reconstruction obtained from the combined studies would increase our understanding or interpretation of the lymph-

FIG. 9. **Top:** CT scan of a 60-year-old patient after A-P resection of the rectum who complained of severe pressure and pain in the sacral area; see presacral area. **Middle:** CT scan of the same patient 1 year later. Patient had intractable pain unrelieved by morphine; see presacral area mass. **Bottom:** CT scan of the same patient after radiation therapy, showing increasing calcification of presacral tumor mass.

angiographic findings. Each test added information, but seeing the nodes with opaque contrast material on CT did not improve interpretation of the lymphangiography. A literature review corroborates these findings. The overall accuracy of CT in the series of Walsh et al. (40) and Lee et al. (22) "does not yet match that of lymphangiograms in the staging of pelvic malignant disease" (22). For a node to be abnormal on CT, it must be greater than 2 cm (40). It was once anticipated that those nodes not filled at lymphangiography would show on CT, e.g., the obturator nodes of the pelvis. For the most part, however, this has not been our experience. Costellino et al. (6) found celiac and renal pelvic nodes in the abdomen that were not seen by lymphangiography. Ginaldi et al. (10) reported two out of seven abnormal CT scans that showed lymph nodes which were not opacified on lymphangiography. Enlarged iliac nodes may be easily seen without previous lymphangiography. If there is no enlargement, however, abnormalities may still be present and determined only by a staging laparotomy or lymphangiogram. Thus George, Asbell, and Pilepich, chairmen of the National Radiation Therapy Oncology Group (RTOG) protocols, do not accept CT findings alone as proof of lymph node involvement (9). The CT scan is not a foolproof diagnostic tool for determining the extent of lymph node disease but can be extremely helpful for identifying gross metastasis. As radiation may also be utilized to treat the lymph node draining areas, including the para-aortic regions, it is important to identify the extent of the metastasis.

Radiation is used to palliate by diminishing the obstruction of tumor-laden lymphatics or tumor itself when it blocks drainage of the leg or surrounds the ureteral orifices. Tumor or lymph node extension can be visualized with CT, and appropriate palliative dosimetry established (Fig. 8).

CT scans show if there is regression of nodal disease after hormones and/or radiation therapy (12). The radiation oncologist may choose to use CT scanning for follow-up after treatment of involved nonopacified lymph nodes.

RECURRENT RECTAL CARCINOMA

Fifty percent of rectal carcinomas, stages B and C, recur in the pelvis. When there has been a recurrence of rectal carcinoma in the pelvis or presacral area after A-P resection, all other diagnostic tests may fail to show disease. The patient may present with pain, obstruction of the ureter, neurologic deficit, or alteration in urinary habits. In this case, sometimes the only test which shows the extent of disease and its exact location is the CT scan.

For example, a patient seen 1 year after an A-P resection complained of pain. A bone scan, sigmoidoscopy, and IVP were negative. A CT scan was done, and no diagnosis of recurrence was established (Fig. 9, top). Because this pain persisted for a year, all tests were repeated. At this point, the recurrence was obvious on the CT scan (Fig. 9, middle).

This example demonstrates the need to establish a normal baseline CT scan of the pelvis after A-P resection. It may be only with comparative studies that the confusion between postsurgical changes and tumor recurrence can be avoided. Regardless of whether patients receive radiation therapy postoperatively, they should be studied every 6 months. Slow regression and sometimes calcification (3,20) (Fig. 9, bottom) are noted on follow-up. Abdominal and pelvic scans should be done for 3 years in all patients who are at risk for recurrence, as it was in this group that para-aortic disease was often noted in our series of 56 patients (3).

CT is an essential part of treatment planning for recurrent colorectal carcinoma, as the sites of metastasis are frequently the nodes and soft tissues (16,24). Sites outside the true pelvis are not ordinarily considered for irradiation, although they may show involvement and therefore require a change of portals. For example, iliac nodes which were enlarged and caused pain in an elderly male after A-P resection were clearly demonstrated on CT (Fig. 10). Other investigators have found CT to be of similar value in this disease (23,42).

CONCLUSIONS

The accuracy of radiotherapeutic treatment planning has improved with the availability of CT scanning. As we continue to investigate the usefulness of CT scanning in tumors of the pelvis, we will be able to refine our treatment plans as we have already done for cancer of the prostate, bladder, and rectum as well as lymphoma. Only in more advanced disease has CT been helpful in gynecologic malignancies. Techniques of CT scanning will need to be altered to improve its usefulness in early and central gynecologic disease.

SUMMARY

CT scans can locate normal structures in the pelvis in normal and disease states. They can demonstrate the sites of primary tumors and metastases in the pelvis, thereby improving tumor localization for treatment planning for many pelvic malignancies. The appropriateness of a curative or a palliative approach can be more accurately ascertained after CT scanning. This has been particularly true in cases where CT is the only test that provides the location, size, and extent of the tumor, e.g., prostatic or bladder carcinoma.

The choice of the plan to be utilized—three- or four-field technique, rotation— can be more accurately and appropriately ascertained after noting the tumor volume on CT scan. Thus most of our patients with pelvic disease undergo this form of diagnostic evaluation prior to treatment in order to ensure completeness.

The CT has not provided us, however, with the assistance we had expected in gynecologic malignancy. Often the disease, clinically found to extend to the pelvic wall, cannot be seen on the CT scan. Frequently disease extending inferiorly toward the vagina goes unrecognized. The presence of a uterus makes evaluation of a tumor in the region of the cervix very difficult, even if it is extensive. The presence of the uterus also makes presacral evaluation in patients after A-P resection for carcinoma of the colon more difficult, as a presacral mass may be either a tumor or the uterus.

CT has provided better palliation in the cases of some tumors where large iliac nodes are found unexpectedly extending out of the true pelvis. After the treatment was changed to include these areas, the pain was relieved. We found CT scanning valuable in the treatment of most pelvic malignancies and strongly recommend its use.

REFERENCES

1. Amendola, M. A., Walsh, J. W., Amendola, B. E., Tisnado, J., Hall, D. J., and Goplerud, D. R. (1981): Computed tomography in the evaluation of carcinoma of the ovary. *J. Comput. Assist. Tomogr.*, 5:179–186.
2. Asbell, S. O., Schlager, B. A., and Baker, A. S. (1980): Revision of treatment planning for carcinoma of the prostate. *Int. J. Radiat. Oncol. Biol. Phys.*, 6:861–865.
3. Asbell, S. O., Schlager, B. A., and Ostrum, B. J. (1980): CT scanning in the evaluation of patients with primary and recurrent rectosigmoid carcinoma. Presented at the American Radium Society, Philadelphia.
4. Bernardino, M. E., and Dodd, G. D. (1981): Imaging of the pelvic contents in the female oncologic patient. *Cancer*, 48:504–510.
5. Brizel, H. E., Livingston, P. A., and Grayson, E. V. (1979): Radiotherapeutic applications of pelvic computed tomography. *J. Comput. Assist. Tomogr.*, 3:453–466.
6. Castellino, R. A., Marglin, S. I., Carroll, B. A., Young, S. W., Harell, G. S., and Blank, N. (1980): The radiographic evaluation of abdominal and pelvic lymph node in oncologic practice. *Cancer Treat. Rev.*, 7:153–160.
7. Chiu, L. C., and Schapiro, R. L. (1977): A primer in computed axial tomographic anatomy: the lower abdomen and female pelvis. *Comput. Axial Tomogr.*, 1:137–144.
8. Doubleday, L. C., and Bernardino, M. E. (1980): CT findings in the perirectal area following radiation therapy. *J. Comput. Assist. Tomogr.*, 4:634–638.
9. George, F. W., III, Asbell, S. O., Pilepich, M. V., and Miljenko, V. (1981): Personal communication.
10. Ginaldi, S., Wallace, S., Jing, B. S., and Bernardino, M. E. (1981): Carcinoma of the cervix: lymphangiography and computed tomography. *Am. J. Roentgenol.*, 136:1087–1091.
11. Goitein, M. (1980): Benefits and cost of computerized tomography in radiation therapy. *JAMA*, 244:1347–1350.
12. Green, N., Broth, E., George, F. W., Goldstein, A., Melbye, R. W., Morrow, J., Onofrio, R., Polse, S., and Skaist, L. (1979): Prostate carcinoma: therapeutic considerations in the management of gross lymph node metastases. *Int. J. Radiat. Oncol. Biol. Phys.*, 6:891–897.
13. Hamlin, D. J., and Cockett, A. T. K. (1979): Computed tomography of bladder: staging of bladder cancer using low density opacification technique. *Urology*, 13:331.
14. Hamlin, D. J., and Cockett, A. T. K. (1980): Modification for computerized tomographic staging of infiltrative bladder carcinoma. *J. Urol.*, 123:489–491.
15. Hodson, N. J., Husband, J. E., and MacDonald, J. S. (1979): The role of computed tomography in the staging of bladder cancer. *Clin. Radiol.*, 30:389–395.
16. Husband, J. E., Hodson, N. J., and Parsons, C. A. (1980): Use of computed tomography in recurrent rectal tumors. *Radiology*, 134:677–682.
17. Jacques, P. F., Staab, E., Rickey, W., Photopulos, G., and Swanton, M. (1978): CT assisted pelvic and abdominal aspiration biopsies in gynecological malignancy. *Radiology*, 128:651–655.
18. Kellett, M. H., Oliver, R. T. D., Husband, J. E., and Fry, I. K. (1980): Computed tomography as an adjunct to bimanual examination for staging bladder tumors. *Br. J. Urol.*, 52:101–106.
19. Kenny, G. M., Hartoner, G. J., Moore, R. M., and Murphy, G. P. (1972): Current results from treatment of stage C & D bladder tumors at Roswell Park Memorial Institute. *Urology*, 107:56–59.
20. Kreel, L., and Bydder, G. (1980): Tumor calcification after radiotherapy demonstrated by computed tomography. *CT*, 4:245–249.

21. Lee, D. J., Leibel, S., Shiels, R., Sanders, R., Siegelman, S., and Order, S. (1980): The value of ultrasonic imaging and CT scanning in planning the radiotherapy for prostatic carcinoma. *Cancer*, 45:724–727.
22. Lee, J. K. T., Stanley, R. J., Sagel, S. S., and McClennan, B. L. (1978): Accuracy of CT in detecting intra-abdominal and pelvic lymph node metastases from pelvic cancers. *Am. J. Roentgenol.*, 131:675–679.
23. Leer, J. W. H., Scholten, E. T., Tjho-Heslinga, R. E., and Binswanger, R. O. (1980): Role of computed tomography in the diagnosis and radiotherapy planning of recurrent rectal carcinoma. *Diagn. Imaging*, 49:208–213.
24. Levitt, R. G., Sagel, S. S., Stanley, R. J., and Evens, R. G. (1978): Computed tomography of the pelvis. *Sem. Roentgenol.*, 3:193–200.
25. Lipshitz, H. I. (ed.) (1979): *Diagnostic Roentgenology of Radiotherapy Change*, Chap. 10. Williams & Wilkins, Baltimore.
26. Paquette, F. R., Ahuja, A. S., Carson, P. L., Mack, L. S., Ibbott, G. S., and Johnson, M. L. (1979): A comparative study of computerized tomography and ultrasound imaging for treatment planning of prostatic carcinoma. *Int. J. Radiat. Oncol. Biol. Phys.*, 5:289–294.
27. Pilepich, M. V., Perez, C. A., and Prasad, S. (1980): Computed tomography in definitive radiotherapy of prostatic carcinoma. *Int. J. Radiat. Oncol. Biol. Phys.*, 6:923–926.
28. Price, J. M., and Davidson, A. J. (1979): Computed tomography in the evaluation of the suspected carcinomatous prostate. *Urol. Radiol.*, 1:39–42.
29. Redman, H. C. (1977): Computed tomography of the pelvis. *Radiol. Clin. North Am.*, 15:441–448.
30. Schlager, B. A., Asbell, S. O., Baker, A. S., Sklaroff, D. M., Seydel, G. H., and Ostrum, B. J. (1979): The use of computerized tomography scanning in treatment planning for bladder carcinoma. *Int. J. Radiat. Oncol. Biol. Phys.*, 5:99–103.
31. Schlager, B. A., Klaus, R., Asbell, S. O., and Baker, A. S. (1979): A comparison of the seminal vesicles on CT scans of the pelvis and seminal vesiculograms in both benign and malignant disease. Presented at the American Radium Society Meeting, Los Angeles.
32. Seidelmann, F. E., Cohen, W. N., and Bryan, P. J. (1977): Computed tomographic staging of bladder neoplasms. *Radiol. Clin. North Am.*, 15:419–440.
33. Seidelmann, F. E., Cohen, W. N., Bryan, P. J., Temes, S. P., Kraus, D., and Schoenrock, G. (1978): Accuracy of CT staging of bladder neoplasms using the gas-filled method: report of 21 patients with surgical confirmation. *Am. J. Roentgenol.*, 130:735–739.
34. Seidelmann, F. E., Reich, N. E., Cohen, W. N., Haaga, J. R., Bryan, P. J., and Havrilla, T. R. (1979): Computed tomography of the seminal vesicles and seminal vesicle angle. *Comput. Axial Tomogr.*, 1:281–285.
35. Seidelmann, F. E., Temes, S. P., Cohen, W. N., Bryan, P. J., Patil, U., and Sherry, R. G. (1977): Computed tomography of gas-filled bladder. *Urology*, 9:337–344.
36. Stern, J., Buscema, J., Rosenshein, N., and Siegelman, S. (1981): Can computed tomography substitute for second-look operation in ovarian carcinoma? *Gynecol. Oncol.*, 11:82–88.
37. Sukov, R. J., Scardino, P. T., Sample, W. F., Winter, J., and Confer, D. J. (1977): Computed tomography and transabdominal ultrasound in the evaluation of the prostate. *J. Comput. Assist. Tomogr.*, 1:281–289.
38. Van Engelshoven, J. M. A., and Kreel, L. (1979): Computed tomography of the prostate. *J. Comput. Assist. Tomogr.*, 3:45–51.
39. Vickery, A. L., and Kerr, W. S. (1963): Carcinoma of the prostate treated by radical prostatectomy. *Cancer*, 16:1598–1608.
40. Walsh, J. W., Amendola, M. S., Konerding, K. F., Tisnado, J., and Hazra, T. A. (1980): Computed tomographic detection of pelvic and inguinal lymph node metastases from primary and recurrent pelvic malignant disease. *Radiology*, 137:157–166.
41. Yu, W. S., Sagerman, R. H., King. G. A., Chung, C. T., and Yu, Y. W. (1979): The value of computed tomography in the management of bladder cancer. *Int. J. Radiat. Oncol. Biol. Phys.*, 5:135–142.
42. Zelas, P., Haaga, J. R., and Fazio, V. W. (1980): The diagnosis of percutaneous biopsy with computed tomography of a recurrence of carcinoma of the rectum in the pelvis. *Surg. Gynecol. Obstet.*, 151:525–527.

Computed Tomography in Radiation Therapy,
edited by C. C. Ling, C. C. Rogers, and
R. J. Morton. Raven Press, New York © 1983

Computed Tomography in Therapy Planning: Bone and Soft Tissue Sarcomas

Jack E. Meyer

Department of Radiology, Massachusetts General Hospital and Harvard Medical School, Boston, Massachusetts 02114

There are 1,900 new cases of primary bone sarcoma and 4,500 soft tissue sarcomas diagnosed annually in the United States, for a total of 6,400. This represents 0.9% of all malignant disease excluding carcinoma *in situ* and nonmelanoma skin cancers (3). Radiation therapy plays an important role in the management of a large proportion of patients with soft tissue sarcomas as well as some primary sarcomas of bone. Computed tomography (CT) provides unique cross-sectional anatomic detail of tumor boundaries as well as defining proximity to or invasion of adjacent normal structures. This information should result in more sophisticated treatment strategies, whether surgery, chemotherapy, and radiotherapy are used alone or in combination. When radiotherapy is utilized, it is essential that the treatment volume be no larger than necessary to cover tissues involved with gross and microscopic tumor. Utilization of CT information in treatment planning should help provide a greater chance for local tumor ablation coupled with the best possible functional and cosmetic results.

SOFT TISSUE SARCOMAS

Soft tissue sarcomas arise from supportive mesenchymal tissue other than bone and include rhabdomyosarcoma, fibrosarcoma, liposarcoma, malignant fibrohistiocytoma, sarcoma of the soft tissue type unspecified, synovial sarcoma, leiomyosarcoma, malignant schwannoma, angiosarcoma, and other types (8).

Possible treatment strategies include radical resection or amputation (7), or radiation therapy plus more conservative surgery and possibly chemotherapy (8,9,11). Radiation therapy alone is not recommended unless surgery is not feasible because of medical or technical considerations.

The staging of soft tissue sarcomas is determined by histopathologic grade, tumor size, lymph node involvement, and distant metastasis, but grade is the primary determinant of stage (8). CT is essentially of no value in determining tumor histopathology; however, malignant lesions often have poorly defined margins and areas of inhomogeneous attenuation, the latter usually secondary to hematoma or necrosis (6). CT can demonstrate bony invasion, but it is uncertain at this time if subtle changes invisible on routine radiography are detectable by CT. Nerve displacement may be visible or inferred from tumor location, and vascular occlusion or displacement is evident after injection of contrast material. Distant metastasis, especially small lung parenchyma nodules located near the pleural surface or in the lower lobes near the diaphragms, may be visible only on CT.

The primary advantages of CT in radiotherapy treatment planning for sarcomas of soft tissue include: (a) a precise outline of tumor volume and relationships with normal structures; (b) the design of boost fields when shrinkage of the initial treatment volume is desired; and (c) follow-up for detection of recurrence.

PRIMARY SARCOMAS OF BONE

Osteosarcoma and Ewing's sarcoma occur predominantly in persons under the age of 20, whereas chondrosarcoma, diffuse histiocytic lymphoma, and fibrosarcoma have a peak incidence in patients 40 to 60 years old. Fibrosarcoma, chondrosarcoma, and osteosarcoma are treated primarily with surgery, whereas Ewing's and reticulum cell sarcoma are most often treated at their primary site with radiotherapy (10). As the goal of treatment is ablation of the primary tumor with retention of musculoskeletal function, a precise definition of anatomic contours and tumor boundaries is essential. The additional information provided by CT includes: (a) more accurate definition of the extent of bony involvement in complex areas such as the pelvis, where overlying gas and feces limit precise evaluation; (b) definition of associated extraosseous soft tissue masses; (c) an evaluation of density changes in the medullary portion of bone as a possible guide to treatment; and (d) follow-up examination after irradiation or chemotherapy (1).

DISCUSSION

Few studies have documented the efficacy of CT in the evaluation of bone and soft tissue sarcomas, although one group reported that CT gave a better indication of tumor location, axial extent, and normal tissue relationships than the conventional imaging procedures in 54% of 50 patients studied (5). CT was considered useful when it provided additional information regarding tumor relationships to bone, muscle groups, large nerves, blood vessels, and joints; and it was particularly helpful in evaluating extraosseous soft tissue extension. The management of 66% of patients was effected by CT data, and 40% of the scans were easier to interpret after the injection of contrast material.

Muscles, nerves, blood vessels, and masses are seen to best advantage when surrounded by fatty tissue of lower attenuation; therefore CT is less helpful in patients who are either young or thin. Comparison with the opposite extremity is imperative in all cases, especially when distinct muscle boundaries cannot be identified. Small lesions located in the distal portion of an extremity are often difficult to define accurately on CT (4).

Other diagnostic modalities are useful alone or in combination with CT in both the pre- and the posttreatment evaluation of patients with sarcoma of bone and soft tissues. In lesions of the extremities, ultrasound accurately determines the size of a soft tissue mass and may be the simplest imaging method for the detection of recurrence after treatment (2). Arteriography is useful when (a) there is a strong suspicion of invasion of an artery or a vein; (b) it is necessary prior to surgery to determine the blood supply of both the tumor and the normal adjacent tissues; and (c) it is necessary to delineate smaller tumors located distally in the extremities (5). Radionuclide scans with ^{99m}Tc-labeled phosphate are of limited value and seem to be most useful in the detection of unsuspected metastatic skeletal lesions.

It is apparent that as experience is accumulated CT will play a more clearly defined and increasingly important role in the pre- and posttreatment evaluation of sarcomas of bone and soft tissue.

REFERENCES

1. Berger, P. E., and Kuhn, J. P. (1978): Computed tomography of tumors of the musculoskeletal system in children. *Radiology*, 127:171–175.
2. Bernardino, M. E., Jing, B. S., Thomas, J. L., Lindell, M. M., and Zornoza, J. (1981): The extremity soft tissue lesion: a comparative study of ultrasound, computed tomography, and xeroradiography. *Radiology*, 139:53–59.
3. Cancer statistics (1980): *CA*, 30:23–38.
4. Heelan, R. T., Watson, R. C., and Smith, J. (1979): Computed tomography of lower extremity tumors. *Am. J. Roentgenol.*, 132:933–937.
5. Levine, E., Lee, K. R., and Neff, J. (1979): Comparison of computed tomography and other imaging modalities in evaluation of musculoskeletal tumors. *Radiology*, 131:431–437.
6. McLeod, R. A., Gisvold, J. J., Stephens, D. H., Beabout, J. W., and Sheedy, P. F. (1978): Computed tomography of soft tissues and breast. *Sem. Roentgenol.*, 13:267–275.
7. Simon, M. A., and Enneking, W. F. (1976): The management of soft tissue sarcomas of the extremities. *J. Bone Joint Surg.*, 58:317–327.
8. Suit, H. D. (1978): Sarcóma of soft tissue. *CA*, 28:284–295.
9. Suit, H. D., and Russell, W. O. (1975): Radiation therapy of soft tissue sarcomas. *Cancer*, 36:759–764.
10. Suit, H., Kaufman, S., and Mankin, H. (1978): Sarcomas of bone and soft tissue. In: *Cancer—A Manual for Practitioners*, edited by B. Cady, pp. 239–248. American Cancer Society, Massachusetts Division.
11. Suit, H. D., Proppe, K. H., Mankin, H. J., and Wood, W. C. (1981): Preoperative radiation therapy for sarcoma of soft tissue. *Cancer*, 47:2269–2274.

Computed Tomography in Radiation Therapy,
edited by C. C. Ling, C. C. Rogers, and
R. J. Morton. Raven Press, New York © 1983

Computed Tomography and Dose Optimization: Brain Tumors

James E. Marks

Washington University School of Medicine, The Edward Mallinckrodt Institute of Radiology, Division of Radiation Oncology, St. Louis, Missouri 63110

Since 1974 the author has routinely used CT scans to plan optimum dose distributions for the irradiation of brain tumors. Requisites for dose optimization, or concentration of radiation in the tumor with relative sparing of surrounding brain, are: a CT scan to demonstrate the spatial relationship between tumor and surrounding brain; a high-energy x-ray beam, 10 MeV or greater; and the ability to reconstruct the dose distribution onto the CT image. To establish a rationale for dose optimization, the author reviews the known dose-response information for glioblastoma multiforme and cerebral radionecrosis within the range of radiation doses most commonly used. Theoretically, dose optimization maximizes the effects of radiation on the tumor and reduces the chance of radiation injury to the surrounding brain. Practically, it is used to spare hair and reduces the incidence of radiation damage to cranial soft tissue.

BACKGROUND

Before discussing advances in the technology of irradiating brain tumors, it is well to set forth some theoretical concepts about the relationship between radiation dose and its biological effects on tumors and normal tissues. The graphic representation of this relationship is typically a sigmoid dose-response curve, labeled Pa_1 in Fig. 1; this curve shows a threshold dose beyond which there is a rapid increase in biological effect on tumor or normal tissue with relatively small increases in radiation dose. The sigmoid dose-response curve has been so thoroughly publicized by the writings of Moore and Mendelsohn (3) that many assume it is the standard curve for all tumors and normal tissues when, in fact, any one of a variety of curves may apply (e.g., Pa_2 and Pa_3 in Fig. 1). Dose-response data for any particular tumor or normal tissue are generally lacking. The reasons for our lack of clinical dose-response information are several and are illustrated quite nicely by brain tumors and the normal tissue in which they originate, the brain.

Firstly, *endpoints used to measure the biological effects of radiation are poorly defined and often confusing*. One cannot look at tumor control for a glioblastoma multiforme because the tumor is seldom eradicated, it predictably regrows, and

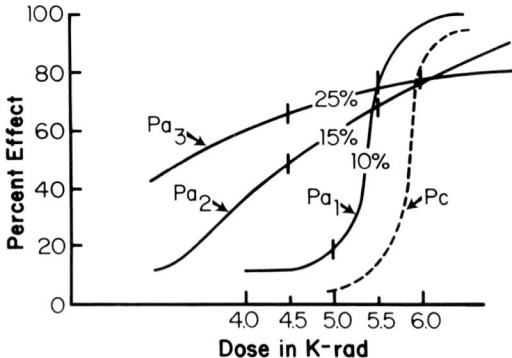

FIG. 1. Theoretical dose-response curves for three tumors and one normal tissue, demonstrating the probabilities for ablating the tumors (Pa_1, Pa_2, and Pa_3) and the probability of producing a normal tissue complication (Pc) as a function of radiation dose. Note that 10%, 15%, and 25% increases in radiation dose have less effect on the tumor as the slope is successively reduced for the dose-response curves. Note also the "single optimum dose" of 5,500 rads.

unlike a cancer of the tonsil it cannot be directly visualized because of its location within the cranium. The only reliable endpoints for assessing the effects of radiation on this tumor are the interval between the relief of neurological signs or symptoms and subsequent neurological deterioration or the death of the patient. The effects of radiation on the brain surrounding the tumor are just as difficult to examine as the effects on the tumor. Again, the only reliable endpoints are the interval free of neurological signs and symptoms or the death of the patient. It is an unfortunate coincidence that the endpoints for the effects of radiation on tumor and brain are the same, for this makes it impossible to differentiate one from the other. Many brain tumor patients are irradiated, improve, and subsequently deteriorate and die without the benefit of autopsy to determine if the cause of death was due to regrowth of the tumor or necrosis of the brain.

The second reason there is limited dose-response information about brain tumors and tumor-containing brain is the *narrow range of radiation doses* commonly employed. Most patients receive between 4,500 and 6,000 rads, so there is a great deal of information within these limits but very little above or below. Consequently one is unable to reliably reconstruct clinical dose-response curves for those regions of dose above and below the range commonly used. Historically, many patients were not irradiated or were irradiated with low doses, but follow-up and recording of neurological signs and symptoms were so poor that much of that information has been lost. It also seems unlikely that the upper regions of dose will be explored in view of the increasing number of recent reports of cerebral radionecrosis (2). Thus the radiotherapist is often forced to decide how much radiation to deliver to tumors and normal tissues without the benefit of reliable dose-response information on which to base his decision.

With the theory of sigmoid dose-response there arose the concept of an "optimum single dose" of irradiation that would maximize tumor effect with an acceptable risk of normal tissue damage. This concept is illustrated in Fig. 1 by the solid dose-response curve for tumor (labeled Pa_1) and the dotted curve for normal tissue (labeled Pc). By increasing the dose 10%, from 5,000 to 5,500 rads, one greatly increases the tumor effect and produces a small percentage of radiation complications to normal tissue. Tokars and Griem (4) give a classic example of this concept of "single optimum dose" in a publication dealing with carcinoma of the nasopharynx and adjacent spinal cord. They advocate greater doses of radiation to improve tumor control and accept a small but significant number of spinal cord injuries. For most radiotherapists and referring physicians, any radiation injury to brainstem, spinal cord, and cerebrum is unacceptable because the neurological consequences are great and frequently lead to death. Iatrogenic death, unlike death due to tumor, carries with it the stigma of wrongdoing and the judgment that the patient was excessively irradiated. It would be better if the radiotherapist avoided radiation injury to the central nervous system and found ways of increasing the dose to the tumor with relative sparing of these normal tissues. The resulting concept of "dose optimization by concentration" is preferable to the concept of "single optimum dose" because it maximizes the effect on the tumor and reduces to the lowest possible level the risk of radiation damage to normal tissues. Those who practice "single optimum dose" radiotherapy accept a degree of risk to normal tissues so long as the effect on the tumor is maximized. Those who practice "dose optimization by concentration" attempt to prevent risk to normal tissues while simultaneously maximizing the effects of radiation on the tumor. The technology necessary to achieve "dose optimization by concentration" is available in select institutions and is discussed in the following section.

TECHNOLOGY

The ability of a radiotherapist to concentrate radiation dose within a brain tumor with relative sparing of surrounding brain has a number of technical prerequisites; these include high-energy x-rays, 10 MeV or greater, computed tomography (CT) scans, and computed dose distributions. This technology is expensive and hence is not universally available. The issue, however, is not whether the technology should be universally available, but if it can be justified in terms of improved benefits to the patient.

Before addressing these important issues, I will review the technology that has been used at our institution since 1974 to achieve "dose optimization by concentration." Preceding the installation of a high-energy 35 MeV linear accelerator in 1974, we had a comparable high-energy x-ray beam generated by a betatron, but this beam was not used for dose optimization as much as the x-ray beam from the linear accelerator because we lacked CT. With the advent of CT scanning in March 1974, we were suddenly able to visualize the spatial relationship between a brain tumor and surrounding brain. Knowing where the tumor was in relation to the surrounding brain made treatment planning or computed dose reconstruction relatively easy. The tumor from the CT scan was drawn onto a contour of the patient's head, and the resulting contour and tumor were then entered into the treatment planning computer. Using a high-energy x-ray beam alone or in combination with a medium-energy x-ray beam, the dosimetrist would generate an optimized dose distribution such as the one shown in Fig. 2. Generally speaking, gradients of 10

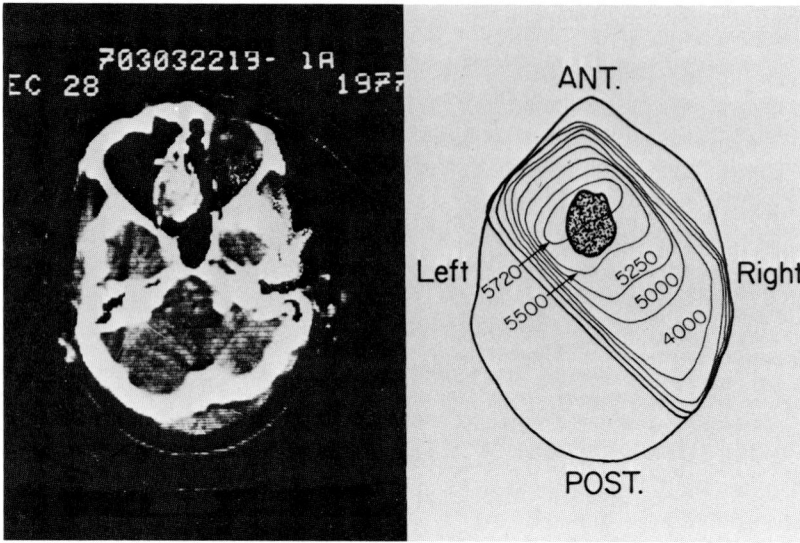

FIG. 2. CT scan of a meningioma that recurred after surgery. At right is an optimized dose distribution using opposed high-energy x-ray beams.

to 15% between tumor and surrounding brain are achieved. Granted, the concentration of radiation dose within the tumor is imperfect, but so too is our knowledge of exactly where tumor ends and normal brain begins. Needed are better correlations between scan morphology and histopathology in the patient.

Radiation therapy treatment planning today is more sophisticated than previously. CT scans can be entered directly into the treatment planning computer, so that dose distributions can be superimposed directly onto the scan. There is also great interest in three-dimensional treatment planning even though the value of two-dimensional treatment planning and "dose optimization by concentration" remains to be proved. The radiotherapist still does not know if this sophisticated technology actually improves survival and lessens the incidence of radionecrosis for patients with brain tumors. However, we do know that retrospective study of two-dimensional dose reconstruction allows us greater insight into the relationship between dose and damaged normal tissues or tumor regrowth in specific anatomical locations.

DOSE RESPONSE FOR TUMOR AND BRAIN

Having examined theoretical dose-response curves for tumor and normal tissues, I next examine known dose-response information for a specific brain tumor as well as tumor-containing brain, and integrate this information with the concept of "dose optimization by concentration." The brain tumor for which we have the best dose-response information is glioblastoma multiforme (GBM). This is a tumor for which patient survival has been documented for doses ranging from 0 to 7,000 rads. A segment of the dose-response curve for GBM (survival in weeks versus dose) has been reported by the Brain Tumor Study Group (BTSG) (5) and is shown in Fig. 3. Below the dose-response curve for GBM is the dose-response curve for tumor-containing brain, depicting the probability of developing cerebral radionecrosis as a function of radiation dose (2). Obviously, whenever the radiation dose is raised to increase the effect on the tumor, there is a simultaneous increase in the risk of radionecrosis to surrounding brain; there is no "single optimum dose" that would be advantageous in this circumstance. Theoretically, there is a point beyond which further increases in dose would cause a plateau or decline in survival as the risk of dying from radionecrosis paralleled or exceeded the relative benefit from irradiating the tumor. The only way to favorably alter this circumstance would be to give a higher dose to the tumor than to the surrounding brain by the process of "dose optimization by concentration." As shown in Fig. 3, a simultaneous increase in dose to the tumor and decrease in dose to surrounding brain of 175 NSD units, or 10% of the total, improves benefit as it reduces risk.

Ironically, "dose optimization by concentration" has been routinely implemented in our institution for low-grade astrocytomas (LGA) but is seldom used for GBM even though GBM is the tumor for which we have the best dose-response information from which to construct a treatment rationale. Dose-response information for LGA (other than comparison of irradiated to unirradiated historical controls) is generally lacking. Patients with LGA generally live longer than those with GBM and thus are more likely to reach the period of risk for cerebral radionecrosis (2); LGAs have therefore been selected for "dose optimization by concentration." Despite the use of sophisticated treatment planning for this group of brain tumors, we have no evidence that these patients survive significantly longer than historical controls in

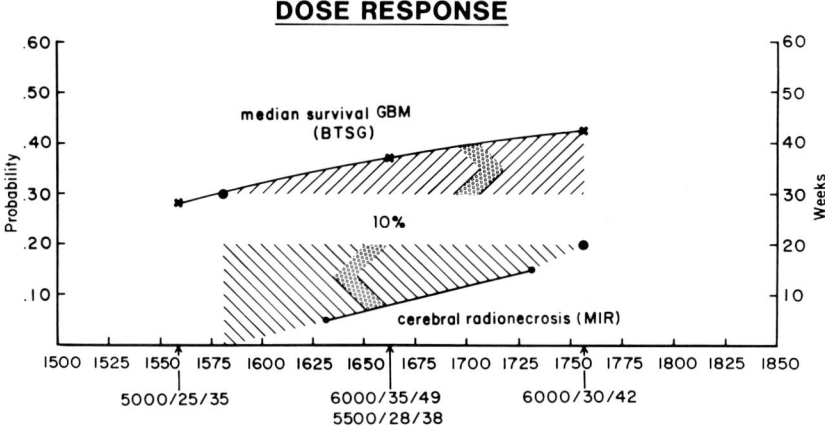

DOSE RESPONSE

FIG. 3. Demonstration of "dose optimization by concentration" as it relates to published dose-response information for GBM (5) and tumor-containing brain (2). Shaded areas with arrows pointing to the right and left show that a 10% increase in tumor dose and a 10% decrease in dose to the brain can improve survival of patients with GBM and reduce the risk of cerebral radionecrosis.

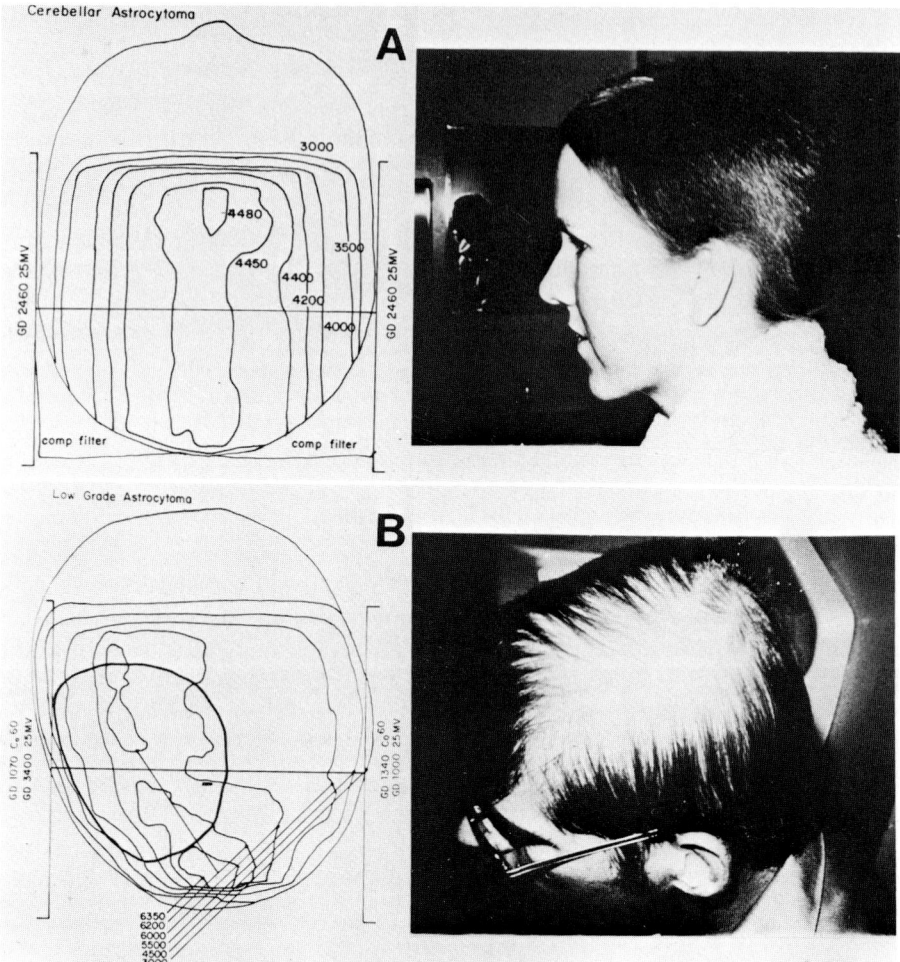

FIG. 4. Regrowth of hair and the dose reconstructions for two patients irradiated by high-energy x-rays alone **(A)** and by high-energy x-rays in combination with 4 MeV x-rays **(B)**.

our own institution or LGA patients in other institutions. We have documented that the incidence of radionecrosis of brain is similar for different populations of brain tumors irrespective of the technique used (2). There are probably too many biological variables within a given population of patients for that population to be a sensitive barometer of 10 to 15% increases in radiation dose to a particular tumor relative to surrounding brain. This complexity is further complicated by the fact that cerebral radionecrosis does not always appear within the zone of greatest radiation dose (2).

ADVANTAGES

If we are unable to document an improved effect of irradiation on the tumor and a reduced effect on the brain, are there then any advantages of "dose optimization by concentration"? It was not until we examined the effects of variable doses of radiation 5 mm below the surface of the scalp that we were able to document an advantage to this technique (1). In this anatomical region there is a steep gradient in dose between skin, hair, soft tissues, cranium, and tumor due to the buildup region from the high-energy x-ray beam; these gradients in dose exceed those generally obtained between tumor and brain and make it possible to discriminate a reduction in radiation effect on the normal tissues in this region as dose is reduced. Specifically, we discovered that hair was more often spared and that radiation effects on cranial soft tissues were reduced as a result of dose reductions from the use of the high-energy x-ray beam (1). Figure 4 illustrates the regrowth of hair that occurs after high-energy x-rays are used entirely or partially for the irradiation of brain tumors.

Hair-sparing along with a reduction in soft tissue damage are thus far the only documented practical advantages of "dose optimization by concentration." The technology required to achieve this small gain might be judged too expensive by some, but not by the individual brain tumor patient whose hair regrows. As we gain additional experience with "dose optimization by concentration," it is possible that we may be able to discriminate an improved therapeutic effect as we increase tumor lethality and decrease the risk of radiation damage to brain.

REFERENCES

1. Baglan, R. J., and Marks, J. E. (1981): Soft tissue effects following irradiation of primary brain and pituitary tumors. *Int. J. Radiat. Oncol. Biol. Phys.*, 7:455–459.
2. Marks, J. E., Baglan, R. J., Prasad, S. C., and Blank, W. F. (1981): Cerebral radionecrosis: incidence and risk in relation to dose, time, fractionation, and volume. *Int. J. Radiat. Oncol. Biol. Phys.*, 7:243–252.
3. Moore, D. H., II, and Mendelsohn, M. L. (1972): Optimal treatment levels in cancer therapy. *Cancer*, 30:97–106.
4. Tokars, R. P., and Griem, M. L. (1979): Carcinoma of the nasopharynx: an optimization of radiotherapeutic management for tumor control and spinal cord injury. *Int. J. Radiat. Oncol. Biol. Phys.*, 5:1741–1748.
5. Walker, M. D., Strike, T. A., and Sheline, G. E. (1979): An analysis of dose effect relationship in the radiotherapy of malignant gliomas. *Int. J. Radiat. Oncol. Biol. Phys.*, 5:1725–1731.

Computed Tomography in Radiation Therapy,
edited by C. C. Ling, C. C. Rogers, and
R. J. Morton. Raven Press, New York © 1983

Computed Tomography in Therapy Management: Tumors of the Head and Neck

R. J. Berry, Beate Planskoy, L. Loverock, and A. M. Bedford

Departments of Oncology and Physics as Applied to Medicine, Middlesex Hospital Medical School, London, England

Although malignancies of the head and neck are relatively infrequent in Europe and the Western world, they form a significant and rewarding part of the work of most departments of radiotherapy and oncology. In the South Thames metropolitan regions, for which a good cancer registry (4) allows reliable information on cancer incidence, during 1975 only 717 of 25,125 (2.9%) patients presenting with new malignancies for treatment had tumors of the head and neck. However, of these, 78% were treated by radiotherapy as part of their primary management, in contrast with an average of only one-third of patients with cancers in all sites receiving radiotherapy as initial treatment. At our hospital during 1980, approximately 2,700 patients were treated by radiotherapy and cytotoxic chemotherapy, of whom about 1,500 presented for the first time. Of these, 144 had malignancies in head and neck sites, 10 being pituitary tumors, which are of special interest to our department.

In common with the majority of centers in the United Kingdom, and in contrast to practice in North America, radiotherapy is employed as the primary treatment modality for attempting cure, even in advanced disease, of almost all head and neck malignancies, with salvage surgery reserved for treatment failures. Such failures, when they occur, present two major problems:

1. If the failure is within the high dose planned treatment volume, this must be regarded as a radiobiological failure. The proportion of such local failures depends on the choice of dose, the dose fractionation, and the level of normal tissue damage accepted as tolerable. Such failures are beyond the scope of this discussion, as hope for improvement in tumor control must involve (a) modified dose fractionation; (b) physical adjuncts, e.g., hyperbaric oxygen or heat; (c) the use of densely ionizing radiation, e.g., fast neutrons whose effects are less dependent on the presence or absence of oxygen and less dependent on tissue repair; or (d) the use of pharmacological adjuncts such as selective radiosensitizers for hypoxic cells.

2. If the failure to control primary tumors of the head and neck occurs at the margins of the irradiated volume, this must be regarded as a failure to adequately assess the spread of the tumor at the time of initial treatment planning. It is to the latter failures that improvements in tumor imaging are directed, and it is here that

89

computed tomography (CT) plays a role. In tumors of the head and neck, more than perhaps any other, the ultimate survival of the patient depends on the achievement of permanent cessation of tumor growth at the primary site.

At our hospital the EMI 5005 body scanner—situated in the Department of Radiotherapy and Oncology but operated jointly by a team comprising radiodiagnosticians, radiotherapists, medical physicists, and radiographers—has been in operation since December 1977. Up to September 1, 1981, more than 6,100 patients had been scanned. Approximately 200 had tumors in head and neck sites, and scans were undertaken in these patients to establish the initial extent of disease, specifically to help plan their radiotherapy, and to assess the posttreatment responses of their tumors. At present, 55% of all scans carried out on this general purpose machine are of the head and 45% of the body. On average, 280 examinations are carried out per month on about 150 patients, a total of over 2,000 scans per month. During

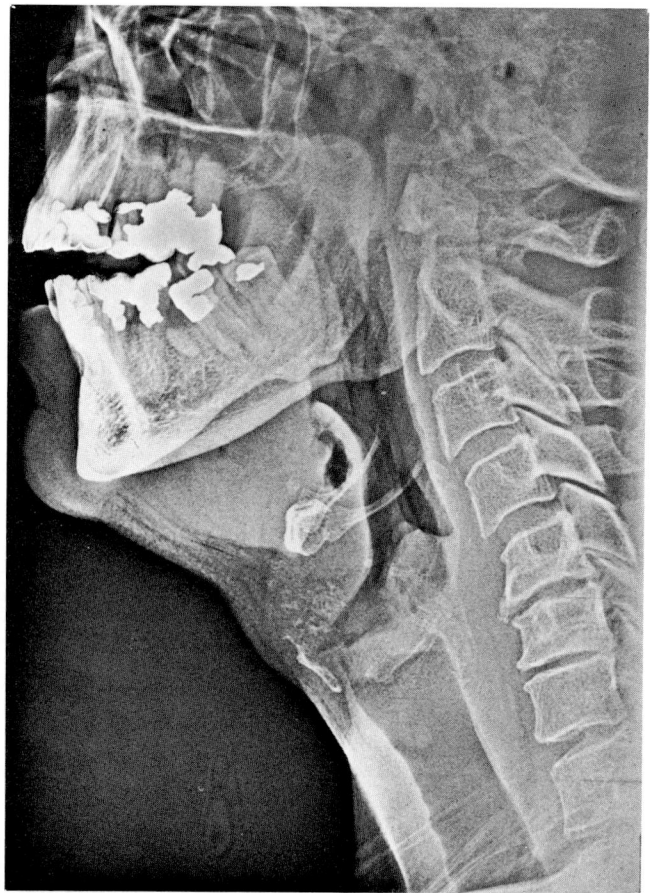

FIG. 1.   Lateral xeroradiograph of the neck in a patient with carcinoma of the larynx.

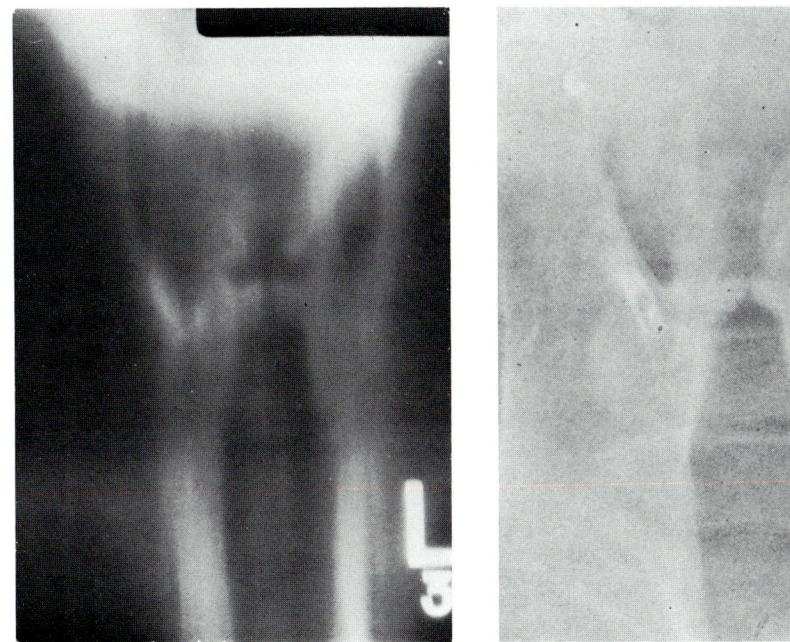

FIG. 2. Frontal tomogram of the larynx in a patient with carcinoma. **Left:** Conventional film tomogram, linear blurring. **Right:** Xerotomogram, elliptical blurring.

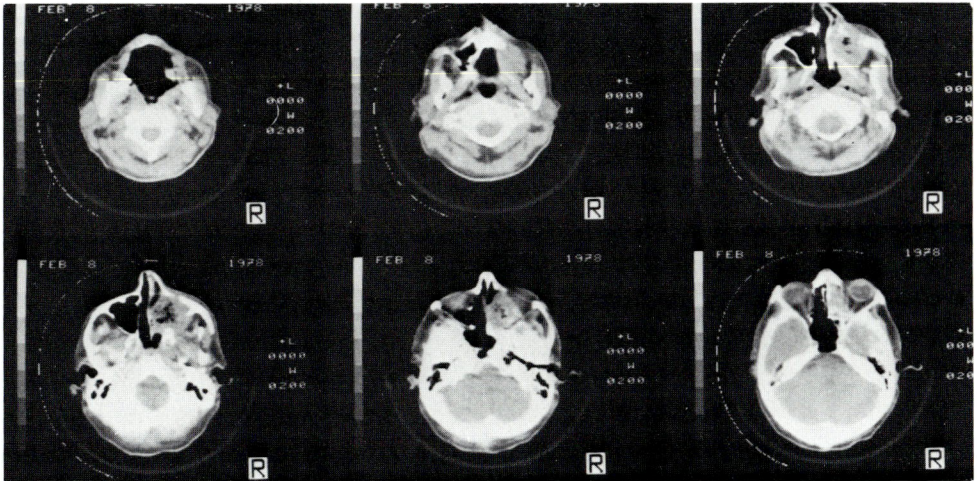

FIG. 3. Extensive carcinoma of the right antrum. Note penetration superiorly into ethmoid air cells, inferiorly through the palate, and anteriorly through the zygoma.

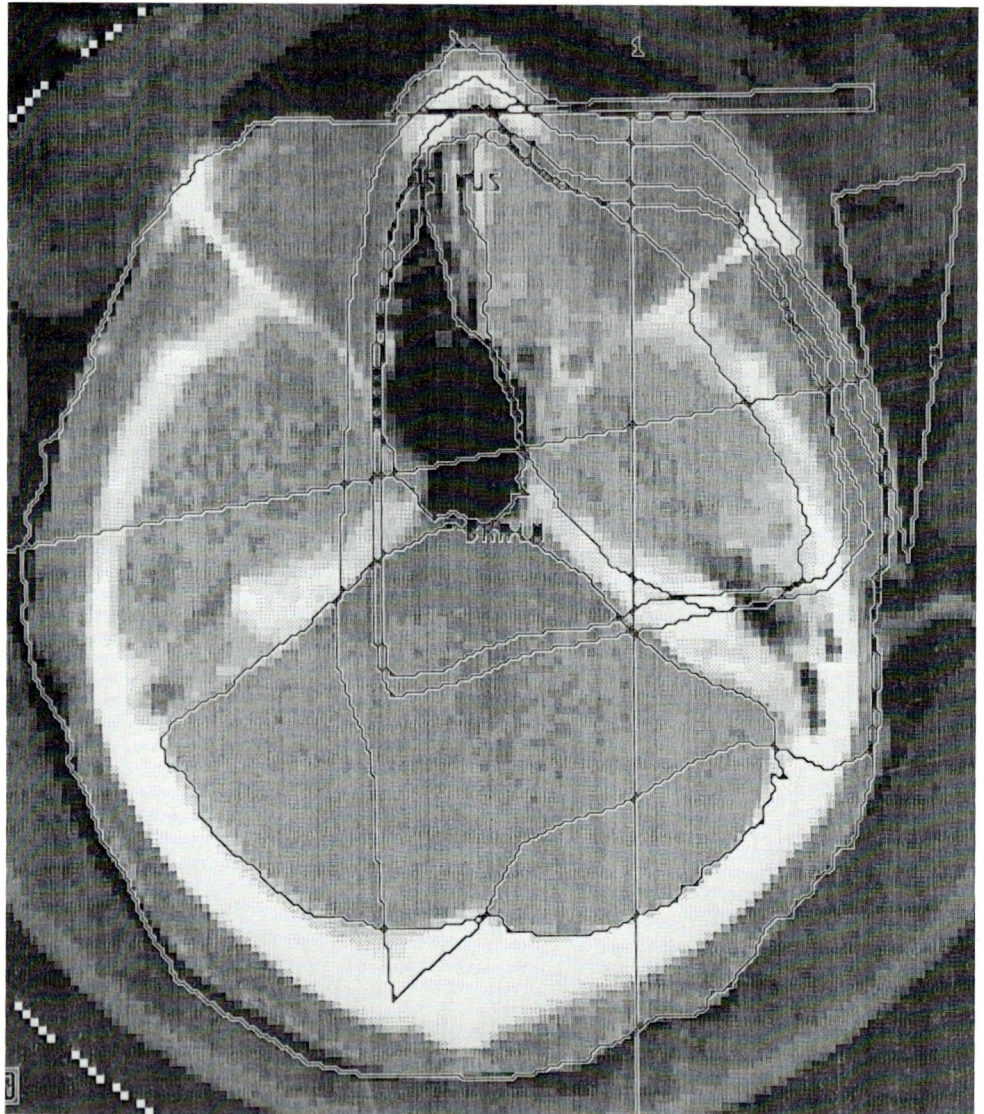

FIG. 4. Hard-copy printout of treatment plan superimposed on CT image of carcinoma of the antrum—the radiotherapist's copy for "thinking and scribbling."

the autumn of 1979 we installed the production prototype EMIPLAN 7000, which allows anatomical information from the CT scanner to be transferred directly (by tape or floppy disc) to a computerized radiotherapy planning system. This free-standing system, based on the Data General Eclipse Computer coupled to an extended intelligent console, provides rapid and extensive operator interaction. The

RDOS operating system supports FORTRAN, BASIC, BCPL, and Assembler Compilers together with a number of editors, which allows considerable programming flexibility for system updates and user development. The installation of this sophisticated planning system and the arrival of the CT scanner at our institution coincided with a project being carried out jointly by the Departments of Oncology and of Physics as Applied to Medicine on optimizing image quality and reducing patient dose in the use of xeroradiography and xerotomography for the localization of head and neck tumors. We were therefore in the privileged position of having exceedingly high quality "conventional" images against which to compare the new information provided by the CT scans (1–3).

Roughly one-fourth of all new head and neck tumors seen at our hospital are of the larynx, and a further one in five are pharyngeal tumors. Here the conventional techniques of inspection, palpation, and indirect and direct laryngoscopy, complemented by good-quality conventional radiography, provide all the information necessary for radiotherapy treatment planning. So long as radiographic examination is undertaken *before* surgical interference, xeroradiography provides high-quality diagnostic information (Fig. 1). Frontal xerotomograms give good definition of the extent of gross disease in soft tissue; and because the xerotomogram visualizes a rather deeper image due to its high resolution for the "out of focus" portion, sufficient bony anatomical detail can be superimposed on the soft tissue image to allow precise anatomical delimitation of the radiation treatment field. A comparison between a conventional film tomographic image of good diagnostic quality and a xerotomogram is shown in Fig. 2. The financial cost of such investigation is trivial compared with that of CT scans. In addition, in terms of radiation dose to a patient, the dose from complete xerotomographic examination is modest compared with the doses of up to 60 mGy (6 rads) per slice for high-resolution CT scans in the head region. This radiation dose is, of course, of no importance in a region which is to receive high-dose radiotherapy, but it must be a consideration if repeated examinations are to be carried out during and after treatment to monitor tumor response.

The extent of gross tumor is less easily visualized in many other head and neck sites, even if one accepts the difficulty of then predicting the direction and magnitude of microscopic tumor spread. For example, assessment of disease in the middle third of the tongue is often no more than an educated guess, and assessment of spread in the posterior third of the tongue must depend on such indirect evidence as the presence or absence of tethering. Such assessment is particularly difficult when prior surgery has made the normal anatomy difficult to unravel. In such sites, CT has become an invaluable adjunct to the palpating finger for assessing deep tumor extension. Adequate encompassing of tumor in planned radiation fields should lead to a significant increase in local control of tumors, particularly when radiotherapy is given in conjunction with hyperbaric oxygen, with the hypoxic cell sensitizers, or using the superior physical localization of charged particle beams or the potentially superior biological effects of fast neutrons.

One site where CT has proved an outstanding improvement in imaging the extent of gross disease is in tumors of the nasopharynx and paranasal sinuses. These tumors occur in areas where the positions of the dose-limiting normal tissues (e.g., the lens of the eye and the brainstem) need to be known with a precision of millimeters if they are not to receive unacceptable damage. Figure 3 shows a series of CT scans through an advanced squamous carcinoma of the antrum in which the bony destruction and extension of the tumor toward the skin show the need for external buildup to achieve secondary charged particle equilibrium and hence uniform dose throughout the tumor volume. However, there is no gain in knowing the position of the tumor in terms of millimeters if the position of the patient cannot be reproduced accurately at each treatment session. High-precision tumor imaging is only part of the complete system of good treatment planning.

We have now begun to appreciate the value of direct superimposition of anatomical information from the CT scan and the computed treatment plan using the EMIPLAN system 7000. Figure 4 shows the hard-copy printout of such a plan. The particular value of such hard copy, which is nearly full-sized when received, is that the radiotherapist can consider the volume being treated and its relation to limiting normal structures in the peace and quiet of his room, not in the hurly-burly of the planning department.

In addition to the diagnostic CT scan, it is clearly necessary to image the patient in the treatment position, particularly at the superior and inferior limits of the initially planned treatment field, in order to ensure clearance of areas of gross tumor and to determine the position of all limiting normal structures. A major shortcoming of the EMI 5005 is its lack of a "scout film" capability to identify the position of individual sectional views. To overcome this, external marks on the PVC cast must be used; we have found ordinary child's plasticine rolled to millimeter-sized tubes to be suitable. Good-quality CT images can be obtained with the patient scanned in the PVC treatment shell, which is used for immobilization. It is further important that correction is made for tissue heterogeneity as seen in comprehensive CT scans. Of particular importance are the air-containing cavities. If beam energies higher than ^{60}Co are being used, lack of secondary charged particle equilibrium at the far photside of air-containing spaces may be a major cause of inadequate tumor dose and/or dose inhomogeneity.

Conventionally, tumors of the antrum are treated by a wedged pair of fields at right angles. However, bulk correction for the air contained in the nose and nasopharynx shows that such a plan may give an excessively high dose in the region of the brainstem. For such a plan the anterior field is a straight and not a wedged one (Fig. 5).

Even with the superlative images of CT, some sites are still difficult to visualize. Extensive surgery often renders the anatomical landmarks unrecognizable, as in the case of carcinoma of the mastoid (Fig. 6).

After nearly 4 years of experience with the use of CT scanning in head and neck tumors, we find it has become an essential adjunct to both the initial assessment of tumor volume and the monitoring of changes in tumor volume during treatment for those head and neck sites where modern conventional radiographic techniques (including xeroradiography and xerotomography) are not helpful. Specific advan-

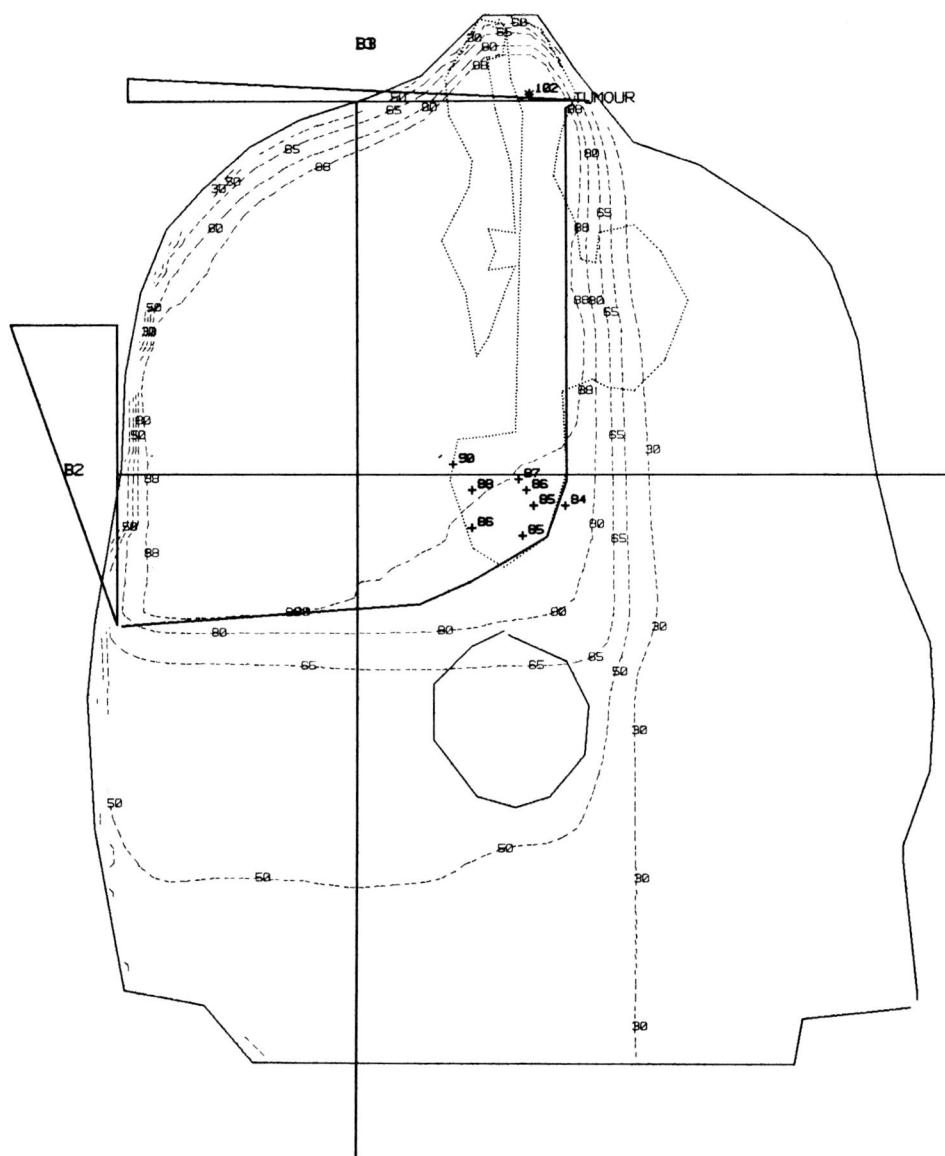

FIG. 5. (*above and following pages*) Carcinoma of the antrum. **A:** Planned without correction for heterogeneity of tissue density.

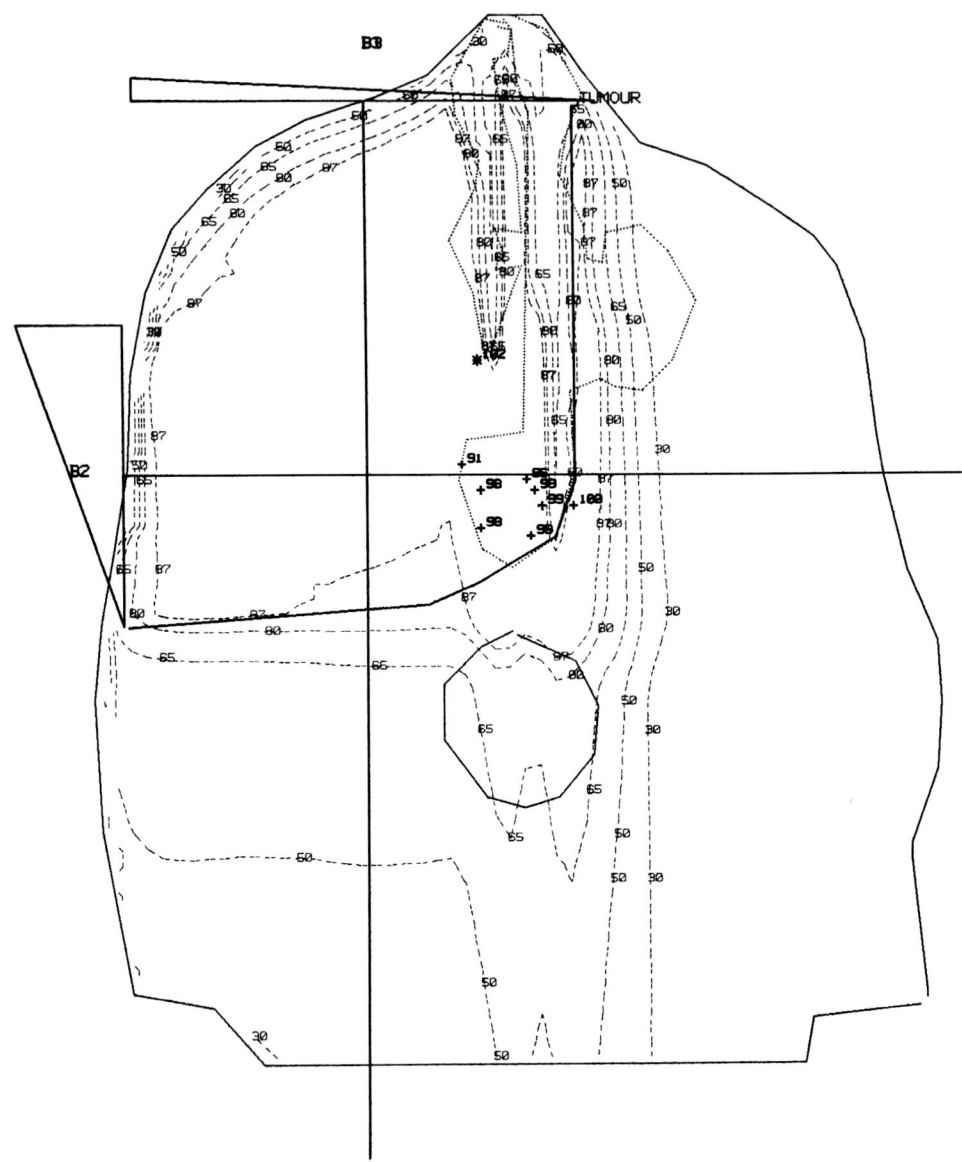

FIG. 5B. Tissue (and air space) heterogeneity included; note high dose to brainstem.

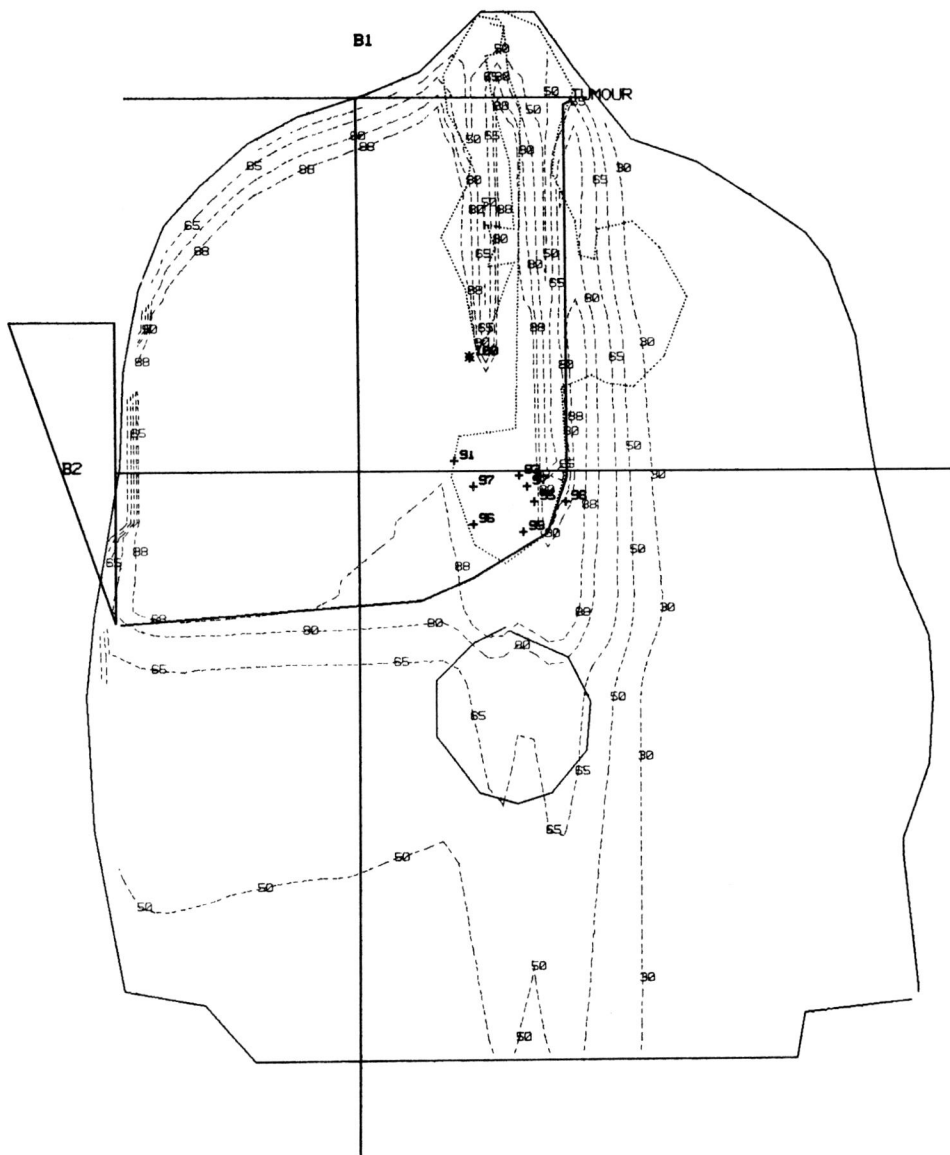

FIG. 5C. Plan modified to bring brainstem dose below tolerance.

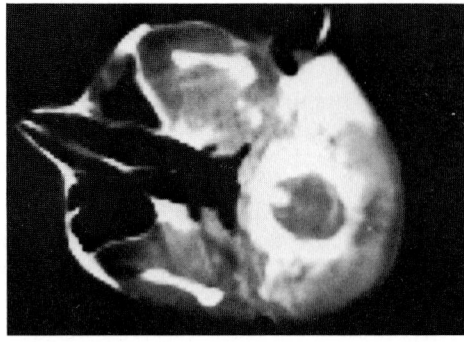

FIG. 6. Recurrent carcinoma of the left mastoid. This is a difficult image to assess due to extensive surgery.

tages are the ability to scan the patient within the immobilizing shell that is to be used for actual treatment and the possibility of directly transferring anatomical information from the scan to the EMIPLAN computerized planning system. The cost of CT in money terms and radiation dose is high, but it is totally justified when patient survival depends on achieving local control of tumor; alternative imaging techniques fail to demonstrate adequately the extent of tumor and the exact position of limiting normal structures.

REFERENCES

1. Bryant, T. H. E., and Julian, W. L. (1978): Reduction of radiation dose to patients in xeroradiography. *Br. J. Radiol.*, 51:974–980.
2. Julian, W. L., Noscoe, N. J., and Berry, R. J. (1981): Xeroradiographic tomography of the larynx. *Clin. Radiol.*, 32:577–583.
3. Noscoe, N. J. (1980): Xerotomography of the larynx—an aid to radiotherapy planning. *Radiography*, 46:199–205.
4. South Thames Cancer Registry (1975): Evidence presented to London Health Planning Consortium, Study Group on Radiotherapy and Oncology.

Computed Tomography in Radiation Therapy,
edited by C. C. Ling, C. C. Rogers, and
R. J. Morton. Raven Press, New York © 1983

Computed Tomography in Treatment Planning: Primary Breast Cancer

*Allen S. Lichter, *Benedick A. Fraass, **Hal A. Fredrickson,
*†Peter L. Roberson, and *Jan van de Geijn

*Radiation Oncology Branch, Division of Cancer Treatment, National Cancer Institute,
Bethesda, Maryland 20205; **Computer Systems Laboratory, Division of Computer
Research and Technology, National Institutes of Health, Bethesda, Maryland 20205;
and †Battelle Pacific Northwest Labs, Richland, Washington 99352

The goal of treatment planning in primary breast irradiation is to treat the breast and surrounding regional nodes with a uniform cancerocidal dose while sparing adjacent normal tissue as much as possible. The three critical normal structures nearby are the underlying lung, the mediastinum, and the opposite breast. These structures and their exact anatomic relationships are readily displayed on computed tomography (CT) scans of the torso (Fig. 1). We have used such scans as a basis for treatment planning in primary breast cancer. Specifically, we have used the CT scan to (a) superimpose dosimetric calculations of isodose curves both on and off the central plane; (b) confirm adequacy of internal mammary lymph node (IMLN) coverage; (c) choose between different field configurations; (d) compute volume

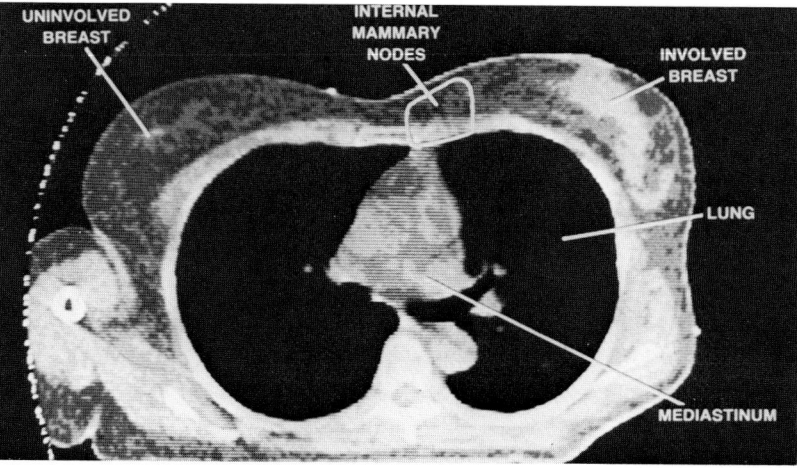

FIG. 1. A CT scan through the breast readily displays the areas to be treated (breast and regional nodes) and the areas to be spared (lung, mediastinum, and opposite breast).

of lung irradiated and dose to that lung volume; and (e) compute the dose to the contralateral breast. This chapter summarizes our experience with CT scanning in primary breast irradiation.

PATIENTS AND METHODS

From June 1979 to August 1981, 40 patients with primary breast cancer were CT scanned and irradiated in the Radiation Oncology Branch of the National Cancer Institute. The patients were scanned on an EMI 5005 whole-body scanner fitted with a flat couch surface. One or both arms of the patient were raised overhead to duplicate as closely as possible the treatment position and to facilitate entry into the scanner's 40-cm aperture. Patients were scanned in quiet respiration so that the thoracic anatomy was not distorted as it is during deep inspiration (1). No bolus was used after January 1980. Points were marked on the patient's skin with radio-opaque catheters and were used as reference coordinates in treatment planning.

The CT data were stored on magnetic tape and then transferred to a DEC PDP 11/70 computer. Programs written by one of the authors (H.A.F.) allowed the CT scans to be displayed on the video screen of the treatment planning system. External and internal contours were entered, and treatment planning was performed super-imposed on the CT scans.

Calculations of dose were performed using the treatment planning system of two of the authors (J.V.D.G. and H.A.F.) (6). Calculations were corrected to account for position and density of lung using the equivalent unit density path length concept (5). A density of 0.35 relative to water was used for all lung tissue.

The relative dose to lung was investigated by a computer program which calculated the area of the lung displayed on the scan of the central plane and the area of lung between isodose lines in increments of 10%. These results were expressed as a percentage of ipsilateral lung receiving a specified dose level or higher.

The dose to the opposite uninvolved breast was determined in four ways: (a) direct patient measurements during therapy with thermoluminescent dosimeters (TLD); (b) measurement of scattered dose from breast field configurations using a water phantom; (c) TLD measurements in a solid phantom with cork lung inserts using breast field configurations; and (d) calculations by the CT scan–treatment planning system.

RESULTS

Dosimetry—Treatment Planning

CT scans taken through the chest lend themselves well to the treatment planning process. Figures 2 through 4 are taken directly from our treatment planning video monitor. In Fig. 2 the scan through the central plan of the treatment volume is displayed. The entrance and exit points for the tangential breast fields are marked with radio-opaque catheters. The beams are positioned in Fig. 3 and are seen to enter and exit through the catheter markings. At this step one can also verify the

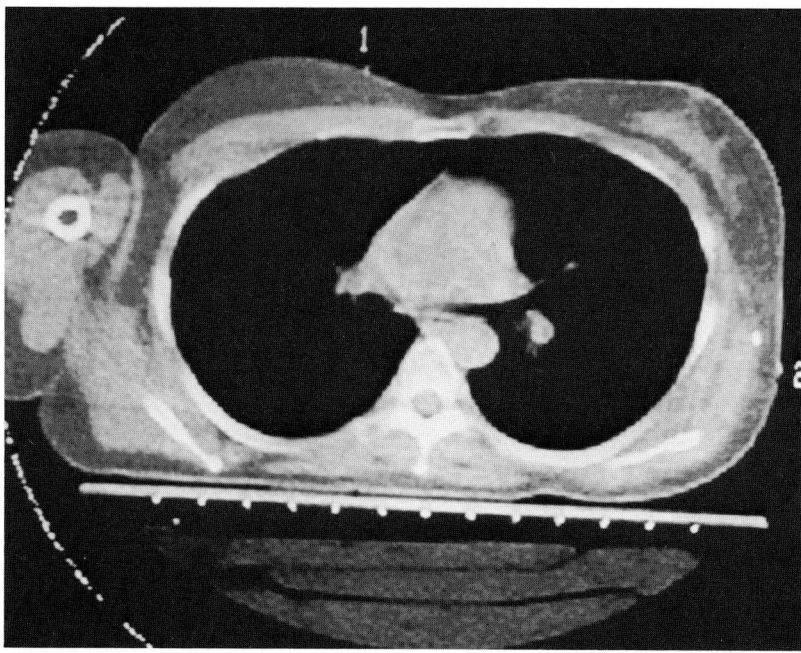

FIG. 2. Central axis scan of a patient with breast cancer. The medial and lateral entrance points taken from the simulator are marked on the skin (1 and 2).

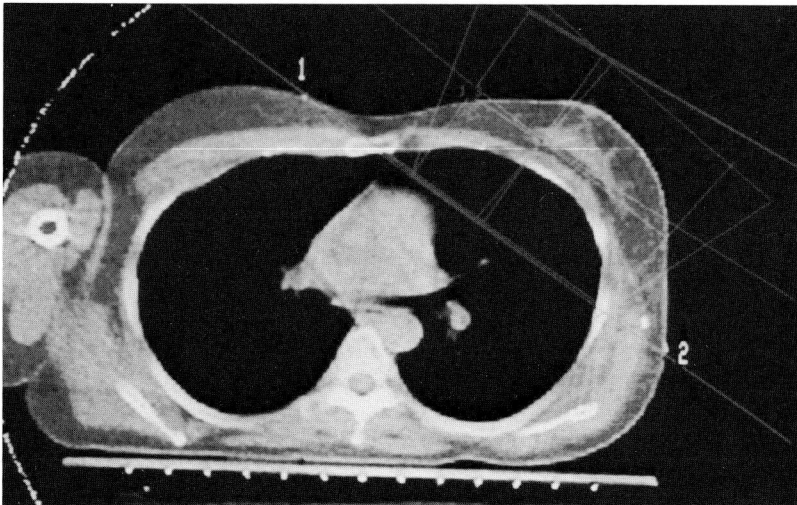

FIG. 3. The beams are angled to enter and exit through the indicated points. All divergence is directed into air, and the beams are opposed within the lung. Wedge filters are necessary in this case.

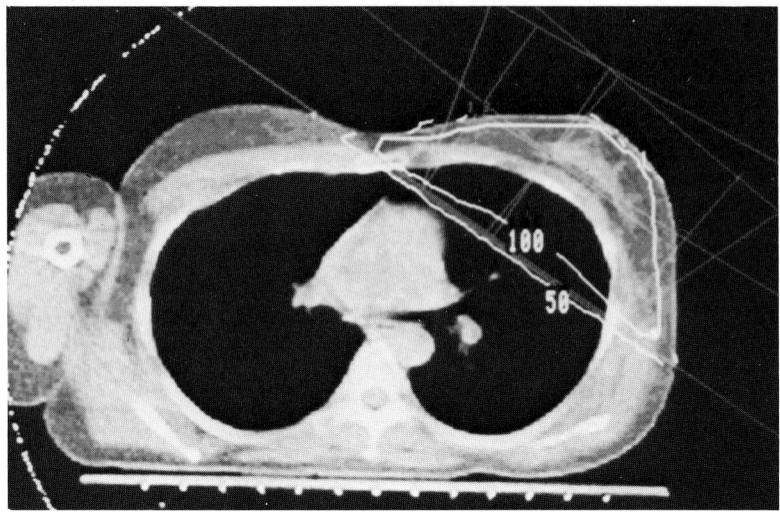

FIG. 4. Isodose curves are displayed directly on the scan.

coverage of IMLNs. These nodes may lie as deep as the pleural surface and as medial as the sternal edge (3). By including the point where the pleura and sternum meet, one is certain to cover the *region* of the IMLN. If the nodal region is not inside the beam edge by at least 0.5 cm, the entrance and exit points are moved to allow for coverage within the tangential beams, or the plan is changed to include a separate *en face* IMLN field. The isodose curves are then calculated and displayed superimposed on the scan (Fig. 4). Dose distributions in parallel planes near the superior and inferior edges of the treatment volume are also checked to ensure that no unacceptable dose nonuniformity exists.

Comparison of Different Field Configurations

Most treatment plans for primary breast cancer are of two types: (a) two-field plans, where opposed tangential breast fields enter and exit contralaterally from the involved breast and are angled so as to encompass the IMLN area; and (b) three-field plans, where a separate *en face* IMLN field is matched to smaller tangential fields. In our opinion, an IMLN that can be encompassed by the tangential breast fields represents an advantage in that it offers homogeneous irradiation of the treatment volume without treatment to the mediastinum and spinal cord. However,

FIG. 5. Top: Two standard tangential fields do not irradiate the IMLN region in this thin patient. **Middle:** Angling the fields deeper to irradiate the IMLN would encompass excessive lung. Fields could be made deeper by moving both the medial and lateral entrance points, but too much contralateral breast would receive treatment. **Bottom:** A three-field technique is best suited for this patient. Notice the small wedge-shaped piece of tissue at the deep junction of the *en face* and medial tangential fields that is left untreated.

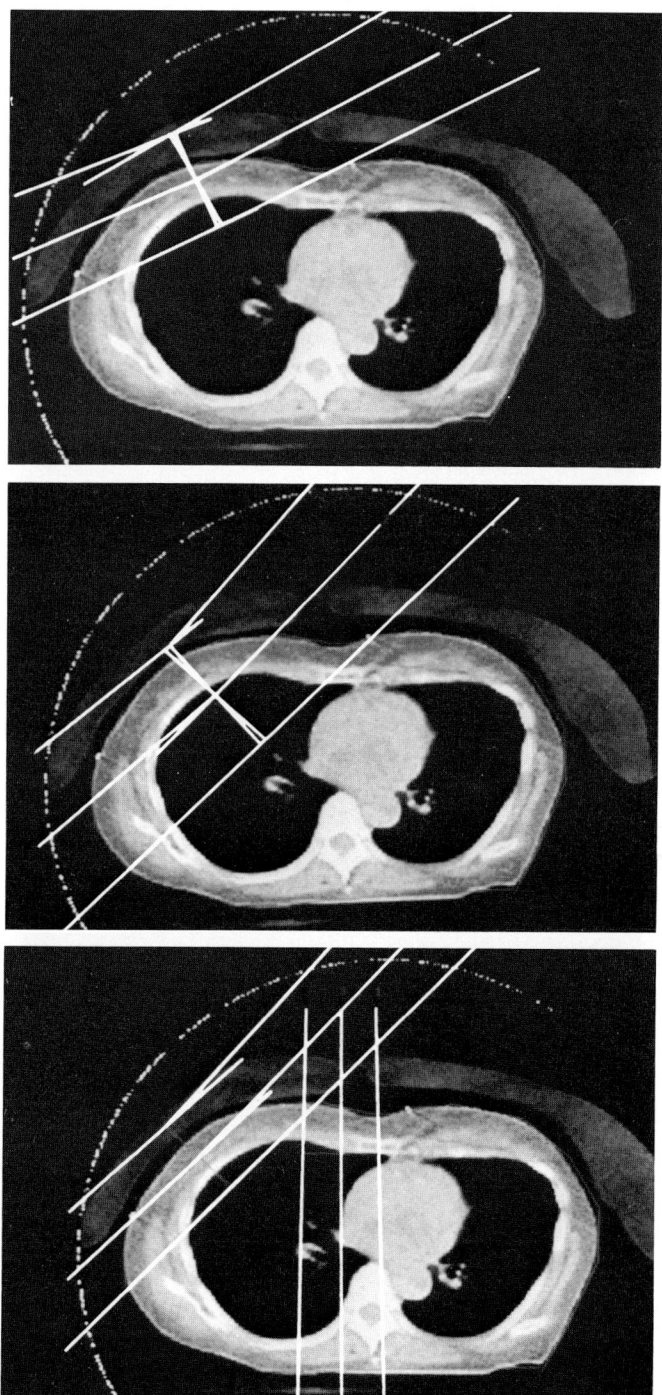

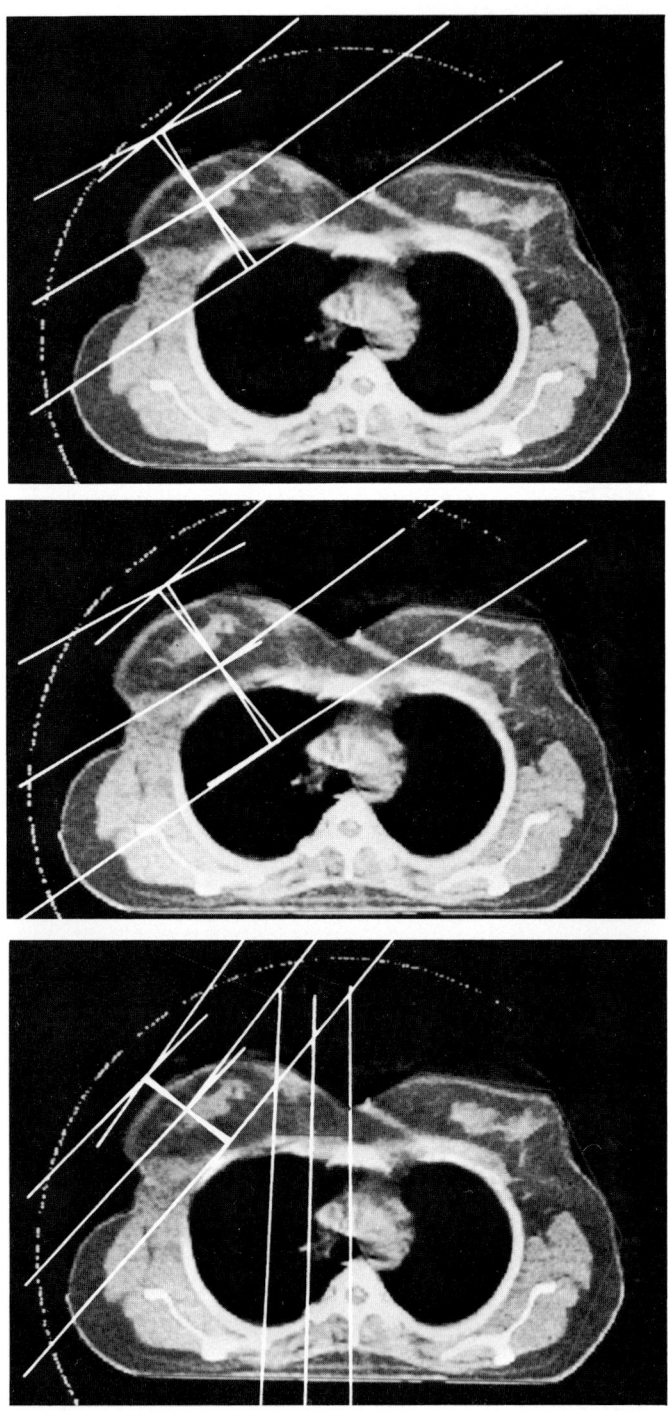

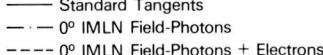

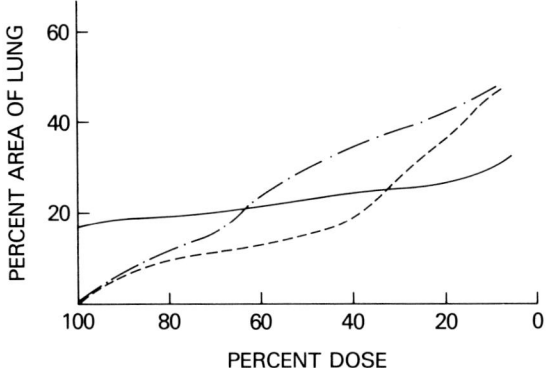

FIG. 7.   Dose to ipsilateral lung as a function of a radiation technique (13 patients). The percent dose is plotted versus the percent area of ipsilateral lung given this dose or greater.

TABLE 1. *Dose to contralateral breast for a dose of 5,000 rads to ipsilateral breast*

Technique[a]	Dose (rads) at 3 to 15 cm[b] from midline				
	3 cm	6 cm	9 cm	12 cm	15 cm
Opposed tangentials (medial field 3 cm across midline)	600	260	170	120	80
Three-field plan (separate direct internal mammary field plus two tangentials)	190	120	90	70	50

[a]6 MeV photons, 11 MeV electrons.
[b]At 1 cm below the surface on the central plane (the major volume of breast tissue is located 6 to 15 cm from the midline).

in some cases tangential fields will not yield an acceptable plan. The thin patient illustrated in Fig. 5 would have too much lung or too much opposite breast irradiated to cover the IMLN region with tangential fields alone (Fig. 5, top and middle). An additional IMLN field is a better solution (Fig. 5, bottom). However, one immediately notices that a small wedge-shaped area of tissue where the IMLN field joins the medial tangential field is left untreated. In this patient the area is trivially small, but such is not the case in all patients, as illustrated in Fig. 6. This rather large

FIG. 6.   Top: Two standard tangential fields miss the IMLN region in this large patient. **Middle:** Moving the fields deep enough to cover the IMLNs brings the fields into the opposite breast. **Bottom:** An *en face* IMLN field can easily treat the nodes. However, the wedge-shaped underdosed region is quite large and is situated directly within the tumor bed. The patient was treated with the top plan.

patient could not receive adequate IMLN coverage in the tangential fields due to thickness of her chest wall (Fig. 6, top and middle). A three-field plan is clearly needed to treat these nodes. However, this patient's medially placed tumor excision site was directly in the match-line between the tangential and IMLN fields (Fig. 6, bottom), and the wedge-shaped underdosed region would have been large enough to encompass the tumor bed. This patient was treated with tangential fields that entered at midline (Fig. 6, top); the IMLNs were not treated. The CT display of cross-sectional anatomy was of great value in the comparison of different treatment techniques for these two patients.

Dose to Lung and Volume of Lung Treated

It is common practice to "eyeball" the amount of lung contained in a tangential breast field as a rough measure of whether a particular field is safe in regard to pulmonary consequences. As the tangential fields in a three-field plan contain considerably less lung than the tangential fields of a two-field plan, the conclusion has generally been that the three-field plan would be less toxic to lung. This may not be the case. Using CT scans, we determined the fractional lung volume irradiated and the dose to that volume for two- and three-field configurations. Our results, averaged for 13 patients, are presented in Fig. 7. The curve for the two-field tangential plan rises very steeply and then levels off, indicating that a portion of lung receives the full dose, and only a small additional volume of lung is treated to less than full dose. This results from the fact that dose fall-off outside the beam edges is rapid, thus sparing all lung outside the main beam boundaries. The curve for the three-field plan rises more slowly and steadily. The area of lung taken to full dose is smaller than in the two-field situation, but a larger area of lung is irradiated to the lesser dose. This is caused by the slower dose fall-off of the IMLN field as it traverses the lung.

For plans using photons only, the curves for the two- and three-field plans intersect near the 60% dose level. Expressed in a different way: for a prescribed dose of 5,000 rads to the breast, both techniques irradiate the same volume of lung to 3,000 rads or more. A noticeable decrease in dose to lung is achieved if the IMLN field is treated with equal fractions of photons and electrons.

Dose to the Opposite Breast

Anatomic information from CT scans has proved useful in the computation of the dose received by the contralateral breast during primary breast irradiation. As two-field plans that include the IMLN region must cross the midline, there is concern that the dose to the opposite breast might be excessive for this field configuration as compared to three-field plans that have the tangential fields located well away from the opposite breast. Our results are summarized in Table 1.

The two-field plan in general gives the opposite breast more dose than the three-field configuration. For the major part of the gland, a 50% increase is noted. Whether there is a significant difference between the effects of 100 rads and 150 rads cannot be determined from currently available clinical information.

DISCUSSION

Little is available in the literature on the use of CT in breast cancer therapy. The only published data concern the ability of CT to reveal the thickness of the chest wall (4). Although this is certainly useful information, it is a rather expensive and elaborate use of CT to obtain data that in our experience and that of others (2) can be easily obtained by ultrasound. However, CT has uses in breast treatment planning that cannot be easily duplicated by any other technique. By displaying whole lung anatomy one can quantitate with accuracy the volume of lung in a treatment plan and the dose to that volume. One can also verify the adequacy of coverage to the IMLN region, using CT data as an aid in deciding between a two-field and a three-field approach. One can also include lung inhomogeneity corrections in the treatment plan if desired and easily view dose distributions on sections away from the central plane. In summary, CT is useful for (a) individualized treatment planning for both primary and postoperative breast cancer patients, and (b) studies quantifying and comparing the dosimetric aspects of the various field configurations used to treat breast cancer.

REFERENCES

1. Battista, J. J., Rider, W. D., and Van Dyk, J. (1980): Computed tomography for radiotherapy planning. *Int. J. Radiat. Oncol. Biol. Phys.*, 6:99–107.
2. Bernardino, M. E., and Spanos, W. (1981): A simple technique for determining internal mammary chain depth by sonography. *Int. J. Radiat. Oncol. Biol. Phys.*, 7:671–673.
3. Haagensen, C. D., Feind, C. R., Herter, F. P., Slanetz, C. A., and Weinberg, J. A. (eds.) (1972): *The Lymphatics in Cancer*, p. 322. Saunders, Philadelphia.
4. Munzenrider, J. E., Tchakarova, I., Castro, M., and Carter, B. (1979): Computerized body tomography in breast cancer. *Cancer*, 43:137–150.
5. Van de Geijn, J. (1972): EXTDOS 71; revised and expanded version of EXTDOS, a program for treatment planning in external beam therapy. *Comp. Prog. Biomed.*, 2:169–177.
6. Van de Geijn, J., and Fredrickson, H. A. (1981): Computation of multi-slice dose distributions in irregular fields modified by irregular blocks. *Med. Phys.*, 8:560.

Computed Tomography in Radiation Therapy,
edited by C. C. Ling, C. C. Rogers, and
R. J. Morton. Raven Press, New York © 1983

Computed Tomography in Brachytherapy

Carl M. Mansfield, Kyo Rak Lee, Samuel Dwyer,
Darwin Zellmer, and Prakairut Cook

*Departments of Radiation Therapy and Diagnostic Radiology, University of Kansas
Medical Center, Kansas City, Kansas 66103*

Interstitial implantations and intracavitary insertions of radioactive sources continue to be important techniques in the management of patients with malignant disease at certain sites. The success of this technique depends on the ability to fully evaluate the implant in relation to the tumor volume and surrounding normal structures. This evaluation is usually accomplished through visual inspection and conventional localization roentgenograms, which may include orthogonal and stereoscopic views.

Computed tomography (CT) has been shown to play an important role in the treatment planning of patients requiring external beam therapy (1,3,4,6,9). CT can also be of value in patients receiving brachytherapy (5,7,8). At our center the initial experience with CT scanning in brachytherapy was in intracavitary therapy for uterine carcinoma (6). This chapter discusses the use of CT in brachytherapy for the patients with gynecologic, breast, and prostatic carcinoma.

Intracavitary implants involve the use of applicators which are placed in the cavity to be treated. These devices may be "afterloading" in type. If the afterloading type is used, "dummy" sources are placed in the applicators for the purpose of the CT and x-ray examination. Interstitial implants involve the placement of radioactive or afterloading sources into tissue. For example, an afterloading technique is used in the breast by placing plastic tubes in the breast and subsequently loading them with radioactive sources.

As soon as the patient comes from the recovery room, orthogonal views are taken and contrast material is used when necessary. In routine cases, in addition to the conventional views, CT scans are taken at three to six levels of interest through the implanted volume. These studies have been sufficient to make an evaluation of most brachytherapy procedures. If two- or three-dimensional reconstruction is desired, scans must be taken through more levels of the implant.

CARCINOMA OF THE UTERUS

Since 1977 patients with carcinoma of the cervix or endometrium have been examined with CT scanning after insertion of intracavitary applicators. Intracavitary therapy is part of a combined therapeutic approach using external irradiation in patients with cervical carcinoma and hysterectomy in patients with endometrial carcinoma.

An afterloading Fletcher applicator consisting of a tandem and two ovoids is inserted in patients with cervical carcinoma. CT scans are obtained using a General Electric model 8800 CT/T (4.8-sec scan, 10 mm thick slice) body scanner. Before scanning, 150 ml 2% meglumine diatrizoate is instilled into the bladder through a Foley catheter and into the rectum by enema. Three or four scans are made through the pelvis at levels of interest indicated by the physician. When planar (sagittal, coronal, or oblique) or three-dimensional reconstruction is planned, scans are obtained at 1.0-cm intervals from the level of the iliac crest to the symphysis pubis in the supine position. The image quality of the scans was satisfactory in nearly all cases, even though artifacts were produced by the tandem and ovoids. CT scanning adequately demonstrated the tandem in the uterine cavity and the ovoids within the vagina. The CT correctly identified the size, thickness, and shape of the uterus in relation to the applicator, and provided spatial information regarding the surrounding normal structures.

When multiple CT cuts were made through the Fletcher applicator, it was possible to generate a two-dimensional reconstruction in the transverse, sagittal, and coronal planes of the implanted area (Fig. 1). The isodose distributions of the implant in the same planes as the reconstructions can be calculated and superimposed on the corresponding CT reconstructions. As most patients with cervical carcinoma receive external beam treatment in addition to intracavitary therapy, it is possible to combine the isodose curves of the external and the intracavitary therapy. Thus the total doses delivered to the various anatomic sites could be calculated accurately (5,7).

CARCINOMA OF THE BREAST

A number of patients with early breast carcinoma were treated with iridium-192 (^{192}Ir) implants to give an additional "boost" dose to the tumor bed after lumpectomy and external irradiation. All patients had a CT scan of the chest as part of their treatment planning prior to external therapy. The traditional technique of implantation of the breast has been to place the iridium in a transverse fashion. Scanning of such implants, using present CT capabilities, provides little meaningful information.

In order to use the CT for localization of the sources, the implant technique was modified, when possible, by implanting the ^{192}Ir in a cephalocaudad direction (parallel to the body axis). Two or three CT scans of the breast were obtained at levels of interest, usually through the center and halfway between the center and the ends of the implant. This was done with dummy wires loaded in the implanted

FIG. 1. **Top:** Transverse view of the pelvis showing the tandem (T) and sigmoid (S). **Middle:** Sagittal reconstruction of the pelvis with a Fletcher tandem (T) and ovoids (O). The uterus is well outlined *(arrows)*. **Bottom:** Coronal reconstruction shows the tandem (T) and ovoids (O).

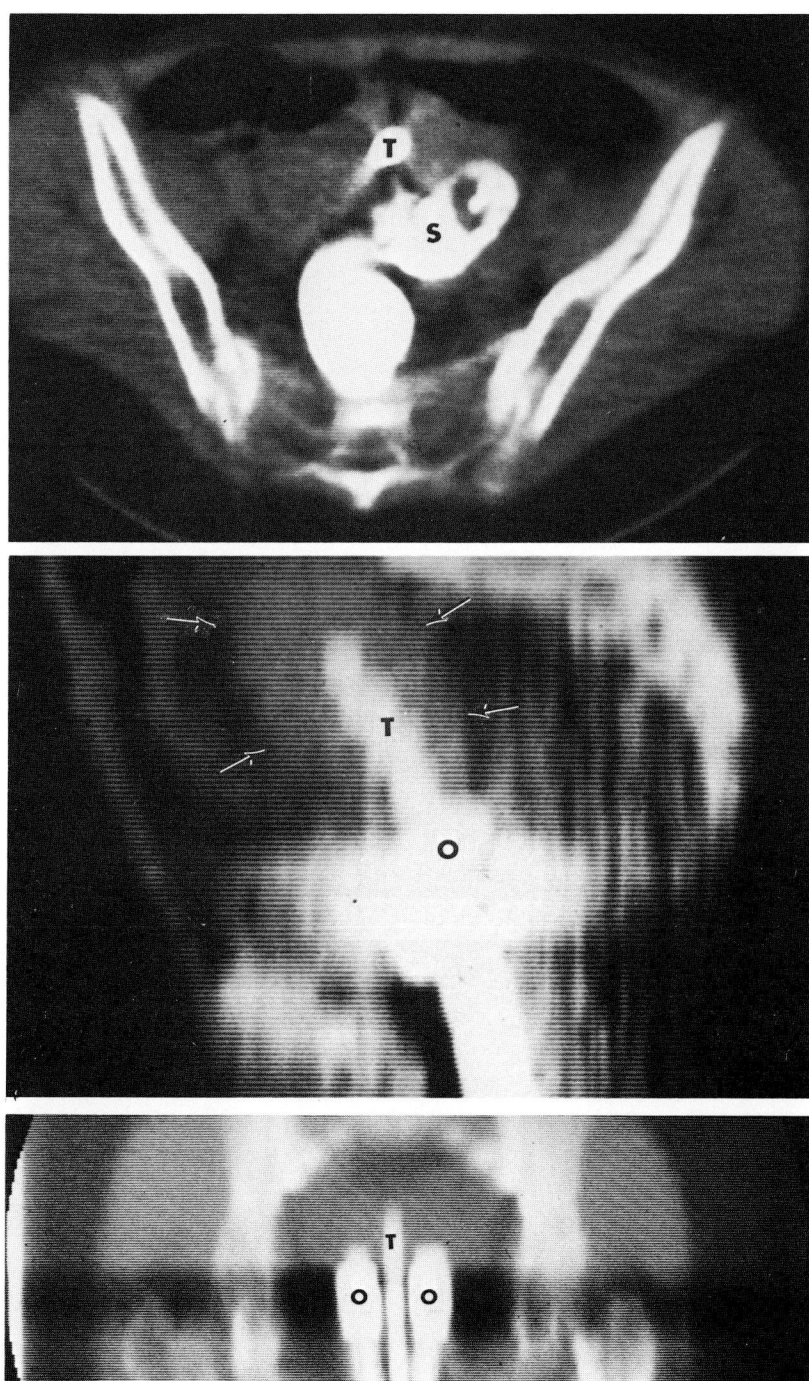

plastic tubes. If two- or three-dimensional reconstruction is planned, multiple scans were made in 10 mm thickness at 1-cm intervals. All patients had conventional orthogonal films. The CT scans clearly demonstrated the implanted wires as point sources without artifacts (Fig. 2). It provided a direct view of the implant in the transverse plane of the breast at multiple levels and of the relationship of the implant to adjacent structures. Direct calculations of the isodose distribution can be made from the scan, or the scan information can be entered into a computer in terms of X-Y coordinates for more detailed manipulations. It is possible to combine the implant and external beam dosimetries as described previously in this chapter.

In order to compare the ability of CT scans and orthogonal films to determine the position of interstitial sources, tissue equivalent material was implanted with plastic tubes and loaded with dummy wires (Fig. 3, top). In many instances the orthogonal films did not accurately represent the position of the implanted wires in the central transverse axis of the implant, because a straight line is drawn between the two ends of the implant as seen on the orthogonal film. If there is any curvature of the implant, it would not represent the real position of the sources (Fig. 3, bottom). (It should be noted that the real position of the implant can be determined from orthogonal films, although this would involve considerable time and effort, whereas the CT scan can provide this information accurately and quickly.)

CARCINOMA OF THE PROSTATE

The majority of the patients with stage B prostatic carcinoma were treated with surgical dissection of the pelvic nodes followed by iodine-125 (^{125}I) seeds implanted in the prostate. When CT was used in these patients for assessing the implanted volume, scans were obtained at 1-cm intervals with 1 cm slice thickness after intravenous infusion of 300 ml 30% meglumine diatrizoate.

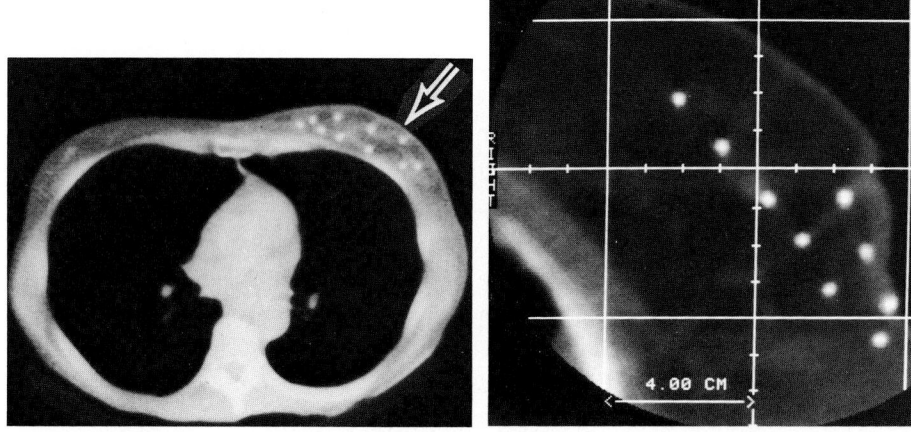

FIG. 2. Left: Transverse section through the center of an implanted breast *(arrow)*. **Right:** Enlarged view with a grid **(left)** demonstrates the correct anatomic relationship of the individual implanted sources and the surrounding structures.

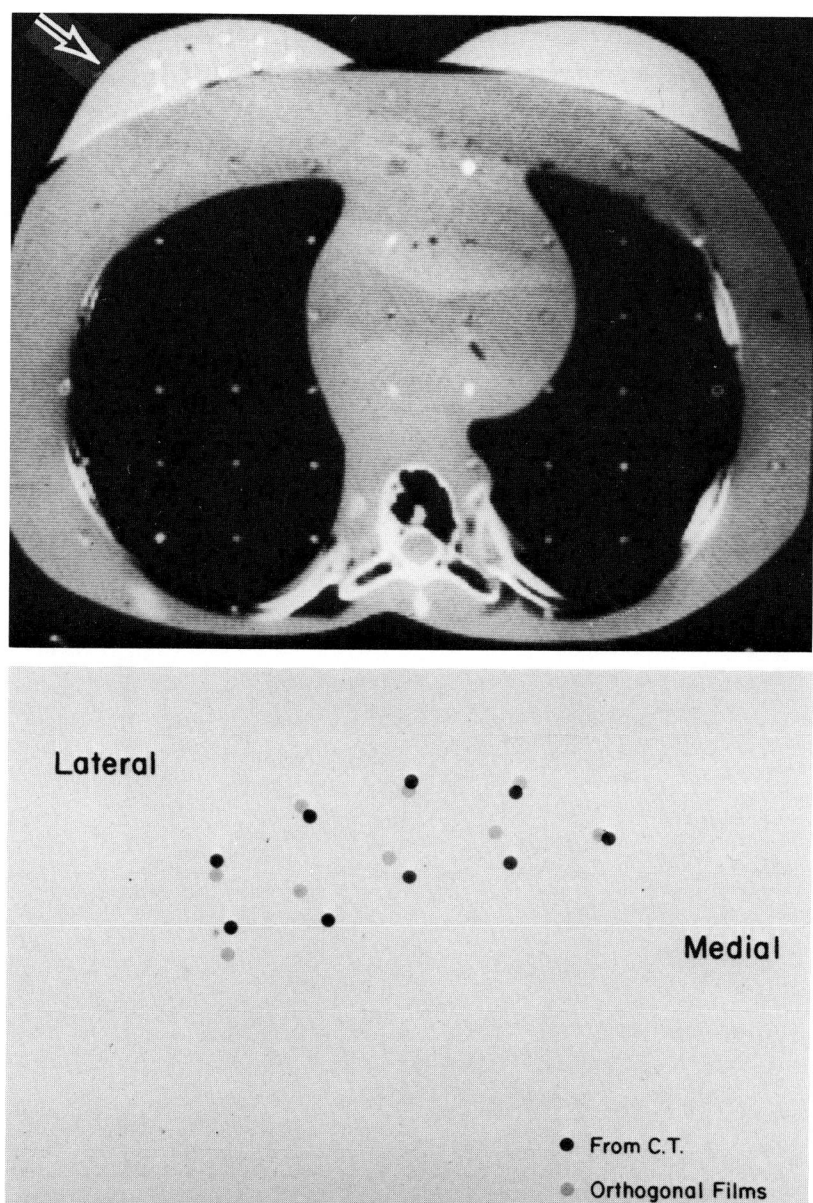

FIG. 3. Top: Transverse CT scan demonstrates implanted dummy sources with the breast of a phantom made of tissue equivalent material. **Bottom:** The position of the dummy sources in **top** localized by using orthogonal views *(light dots)* compared to their position localized by CT *(dark dots).*

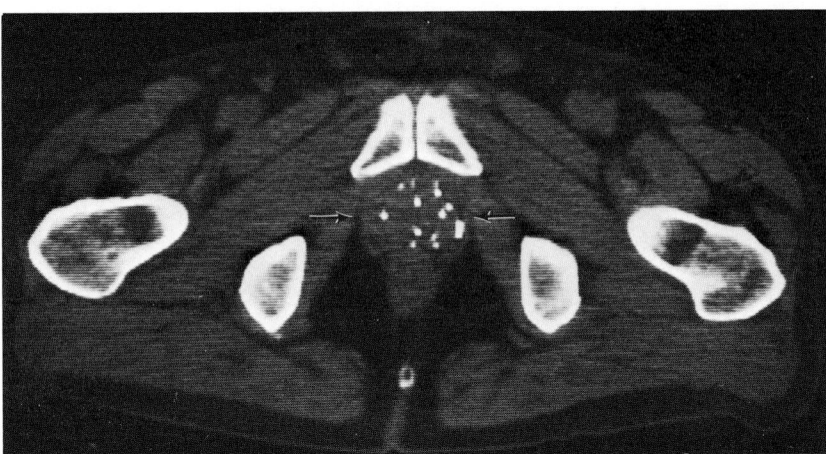

FIG. 4. Transverse section of a prostate implant with seeds in the prostate *(arrows)*.

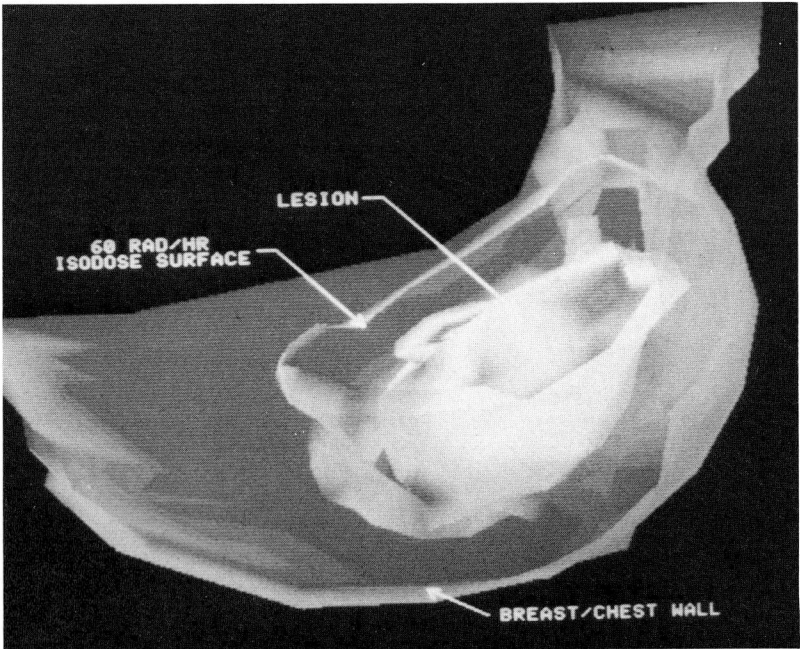

FIG. 5. 3D reconstruction of a breast demonstrates the tumor and the 60 rads/hr isodose surface.

The scans in the first patients were disappointing in terms of delineating the tumor volume and identifying the individual seeds. The slice thickness and intervals were too thick, and the contrast material within the bladder obscured some of the implanted seeds and gland. The most recent patient had CT without contrast material

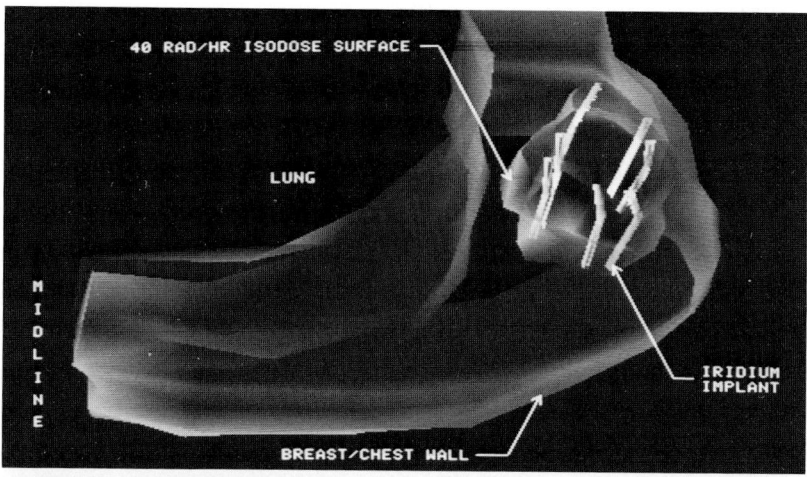

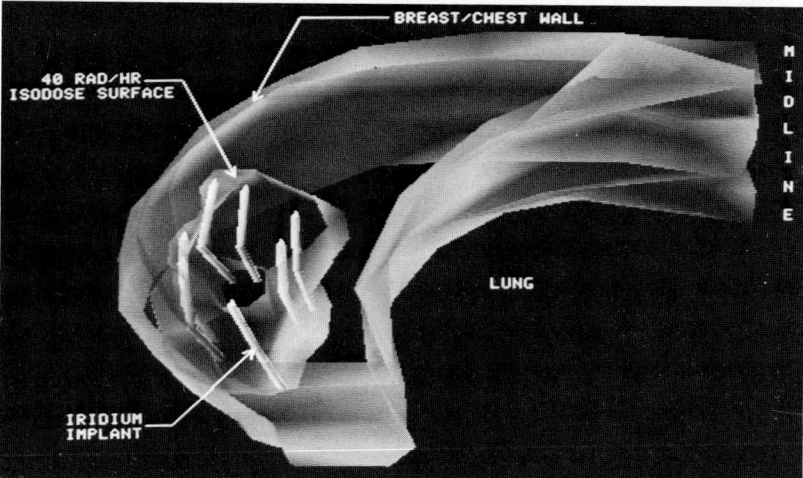

FIG. 6. Top: The implanted tumor volume, iridium wires, and 40 rads/hr isodose surface are shown by 3D reconstruction. **Bottom:** 3D reconstruction can be rotated for viewing at any angle.

in the bladder. Scans were obtained at 0.5-cm intervals and with 0.5 cm slice thickness. The thinner slices obtained in the last patient without contrast material in the bladder better demonstrated the seeds (Fig. 4). Although individual seeds were difficult to identify, approximately 50 of 55 seeds were identified with reasonable accuracy when the CT and orthogonal films were used together. CT scanning did delineated the entire implanted volume.

THREE-DIMENSIONAL VOLUME DISPLAY

By taking multiple cuts through the implanted volume, the distribution at multiple points within the volume can be determined. It was possible to combine these cuts

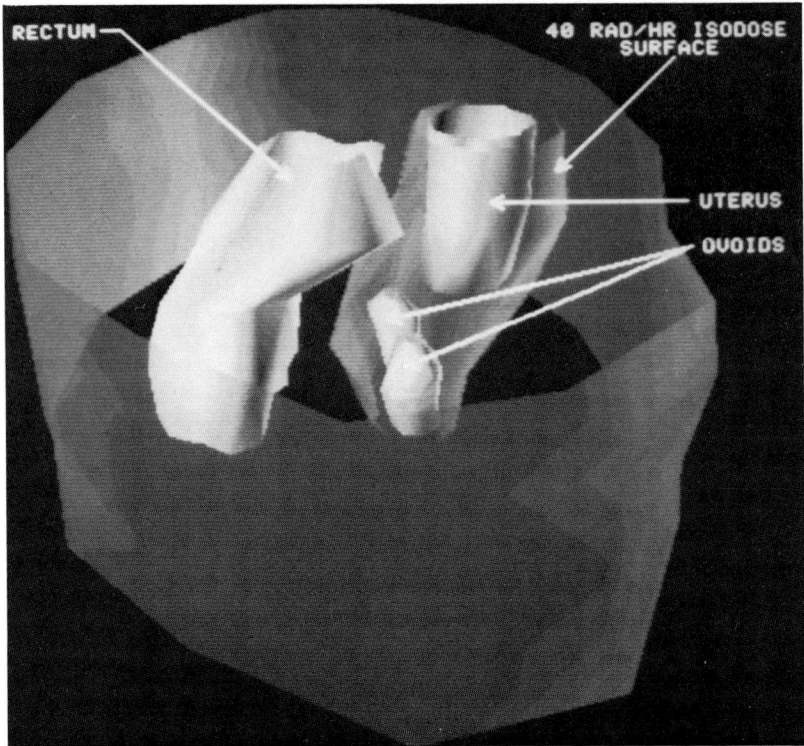

FIG. 7. 3D reconstruction of a Fletcher implant.

and make a three-dimensional (3D) reconstruction of the treatment volume. In order to construct and display the 3D representation of the anatomic sites and dosimetry surfaces, the anatomic sites of interest must be identifiable on the CT scan. In addition, the contours of the anatomic structures and dosimetry surfaces must be manifested as simple closed curves; i.e., each surface contour must be specified by a finite sequence of points. The algorithms have been described elsewhere (2).

Figure 5 is a 3D reconstruction of a breast and its tumor using this technique. The reconstructed implant can be rotated and viewed from any desired angle (Fig. 6). Figure 7 shows a reconstructed Fletcher implant and Fig. 8 a vaginal implant. A prostatic implant volume is shown in Fig. 9.

SUMMARY

CT scanning adds to the ability to evaluate brachytherapy techniques. It provides an additional method in the assessment of patients who are candidates for or who are being treated by brachytherapy. The CT scan can give information regarding the position of the sources and their relation to the tumor and normal structures with greater ease than do orthogonal views. This makes it possible to accurately

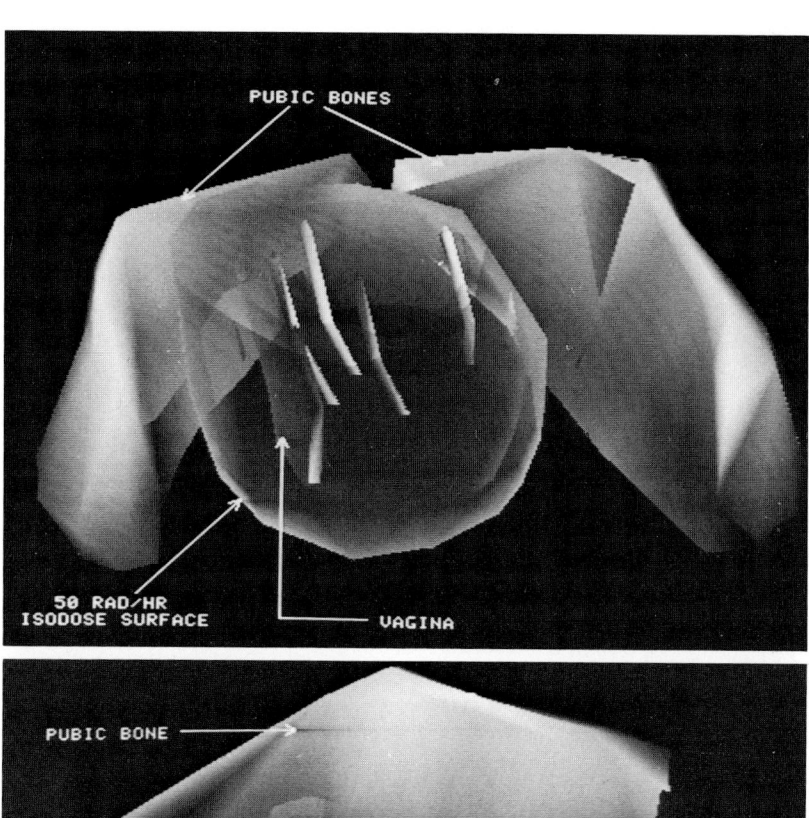

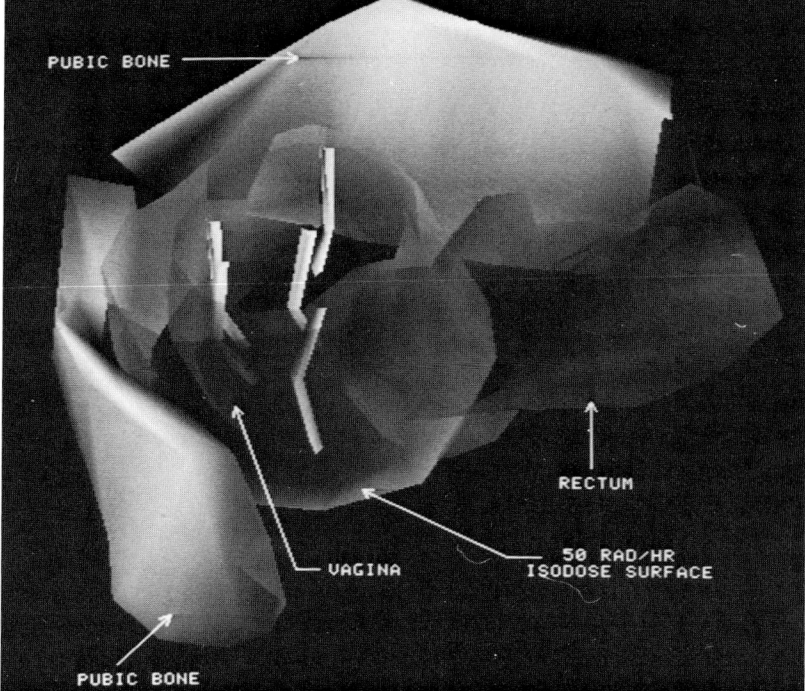

FIG. 8. 3D reconstruction of a vaginal implant viewed at different angles.

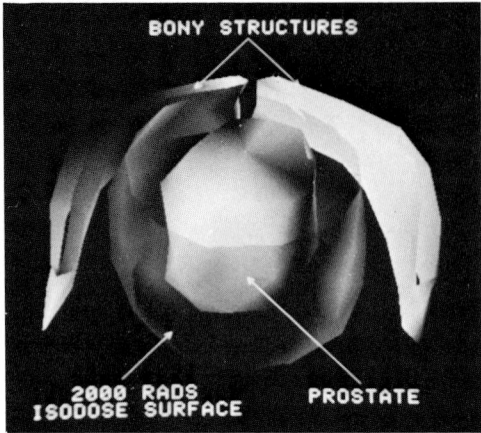

FIG. 9. 3D reconstruction of an ^{125}I prostate implant volume.

calculate areas of high or low dose. Potential areas of overdose can be recognized, thereby decreasing the chances of postbrachytherapy complications.

CT scanning can be used at various levels of complexity in dosimetry evaluation. Adequate brachytherapy dosimetry information is obtainable from CT slices through one or more levels of the implanted volume. In some instances it is possible to obtain additional information by reconstructing the scans in other planes, e.g., coronal or sagittal.

Three-dimensional viewing of the implant is desirable, but it should be pointed out that this approach is time-consuming and beyond the capabilities of most institutions at present. It will be necessary to continue work on three-dimensional treatment planning to make it readily available.

REFERENCES

1. Abrams, H. L., and McNeil, B. J. (1978): Medical implications of computed tomography ("CAT scanning"). *N. Engl. J. Med.*, 298:255–261, 310–318.
2. Cook, L. T., Cook, P. N., Lee, K. R., Botnitzky, S., Wong, B. S., Fritz, S. L., Ophir, J., Dwyer, S. J., Bigongiari, L. R., and Templeton, A. W. (1980): An algorithm for volume estimation based on polyhedral approximation. *IEEE Trans. Biomed. Eng.*, 27:493–500.
3. Goiteien, M., Wittenberg, J., Mendiondo, M., Doucette, J., Friedberg, C., Ferrucci, J., Gunderson, L., Linggood, R., Shipley, W. U., and Fineberg, H. V. (1979): The value of CT scanning in radiation therapy treatment planning: a prospective study. *Int. J. Radiat. Oncol. Biol. Phys.*, 5:1787–1798.
4. Jelden, G. L. Chernak, E. S., Rodriguez-Antunez, A., Haaga, S. R., Lavik, P. S., and Dhaliwal, R. S. (1976): Further progress in CT scanning and computerized radiation therapy treatment planning. *Am. J. Roentgenol.*, 127:179–185.
5. Lee, K. R., Anderson, W. H., Dwyer, S. J., III, Cox, H. L., Mansfield, C. M., Levine, E., and Templeton, A. W. (1979): An interactive treatment planning using computed tomography for intracavitary radiotherapy. In: *Proceedings: Sixth Conference on Computer Applications in Radiology and Computer/Aided Analysis of Radiological Images*, pp. 56–60. American College of Radiology and the IEEE Computer Society, Newport Beach, CA.
6. Lee, K. R., Dwyer, S. J., III, Mansfield, C. M., Cox, H. L., Levine, E., Templeton, A. W., Cook, N., Anderson, W., Tarlton, M., and Fritz, S. L. (1978): A three-dimensional model for computed display of radiation treatment plans. Exhibited at the 64th Scientific Assembly and Annual Meeting of the Radiological Society of North America, Chicago.

7. Lee, K. R., Mansfield, C. M., Dwyer, S. J., III, Cox, H. L., Levine, E., and Templeton, A. W. (1980): CT for intracavitary radiotherapy planning. *Radiology*, 135:809–813.
8. Mansfield, C. M., Zellmer, D. L., Lee, K. R., Fritz, S. L., Anderson, W. H., Cook, P. N., and Dwyer, S. J., III (1981): Abstract of the XVth International Congress of Radiology, Brussels, Belgium.
9. Munzenrider, J. E., Pilepich, M., Rene-Ferero, J. B., Tchakarova, E., and Carter, B. L. (1977): Use of body scanner in radiotherapy treatment planning. *Cancer*, 40:170–179.

Computed Tomography in Radiation Therapy,
edited by C. C. Ling, C. C. Rogers, and
R. J. Morton. Raven Press, New York © 1983

Introduction to Computed Tomography

David J. Goodenough and Kenneth E. Weaver

Division of Radiation Physics, The George Washington University Medical Center, Washington, D.C. 20037

The mathematical basis of the reconstruction of an object from the data obtained in a number of views around the object was developed as early as 1917 by Radon (20). In 1956 Bracewell developed practical techniques for measuring microwave radiation emitted by the sun by using a series of strip-sun measurements in different measurements (5). In 1975 Gordon et al. cited more than 1,500 references related to image reconstruction (16).

The first published attempt at medical application of reconstruction was carried out by Oldendorf in 1961 using a method called "spin migration" (19). Important experiments were carried out in 1963 by Kuhl and colleagues at the University of Pennsylvania utilizing a tomographic image scanner for radionuclide imaging (18a). The first clinically useful computed tomography system was pioneered by Hounsfield of EMI Ltd. in England, and installed in 1971 in the Atkinson Morley hospital near London (1,18). The full impact of CT on the medical field is difficult to estimate because it is still evolving; however, the profound diagnostic, social, and economic impact of its development has already been sufficient for some to compare the discovery to that of Roentgen's discovery of the x-ray in 1895.

This chapter presents an overview of computed tomography with particular attention given to the construction utilizing x-ray transmission data. It is hoped that the presentation is sufficiently broad that the material can be extrapolated to other energy sources of transmission or emission data.

THEORY

Computed tomography (CT) is the term generally used to characterize the imaging technique in which transmission measurements of a narrow beam of x-rays, made at several angles or projections around a given object, may be used with an appropriate computer program to resynthesize particular slices of interest within the object.

CT differs from the more conventional x-ray tomography in that one uses digital or computer techniques to restore the slice of interest rather than the analog conventional tomographic techniques of deliberately casting unwanted information into "out-of-focus" planes on a film moving in a complex, prescribed, geometric pattern with the x-ray tube. One problem with the older conventional techniques is that the unwanted information is reduced to a general scatter or fog level on the film, thus reducing inherent contrast. Both techniques have in common the desire to isolate a given plane (actually a thin section) of information from the sometimes confusing information arising from the rest of the three-dimensional object and found superimposed on the relevant information when a single projection (e.g., anteroposterior) is obtained on a standard two-dimensional image receptor such as a radiograph.

RECONSTRUCTION TECHNIQUE

If one considers the nature of the x-ray attenuation profiles one might expect from a cube of material scanned across the x and y axes that each profile would be expected to rise and fall in a discrete stepwise manner. If one had only the profile data along the x and y axes, how might it be used to estimate the original object distribution? One's first tendency would probably be to literally throw back the given data for each axis across the whole x/y plane. If one does this, as well as a crude estimate of the cube of interest, one also generates some background information which is not in the original object. This spurious information tends to obscure or diminish the contrast and true nature of the real object of interest. Such a simple operation is usually called *back-projection* (6). Consider what happens when we try to back-project several of the profiles we have obtained from scans of an isolated central pin. One obtains a hot central region somewhat resembling the pin, but we also have an accompanying characteristic star-type artifact which is radiating from the point of interest, obviously greatly degrading the spatial information concerning the point of interest. If it is known how a point is blurred or degraded by a system, then in a sense under certain conditions of linearity and isoplanacity it is possible to exactly characterize the amount of degradation introduced by that point spread function. These conditions of linearity and isoplanacity lead to the assumption that each point in the object plan is imaged the same as every other point up to the local intensity value, which just becomes a weighting factor. In an analogous way, because one knows the way an individual point might be blurred by a simple back-projection operation, one might hope to "deconvolve" or deblur the deleterious effect of simple back-projection. The correction for the blurring function (or deconvolution) can be carried out on each projection by "filter back-projection" wherein each profile datum is corrected for the effect of the simple back-projection operations; however, complicated spatial convolution operations reduce to simple multiplicative relationships in the Fourier spatial plane frequency. Thus another way of dealing with the CT reconstruction is to take the profile data generated from the scanning and data acquisition system and generate the corresponding Fourier transform for each projection (6).

Each angle or view will give us a separate Fourier transform, which may be multiplied by the correction function. In this manner a series of one-dimensional Fourier array transforms may be built up to establish two-dimensional Fourier array.

One may then interpolate between sampled points and inverse Fourier transform to return to the now deconvolved object of interest. Under certain conditions this resynthesis can become exact. Interestingly enough, these so-called analytic or potentially exact types of mathematical reconstructions filtered back-projection or Fourier techniques were not applied in the first CT scanners, i.e., the EMI head scanner. Rather, the original reconstruction techniques involved iterative computer techniques in which the profiles are taken, back-projected, and then successively modified or iterated until the modified data are consistent with all the x-ray profiles. Successive approximation and changes are made after each iteration to make the profile become more and more reasonable. There continues to be some discussion about the efficacy of the various analytic and iterative (arithmetic) techniques (especially in the presence of noise).

RADIATION PHYSICS

It is well known that a beam of monoenergetic x-ray transversing matter is attenuated exponentially. One can note that the attenuation is affected by the composition of the material as represented by the local linear attenuation coefficient (μ) as well as the distance through which the beam traverses. Figure 1 shows the relative mass attenuation coefficient of some substances of biologic interest. Equation 1 shows how the output of an original EMI machine can be related to the effective linear attenuation coefficient characterizing a local region of interest.

$$\text{CT No.} = K(\mu - \mu_w)/\mu_w \doteq 2{,}630(\mu - \mu_w) \tag{1}$$

This local region or volume of interest in a CT scan is often defined as: the voxel

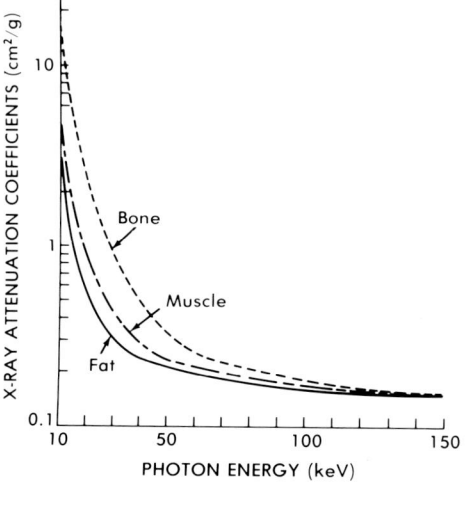

FIG. 1. Mass attenuation coefficients for bone, muscle, and fat.

(ΔV) — the volume element represented by the product of the matrix of pixel size ($\Delta x \Delta y$) times the slice thickness (Δz): $\Delta V - \Delta x \Delta y \Delta z$. Thus for the EMI head scanner, the EMI number found in the 160×160 volume elements of $1.5 \times 1.5 \times 13$ mm is given by the difference between the attenuation coefficient of the region of interest and the attenuation coefficient of water (approximately 0.190 cm^{-1}). This difference is amplified by a factor of approximately 2,630, which is essentially 500 divided by the linear attenuation coefficient of water (μ_w). When this CT scaling is applied to attenuation coefficients encountered within the body, one arrives at a CT scale where $+500$ is bone, 0 is water, and -500 is air. Most tissue is found between approximately -50 and $+50$. Note parenthetically that this scale is often arbitrarily expanded by a factor of 2, in which case $+1,000$ would represent bone and $-1,000$ would represent air. This $\pm 1,000$ scale is often considered the Hounsfield (H) scale. One finds that, for example, gray and white matter are separated by only a few EMI numbers, and thus a CT system offers an extremely fine x-ray probe to distinguish between very small fractional percent changes in tissue density or tissue composition.

In terms of sensitometry, or the meaning of the CT number, one should note that it is not surprising that two types of CT machine, encompassing different design features that impose differing spectral quality of the x-ray beam (e.g., the presence or absence of a water bath), might produce different CT numbers for the same nominal object. Although by and large there is good correlation, there is some variation from system to system; and in particular, objects showing high atomic number properties can be expected to show fairly different results when modulated by the different x-ray energy spectra. The exact relationship between CT number and attenuation coefficient is complicated by the fact that the CT system uses a polychromatic spectrum of x-ray energies (e.g., an x-ray tube operating at 100, 120, or 140 kVp) (see Fig. 2, for example) (10). Because the x-ray photons in this energy spectrum are subject to both photoelectric (μ_{pe}) and compton (μ_c) interactions, the total attenuation coefficient is given by: $\mu = \mu_{pe} + \mu_c$. Then, because μ_{pe} is strongly dependent on atomic number (e.g., Z^3) as well as electron density (N_e), and μ_c is primarily dependent on electron density (N_e), the determined values of the CT number (i.e., μ) represent a complicated dependence on both the atomic number and the electron density of the material attenuating the x-ray spectrum (3,17).

Let us review the various CT systems proposed (Table 1) to obtain such differential linear attenuation coefficient measurements. The second-generation system is usually considered a hybrid or multiple pencil beam scanner. The third-generation machine is often considered a single-motion rotating fan beam scanner. Variations on this design include up to several hundred stationary crystal detectors with a source rotating inside, or "nutating" outside the crystal ring. The pencil beam scanner usually follows the design of an EMI Mark I head scanner in that a single detector and single x-ray source assembly generate the narrow-beam x-ray attenuation coefficient data. The pencil beam scanners are typically characterized by both rotate and translate motions, with a total rotation angle ranging from 180° to

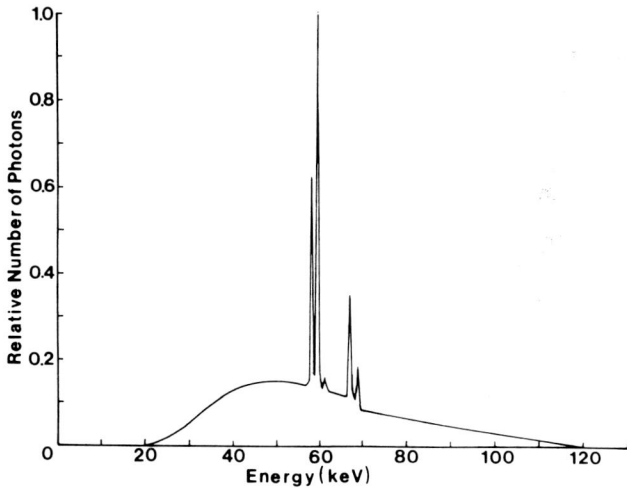

FIG. 2. Typical 120 kVp diagnostic x-ray spectrum.

TABLE 1. *Scanner types*

Pencil beam
Hybrid—multiple pencil beams
Fan beam (rotating detector and x-ray source)
Fan beam (rotating source only)

240°. The type of x-ray tube is usually of continuous emission design. This design uses a combination of linear and rotational motions to generate a series of x-ray transmission profiles. This type of design, although basically slow (several minute scans), offered some built-in redundancy of sampling that makes the reconstruction problem somewhat easier. The design suffers from long scan times, allowing the possibility of patient motion. In particular, the original EMI machine used a water bath to surround the patient's head. Such a water bath provides a number of practical advantages, e.g., reducing the extent of (spectral) beam hardening that results from transmission through varying distances. Then, too, the dynamic range requirements on the detector system may be reduced by this kind of design. In the sense that such scanners utilize a scanning pattern of only about 180°, one will, of course, encounter as uneven deposition of energy throughout the patient's head according to well-known depth-dose distribution with the maximum at about 90° on the x-ray tube side of the scan. The second-generation systems (Fig. 3) (so-called hybrid machines) now use multiple detectors instead of a single detector monitoring a single x-ray source; such a detector source configuration might be described as a limited fan beam. Note, however, that the rotate and translate motions have been preserved.

In the hybrid system, multiple detectors are used to enable the system to rotate a larger angular increment than for a single detector system. The same number of

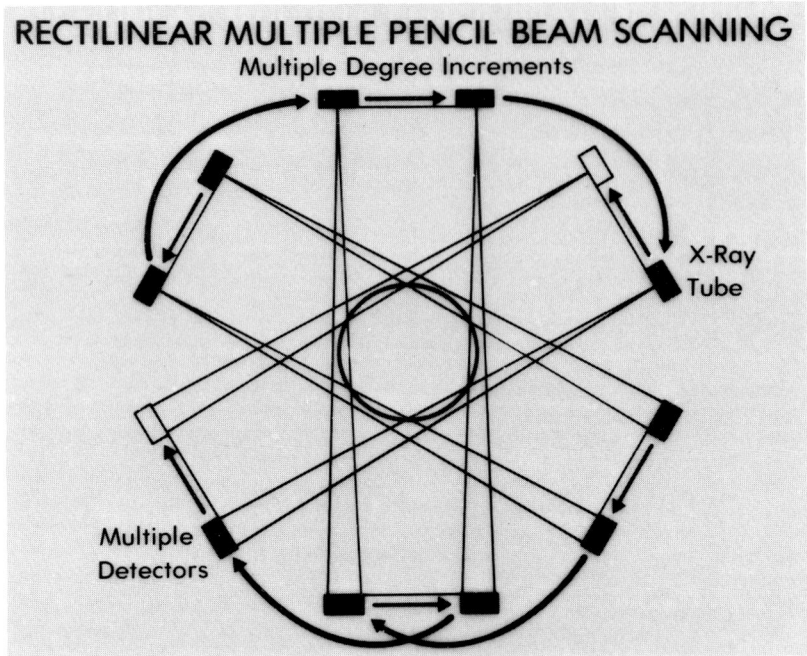

FIG. 3. Second-generation CT scanner retains rotate-translate concept of first-generation scanner, but more detectors allow greater angular increments.

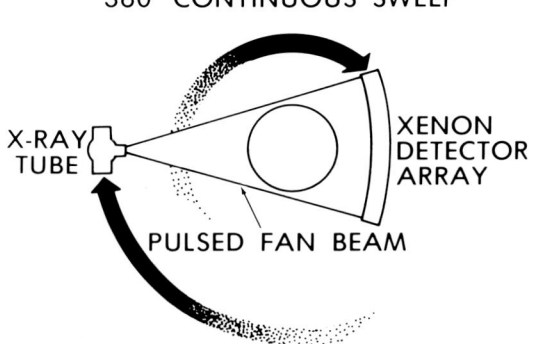

FIG. 4. Third-generation CT design.

rays as the pencil scanner may now be obtained within approximately 20 sec. This type of machine is usually still characterized by a continuous-emission x-ray source.

The so-called third-generation system (Fig. 4) utilizes a fan beam geometry that involves a large number of detectors moving in a single motion, i.e., continuous rotational motion with the bank of detectors looking back at an x-ray source which moves synchronously with the detector motion. In addition, one now encounters pulsed-emission x-ray sources.

An additional variation of the rotate-only geometry is the fourth-generation design, in which there are several hundred detectors which are kept fixed while the x-ray source itself moves on an inscribed circle. Third- and higher-order-generation systems have been advocated because the data may be acquired in times on the order of 5 sec or less, opening up the possibility of significant decreases in motion artifacts.

Third-generation scanners do not need to be view-limited, because they may sample at a large number of angles; however, the basic ray spacing is limited by the detector cell spacing. Fourth-generation systems can develop a detector fan beam and, as such, may not be ray-limited.

ARTIFACTS

There are many types of artifact encountered in CT machines depending on the particular generation and design of CT scanner (Fig. 5). Indeed artifacts may be visually disturbing as well as analytically erroneous. Perhaps the most commonly encountered artifacts are the streaks. These can be caused by movement of the

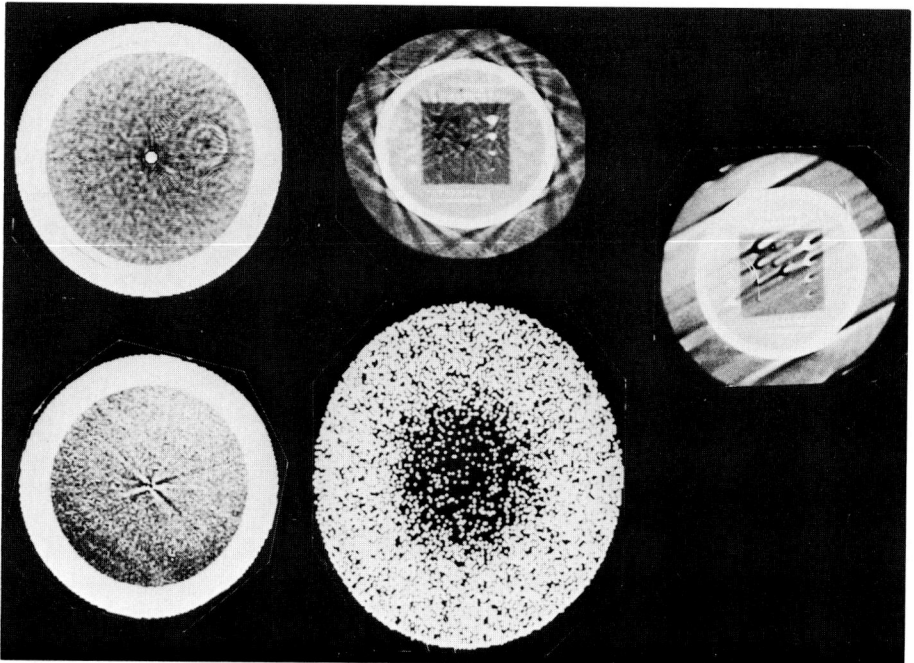

FIG. 5. Examples of CT artifacts include shaping, streaks, and circles.

patient, misalignment or faulty timing of the CT system, or overranging, i.e., the values lying outside the dynamic range of the detector system. One may also find radiating streaks coming from foreign or very dense substances; herring-bone artifacts which may arise from combinations of dense objects, algorithms, discs, or electronic problems; and concentric circle artifacts which have been seen in early third-generation scanners involving certain xenon gas detectors. Circular artifacts have often been claimed to result from detector or, perhaps more correctly, electronic imbalance in third-generation scanners, and may or may not be a significant problem in clinical practice. In addition, erroneous CT numbers can arise from shading due to incorrect treatment of x-ray polychromaticity consideration.

SPATIAL RESOLUTION

There are three basic sources of resolution degradation or unsharpness in screen/film radiography: (a) motion unsharpness—the blurring of a point due to the motion of the patient during the exposure time of the procedure; (b) receptor unsharpness—the inherent blurring operation caused by the transducing or conversion of x-rays into light within the intensifying screen; and (c) geometric unsharpness (focal spot unsharpness)—blurring due to the finite size and x-ray intensity distribution of the x-ray focal spot. Combinations of these sources generally lead to an overall blurring or defocusing effect.

This blurring or unsharpness may be characterized by its spatial extent, which is generally the blur size or "point spread function," or by the modulation transfer function (MTF), which describes how the spatial frequencies that make up an object are transferred by the image recording system (12,22,23).

The overall system point spread function might be considered a gaussian-shaped function. The approximation is convenient in that a rotationally symmetrical gaussian distribution may be fully described by a single parameter, i.e., its standard deviation (u_T), which is a measure of the width of the distribution and the extent of the blurring. A specification of u for each of the three blurring sources mentioned previously may be used to describe the relative blurring effect of each source of unsharpness: motion unsharpness (u_m), receptor unsharpness (u_r), and geometric unsharpness (u_g). In addition, by assuming that the individual blur functions are gaussian, the overall unsharpness or blurring function is given by the root mean square *(rms)* of the individual blur contributions.

$$u_T = \sqrt{u_m^2 + u_r^2 + u_g^2} \qquad (2)$$

These various blur sources combine into an overall general blur or degradation function for radiography, where M is the magnification and t the exposure time. A good estimate of the total overall blur width is given by $4u$, or 95% of the area under the gaussian distribution.

$$u_T = \left[\frac{u_r{}^2}{M^2} + u_m{}^2 t^2 + u_g{}^2\left(\frac{M-1}{M}\right)^2\right]^{1/2} \tag{3}$$

Although difficult to predict, a motion unsharpness value of $4u_m = 5$ mm/sec has been suggested. Certain advantages can be obtained from magnification studies, in that the focal spot, image receptor, and patient motion blur factors may be carefully selected so as to produce some reduced overall unsharpness. Scatter is generally considered independently of MTF and is deemed a contrast reducing factor. Moreover, magnification is often used with an air gap technique which reduces the scatter contribution without the need for grids. Of course it can be noted that the x-ray generator output and the focal spot size (both the nominal and the actual size) are important for determining the practical limits of magnification.

Although some of these same factors encountered in radiography enter into the overall consideration of resolution in CT, some of the factors (e.g., motion) are not as tractable and may manifest differently as artifacts, rather than blurring, depending on the sampling scheme and type of motion encountered. An indication of the spatial frequency transfer capability of a CT system can be obtained by taking a Fourier transform of the average data resulting from several CT scans of a thin wire object aligned with the vertical axis *(z)* of a centrally located volume element. The wire object then constitutes a point source input in the axial scan *(x,y)* plane of the CT system. Typical MTFs for CT scanners are shown in Fig. 6.

In this case, following Eq. 3, and removing u_m from consideration in the sense that it may be artifactual rather than simple blurring, one may consider u_r to be

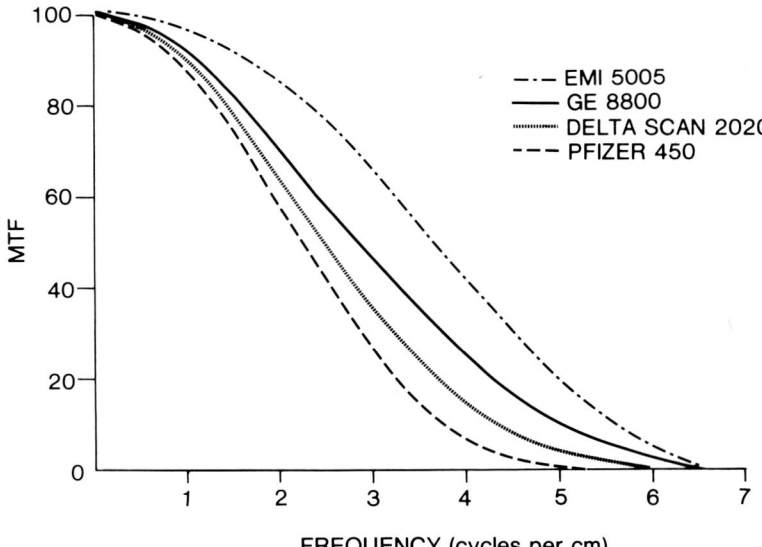

FIG. 6. MTFs for indicated CT systems.

related to the detector aperture width and u_g to be related to the focal spot width. In this case for conventional CT systems, M is the focal spot-to-detector distance divided by the focal spot-to-pivot distance, and is on the order of 1.4 to 2 for conventional systems and up to the order of 2.5 for CT systems offering geometric enlargement. Even first-order consideration of these blurring functions will rapidly reveal that CT systems are greatly challenged to achieve spatial resolution levels much beyond 1 cycle/mm, particularly if one requires a full body section (or head) scan to be obtained within a few seconds. The small focal spot size required for such resolution will be challenged to produce adequate x-ray intensity (and thus "contrast resolution" as dictated by low noise levels) within short scan times. Thus alternate x-ray sources such as an electron beam may need to be sought to produce adequate x-ray flux in short times, e.g., the 50 to 100 msec suggested for cardiac imaging.

Then, too, one must consider a very important aspect of CT resolution which is not usually encountered in conventional radiography, i.e., sampling rate and sampling pattern. Moreover, the sampling rate and sampling pattern are dependent on the type of geometry (generation) utilized in the CT scanner (13). First-, second-, and fourth-generation designs tend to offer a redundancy of spatial sampling because of the ability to interrogate (sample) the detector at an almost unlimited number of times (or spatial positions) for a given "view" or angular position of the scan. Of course a penalty may be paid by total scan time, but artifacts due to undersampling (aliasing) may be essentially removed (4). The third-generation designs, on the other hand, may be ultimately limited by the fact that the fixed source-detector configuration enables a redundancy of "views" (sampling at different angular positions) but a limited number of ray or spatial sampling for a *given* view. The question of the practical limitation of this technique transcends commercial exploitation and depends ultimately on the degree of spatial resolution required by the diagnostician and the limit to which he is able to tolerate aliasing (undersampling) artifacts.

In addition, there is a limit to how small a signal the CT systems will detect because of the volume averaging effect (the influence of slice width as well as the pixel) and the inferior spatial resolution of CT systems compared to that of radiography. Thus for small objects where the contrast (in particular the edge perception) is strongly influenced by MTF (i.e., related approximately to the integral of the square of the MTF), the contrast in CT and radiography is weighted by the

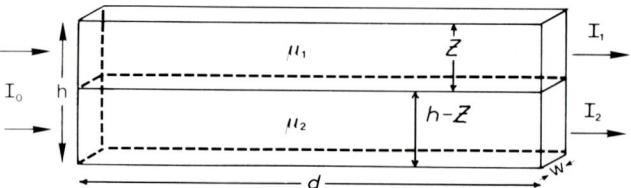

FIG. 7. Transmission of CT x-ray beam through an object stratified into two homogeneous layers, μ_1 and μ_2; *d* is the spatial extent of the stratified layers.

spatial resolution properties of the radiographic system compared to the spatial resolution properties of the CT system in a quadratic or square nature.

The problem of "volume averaging" in CT was recognized early in the scientific literature (14,15,25). It is surprising, however, that the fundamental limitations imposed by volume averaging to the accuracy of CT reconstruction by analytic (noniterative) techniques does not appear to have been documented.

It will be explained that the justification for simple volume averaging is misleading and often erroneous. The errors stem from what might be called an independent voxel model, as developed by Thomas et al. (24). These errors are not significant in the case of tissue averaging considered by Thomas, but are significant in the case of air or bone averaging.

The nature of the problem may be understood by examining Fig. 7, which shows an idealized case of a radially symmetrical CT slice partitioned into two homogeneous layers characterized by linear x-ray attenuation, μ_1 and μ_2, respectively. It should be noted that the situation depicted in Fig. 7 is for a stratified rather than a random mixture.

The transmission source is assumed to be monoenergetic and to have an effectively uniform beam profile in the z-direction. It is straightforward to predict the effective CT attenuation coefficient that would be assigned by routine logarithmic transformation of relative x-ray intensity values. Each of the partitioned regions will attenuate x-rays according to its respective μ value. The intensity of the unattenuated beam is denoted by I_0, and the attenuated intensity as I_1 and I_2 at the exit of the respective regions. The slice width is denoted by h; the fraction of μ_2 is z/h; the fraction of μ_1 is $1 - z/h$.

$$D = I_1 \cdot z \cdot w + I_2 \cdot (h - z) \cdot w \rightarrow \tag{4}$$

$$D_0 = I_0 \cdot w \cdot h \rightarrow \tag{5}$$

where

$$I_1 = I_0 e^{-\mu_1 d} \rightarrow \tag{6}$$

and

$$I_2 = I_0 e^{-\mu_2 d} \rightarrow \tag{7}$$

then

$$\mu_{\text{eff}} = -(1/d) \log_e \left[(D)/(D_0) \right] \rightarrow \tag{8}$$

$$= -(1/d) \log_e \left[I_1 z + I_2 (h - z) \right]/(I_0 \cdot h) \rightarrow$$

$$= -(1/d) \log_e \left[e^{-\mu_1 d} \cdot z + e^{-\mu_2 d} \cdot (h - z) \right]/h \rightarrow \tag{9}$$

$$= \mu_2 - (1/d) \log_e \left[1 + (z/h) (e^{(\mu_2 - \mu_2)d} - 1) \right] \rightarrow \tag{10}$$

The limiting values of the above equation yield the expected values in that for:

Case 1

$$z = 0, \ \mu_{\text{eff}} = \mu_2 \tag{11}$$

Case 2

$$z = h, \ \mu_{\text{eff}} = \mu_1 \tag{12}$$

Case 3

$$(\mu_2 - \mu_1)d \to 0 \quad \mu_{\text{eff}} \to \mu_1 \frac{z}{h} + \mu_2 \left(1 - \frac{z}{h}\right) \tag{13}$$

Case 3 corresponds to the often assumed (first-order) equation for simple volume averaging. This linear equation is true only when the product of the difference in μ values and the spatial extent (d) of the differing regions is small. The exact solution indicates a nonlinear dependence not only on $(\mu_2 - \mu_1)$ but also on the spatial extent of the mixing (d). Note that if the equations are restricted to a single independent voxel, as in the Thomas et al. article (24), then the maximum value permissible for d is dictated by the voxel dimensions—the pixel width and slice width. In the particularly restrictive case of the Thomas model, where the averaging is developed in a sagittal or coronal fashion, d will be no greater than the pixel width (a millimeter or so). Thus the product of $(\mu_2 - \mu_1)d$ will be artificially restricted by the dimensions of the voxel model. When the theory is developed to the actual spatial extent (perhaps many pixel lengths) of mixing, the product $(\mu_2 - \mu_1)d$ can no longer be assumed negligible, and case 3 does not hold. We now proceed to show how serious errors may occur from the simple volume averaging model.

Equation 10 is of more than simple mathematical interest in that it points out a seemingly fundamental limitation to analytic (noniterative) back-projection reconstruction techniques. A single integrated detector reading cannot yield the correct composition of a volumetrically mixed region without first knowing the spatial extent (d) of the mixed volumetric region. Moreover, the "exact" solution is exact only for the prescribed two-compartment stratified model, for a monoenergetic beam, and for a uniform x-ray beam intensity. Appropriate modification to this model for beam profile and spectral composition is not fundamentally difficult, but will not be included in this analysis. Figure 8 shows the use of the solution in Eq. 10 to predict the effective μ_{eff} values for stratified mixing of dense bone ($\mu_1 = 0.4$ cm^{-1}) and tissue ($\mu_2 = 0.2 \ \text{cm}^{-1}$) as a function of the spatial extent (d) of the volume averaging. Similar changes in magnitude for μ_{eff} as a function of spatial extent would be expected for mixing tissue ($\mu_1 = 0.2 \ \text{cm}^{-1}$) and air ($\mu_2 = 0$ cm^{-1}). Large deviations from the simple volume averaging model (the ordinate values) can be seen with increasing d.

Equation 10 and Fig. 8 predict that small, thin discs with a thickness less than that of the slice should have CT numbers dependent on their diameter. This pre-

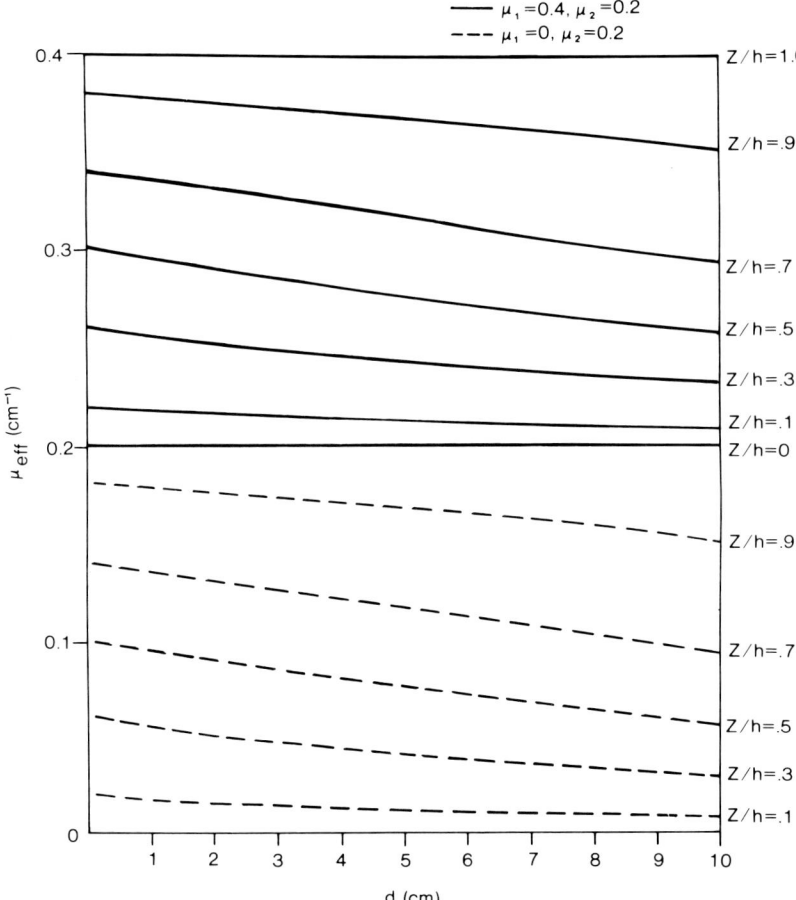

FIG. 8. Predicted change in CT values as a function of spatial extent *(d)*, and the relative fraction *(z/h)* of stratified layers of tissue (μ_2 = 0.2 cm^{-1}) and bone (μ_1 = 0.4 cm^{-1}); and tissue (μ_2 = 0.2 cm^{-1}); and air (μ_1 = 0 cm^{-1}). Note the deviation from the simple volume averaging model (the ordinate values) as a function of increasing *d*.

diction was tested by cutting thin aluminum discs of various diameters from a single sheet of aluminum and scanning them on an EMI 5005 CT scanner. The discs were placed in a water bath in the center of the scan volume (*x*, *y*, and *z*). For the case of thin, small discs in a water bath, it can be shown that differences in CT value of the discs due to differences in beam hardening effects should be minimal because of the small changes in spectral quality and the small changes in net detector signal. Moreover, it can be shown that for discs centered in the middle of the slice thickness, a nonuniform gaussian-type slice profile will yield equivalent changes in μ_{eff} as a uniform beam of slice thickness about equal to the full width half maximum (FWHM) of the gaussian distribution. The excellent agreement of theory and experiment is shown in Fig. 9. The magnitude of the predicted and empirical change in CT

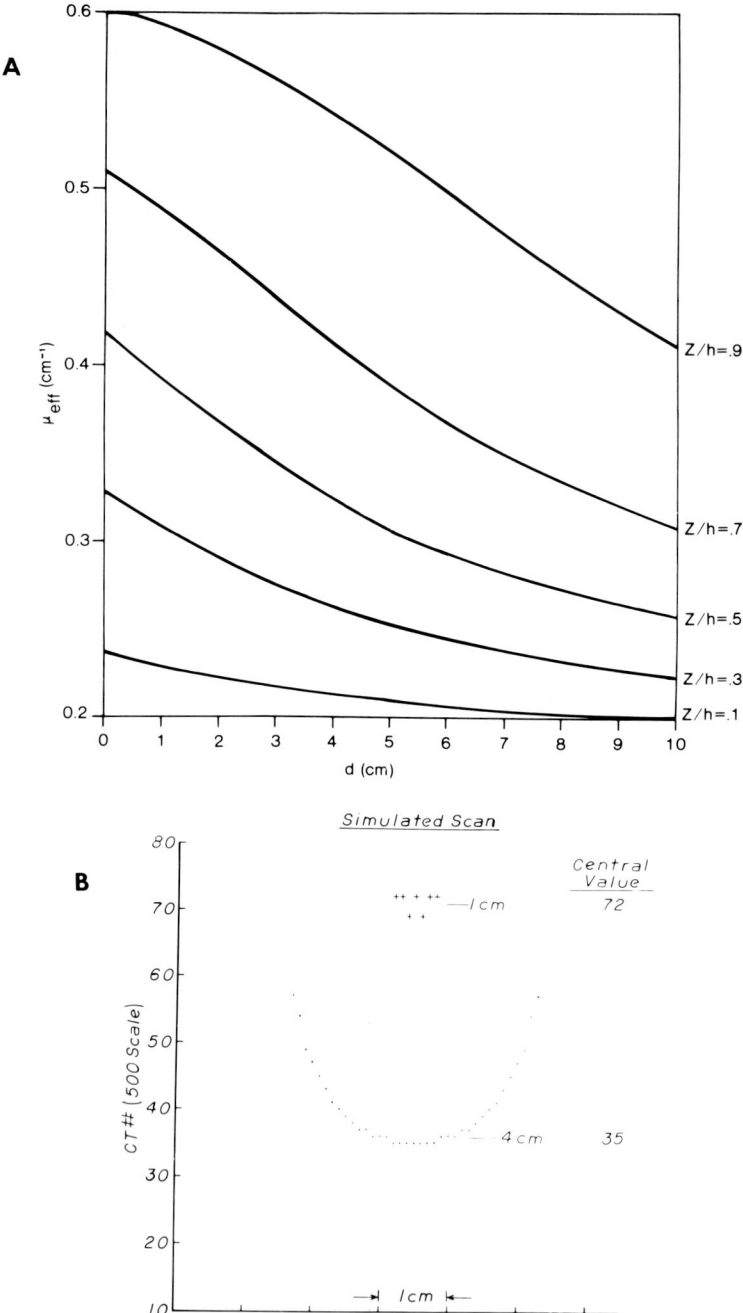

FIG. 9. **A:** Predicted change in CT value of aluminum discs ($\mu' = 0.62$ cm^{-1}) as a function of disc diameter *(d)* and relative fraction *(z/h)* of aluminum to water ($\mu = 0.19$ cm^{-1}). **B:** Output of simulated reconstruction of 1.0 mm thick aluminum discs in a 13-mm slice utilizing filtered back-projection of intensity values derived from Eq. 7. The experimental CT values from scanning 1.3-mm discs with an EMI 5005 scanner with an FWHM of 13 mm and scanning at 120 kVp for the 1-cm disc was 72 ± 2, and the experimental CT value for the 4-cm disc was 33 ± 2.

number as a function of radius is much larger than statistical limitations of a few CT numbers. Note that simply by changing the diameter of the thin aluminum disc from 4 cm to 1 cm, the theoretical predictions and experimental results show that the central CT number has more than doubled. The simple volume averaging model would have predicted no significant change in CT number with disc diameter.

Then too, one can note the interesting cupping of CT values in the larger disc. This theoretically predicted phenomenon is found experimentally and results from the variable path lengths of the aluminum presented to the beam as it crosses the disc, ranging from the disc diameter in the center of the disc to zero at the outside edge of the disc. The phenomenon should not be confused with spatial resolution degradation, which usually results in a more capping-like phenomenon.

Similarly, Eq. 10 predicts that thin (subslice thickness), volumetrically stratified objects which do not have a constant path length in all possible sampling directions should result in inconsistent effective attenuation values. Such predictions may be tested rather simply by cutting several pieces of aluminum with the same net area but different shape. Figure 10 shows the increasing differences in μ_{eff} as one moves from circular symmetry toward a one-dimensional (asymmetrical) area. Again, in contrast to the predictions of the simple volume averaging model, one encounters dramatic differences in CT number resulting from the spatial distribution of the volume averaged object. Then too, such a phenomenon would tend to produce artifacts and is probably related to streaks seen in cranial transverse CT reconstructions at the level of the petrous bones (11).

The final important observation to be made from Eq. 10 is that CT "sensitivity" profiles based on the use of an aluminum ramp are subject to large theoretical errors, particularly as the width (spatial extent) of the ramp becomes large (8). This error can be traced to the variable spatial extent of the averaged layers of aluminum and surrounding material that the ramp presents to the detectors, according to the orientation of the aluminum ramp and the sampling geometry under consideration.

In conclusion, we have shown theoretically and experimentally that the simple volume averaging model leads to significant errors in the CT attenuation values for

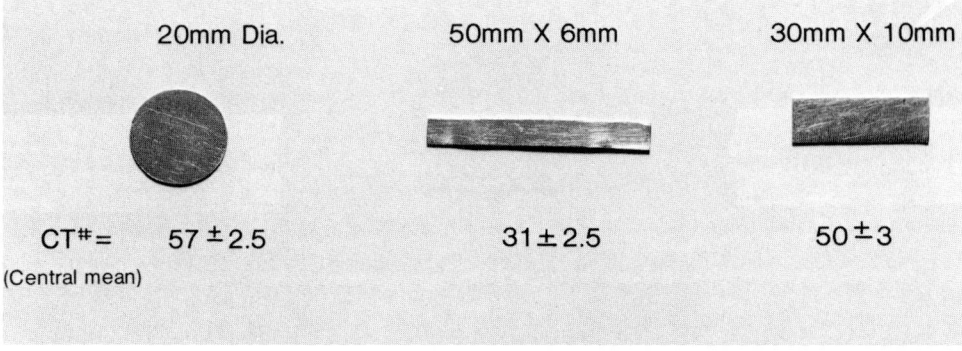

20mm Dia.	50mm X 6mm	30mm X 10mm

CT# =   57 ± 2.5   31 ± 2.5   50 ± 3
(Central mean)

FIG. 10. CT values resulting from scanning 0.5 mm thick aluminum discs of differing shapes but equivalent areas on an EMI 5005 scanner.

averaging (mixing) high- or low-density materials (e.g., bone or air) with tissue. Radiation therapy treatment planning should consider this problem.

NOISE IN CT SYSTEMS

An equation often used to describe the relative standard deviation of the x-ray attenuation values per unit pixel element $\sigma(\mu)/\mu$ in a CT scan with pixel element dimension *(w)*, slice thickness *(h)*, and the patient dose *(D)*, is given by (7):

$$\sigma(\mu)/\mu \propto 1/(D^{1/2} w^{3/2} h^{1/2}) \tag{14}$$

This relationship, however, is simplistic in that it ignores the important question of the character of the noise that results from the combination of photon statistics *and the choice of a filter function.* A rigorous treatment of the noise in a CT scan is similar to that of radiography in that it requires consideration of the autocovariance properties of the noise (or the corresponding noise power spectrum).

Somewhat similar to the phenomenon of quantum mottle, the filter function has a significant effect on the *amplitude and character* of the noise component in CT scanning.

Assume that small changes in light intensity *(T)* reaching the eye from a region of the CT image are approximately linearly related to small changes in the CT values, and therefore to changes in the linear attenuation coefficient. Consider the case where signal area *(a)* is relatively "large" compared to the pixel area *(w²)*. The smoothing factor for CT can be provided an elegant and useful solution for the case of exponential and gaussian filter functions (9). Figure 11 demonstrates how the "large area" noise behaves in a Poisson manner. That is to say, the "large area" relative noise decreases inversely with the square root of the sampled area scaled back to a single pixel noise level about twice its actual value. The expected standard deviation of μ values in area *a*, $\sigma(\mu,a)$, can then be predicted as

$$\sigma(\mu,a)/\mu = 2 K_2/(Dwh\ a)^{1/2} \tag{15}$$

where K_2 is a constant, and the FWHM of the point spread function is assumed to about twice the pixel width (14).

If one considers experimental noise levels in CT scanners, then for D = dose in rads, w = matrix dimension width in centimeters, and a = signal area in square centimeters, than one can estimate K_2 on the basis of early head scanners as approximately 5×10^{-4} cm², and several times that magnitude for body scanners due to increased attenuation.

Let the signal-to-noise ratio *(d')* be defined as the ratio of signal contrast to noise amplitude; then for CT head scans, where $(\mu_S - \mu_B)$ is the differential attenuation contrast between the signal and background

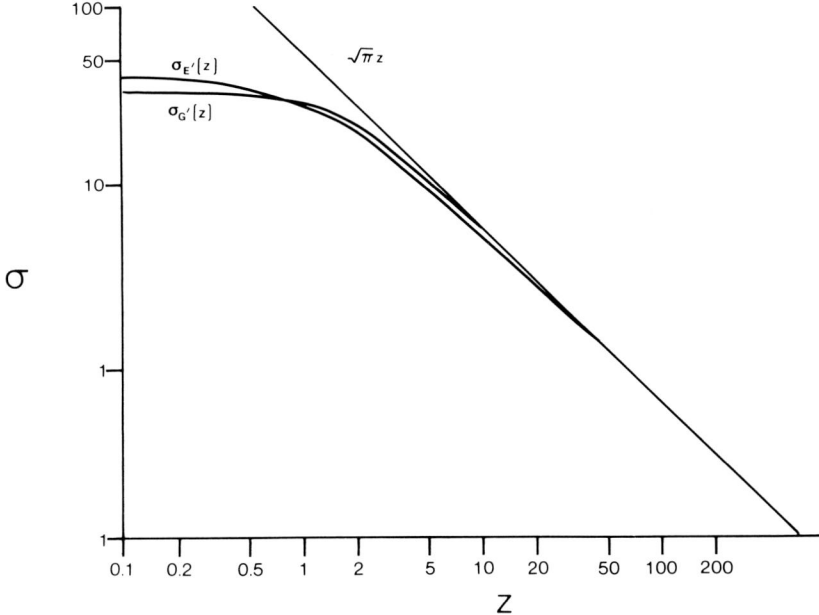

FIG. 11. Relative noise amplitude (σ) as a function of z for two reconstruction filters. E' is an exponential filter; G' is a gaussian filter. z corresponds to the diameter of the circular scanning (viewing) aperture divided by the FWHM of the appropriate filter. For large areas the relative noise amplitude follows a reciprocal square root dependence on area scaled back to a single pixel amplitude of approximately twice its actual value.

$$d'_{CT} \doteq (10^4/2) \, (\mu_S - \mu_B) \, a^{1/2} \, (whD)^{1/2} \tag{16}$$

whereas d' for body scans is reduced according to the additional x-ray attenuation involved.

One can note from inspection of Eqs. 14–16 that the often quoted cubic requirement of increased spatial resolution *(w)* on increased dose *(D)* is true only for the case of requiring a constant noise amplitude *per unit pixel*. If one requires only a constant noise *per unit area* (as, for example, when the pixel size becomes small compared to the integration area of the eye or search aperture), then one requires a much less restrictive linear demand of spatial resolution on dose.

ALTERNATE MODALITIES

If we consider the comparison of the signal/noise ratios for CT versus radiography, we find some interesting relationships. For radiography, we must consider the important image parameters: G = gradient of the radiograph screen-film combinations, d = the diameter of the signal, $\bar{n}_x$ = photon flux, and the differential attenuation between the signal and background = $(\mu_S - \mu_B)$. If the same x-ray spectrum is assumed, then one arrives at a fairly interesting relationship between the signal/noise ratio of CT compared to that of radiography.

Conventional radiography is beset by two major problems: limited dynamic range and contrast-degrading scattered radiation. If one assumes a large-scatter clean-up and a photon information level in radiography of approximately 10^7 photons per square centimeter, then it can be shown that the advantage of CT increases as the diameter of the signal gets *smaller*. Thus at a few centimeters signals might be detected equally; when signals get down to the order of 1 cm or so, the signal/noise ratio of CT might be appreciably better than radiography. However, it should be noted that there is a real limit to how small a signal one might presently hope to find with CT systems because of the volume averaging effect (the slice width as well as the pixel) and the realization that spatial resolution of CT systems is still much inferior to radiography. In addition, as mentioned earlier, improvements in spatial resolution place strong demands on dose (e.g., to have the same pixel noise level in a pixel of one-half size, one might need an eightfold increase in dose). In light of the present dose levels of CT scanners ($\sim$1 to 20 rads), there is obviously some need to pay attention to changes in the upper end of this scale. Thus for small objects where the contrast (in particular the edge perception) is strongly influenced by the spatial resolution of MTF (i.e., related approximately to the integral of the MTF squared), the contrast in CT and radiography is weighed by the spatial resolution properties of the image system in a quadratic or square nature. One should also keep in mind the important questions and differences presented by the two modalities in terms of pattern recognition and anatomic noise, as well as other known parameters of image quality.

DEVELOPMENTS IN OTHER MODALITIES

Success is being reported in terms of reconstruction of the distribution of radioactive emission sources. In particular, commercial instruments have been produced for reconstruction "single" photon emission sources (following the pioneering work of Kuhl et al.) as well as reconstruction of positron coincidence photons. Such developments are important in medicine because of the opportunity to study "quantitatively" physiological processes *in vivo*. Challenges in this modality remain when working with relatively low photon fluence levels (e.g., 1 mCi = 3.7×10^7 dps) and limiting geometric detecting systems. Scan times are thus usually of many minutes' duration. Problems with detecting and quantifying small tumors at depth by conventional single-view LFOV cameras are well established (2).

Other modalities in various stages of development and investigation in terms of reconstruction potential include ultrasound, heavy particle beams, and nuclear magnetic resonance (NMR). Each of these modalities holds its own diagnostic promises and challenges to CT technology.

FUTURE DEVELOPMENTS IN CT

CT scanners have evolved from the earliest scanners operating at scan times of several minutes with iterative reconstructions of several minutes and reconstruction matrices of 80 × 80 (i.e., 3 × 3 mm pixels). The current scanners operate at scan times of only a few seconds with virtually instantaneous (hard-wired or large-array processors) reconstructions and pixel sizes corresponding to 512 × 512 or 1,024 × 1,024 matrices. Additional advances in scan time and/or spatial resolution levels become more and more demanding on "state-of-the-art" electronic circuitry, x-ray tube technology, and mechanical engineering.

It is of interest to consider some possible areas of research and/or optimization of current x-ray CT scanners. One important area of development is the possibility of heart scanning. In terms of the temporal constraints of the beating heart, and the need for adequate spatial and density discrimination levels, it is clear that one needs to develop either high-dose (photon fluence) rates to be delivered in about 50 msec by single or multiple sources, or perhaps adequate "gating" of the cardiac and respiratory cycles with the data acquisition scheme. One very promising development in this area is the work being performed at the Mayo Clinic using multiple ($N = 28$) x-ray sources and image intensifiers to achieve "dynamic" reconstructions of the heart (21).

Another area of current attention is the possible development of the quantitative aspects of CT. The term "tomochemistry" has been used to describe the general attempt to unfold the energy-dependent contributions of the compton and photoelectric contributions of the CT number. In addition, there remain possibilities for filtering the polychromatic x-ray spectrum and/or utilizing monoenergetic sources and photon-counting devices for CT reconstructions aimed at unfolding electron density and atomic number contributions.

CONCLUSIONS

The CT system is not rigorously a linear system in that in certain circumstances the output may be nonlinear or systematically or randomly in error. The nonlinearities can arise from volume averaging errors, beam hardening errors, artifact propagation, and stochastic or systemic sources of noise.

Treatment planning systems should be aware of these sources of deviation from nominal x-ray attenuation (electron density) values. In addition, positioning errors and resolution levels further limit the accuracy to which a given dose may be delivered to a targeted site.

It appears that CT treatment planning systems need to establish the efficacy of the use of present diagnostic scanners as opposed to dedicated CT treatment planning scanners (e.g., replacement or adjunctive to present simulators). Major questions that arise are: reproducibility and accuracy of localization schemes, both intra- and interdiagnostic and therapeutic systems; intrinsic CT information matrix versus treatment planning matrix (e.g., is it efficacious to use a 512 × 512 CT matrix with a 64 × 64 dose treatment matrix?); differences in therapeutic use may allow (or require) cost engineering in terms of relaxed reconstruction times and normal through-put variables; the degree to which nonlinearities (e.g., energy dependencies and volume averaging) might be better approached from therapy-based beam widths and energies, as well as a lessened constraint on patient dose.

SUMMARY

The basic tenets of CT are examined in light of the linear systems theory. The CT system is considered as a reconstruction device attempting to correct for known back-projection degradation through the use of the reconstruction point spread function and corresponding Fourier filter. Deviations from linear systems assumptions were discussed, including position-dependent effects in *xyz* space, as well as artifacts and polychromatic effects which challenge assumptions of linearity and isoplanacity. Current and anticipated levels of spatial resolution, slice thickness (volume averaging), noise (density resolution), polychromatic effects, and data acquisition time (motion artifacts) were reviewed. An effort was made to place CT in perspective with other image modalities such as radiography and nuclear medicine, particularly in terms of the signal-to-noise ratio. Future possibilities for improvements in CT systems were briefly discussed.

REFERENCES

1. Ambrose, J. (1973): Computerized transverse axial scanning (tomography). II. Clinical application. *Br. J. Radiol.*, 46:1023–1047.
2. Atkins, F. B., and Goodenough, D. J. (1981): Simulated uptake ratio requirements for spherical lesions imaged with a conventional scintillation camera. In: *Receptor-Binding Radiotracers*, edited by W. C. Eckelman. CRC Press, Boca Raton, FL *(in press)*.
3. Baker, H. I., Hauser, O. W., McCullough, E. C., and Reese, D. H. (1974): An evaluation of the quantitative and radiation features of a scanning x-ray transverse axial tomograph: the EMI scanner. *Radiology*, 111:709.
4. Barnes, G. T., and Yester, M. V. (1977): Geometrical limitations of computed tomography (CT) scanner resolution. *SPIE Optical Instrumentation in Medicine VI*, 127:296–303.
5. Bracewell, R. N. (1956): Strip integration in radioastronomy. *Aust. J. Phys.*, 9:198–217.
6. Brooks, R. A., and DiChiro, G. (1975): Theory of image reconstruction in computed tomography. *Radiology*, 117:561–572.
7. Brooks, R. A., and DiChiro, G. (1976): Principles of computer assisted tomography (CAT) in radiographic and radioisotopic imaging. *Phys. Med. Biol.*, 21:689–732.
8. Brooks, R. A., and DiChiro, G. (1977): Slice geometry in computer assisted tomography. *J. Comput. Assist. Tomogr.*, 1:191–199.
9. Doi, K. (1969): Investigation of radiological image. In: *Proceedings, Radiologic Image Information*, Vol. 2, pp. 264–270.
10. Fewell, T. R., and Weaver, K. E. (1976): The measurement of diagnostic x-ray spectra with a high purity germination spectrometer. In: *Proceedings of 1974 BRH/SPIE Symposium—Medical X-ray Photo-Optical Systems Evaluation*. Published by SPIE, Vol. 56.
11. Glover, G. H., and Pelc, N. J. (1979): The nonlinear partial volume artifact. *J. Comput. Assist. Tomogr.*, 3:573–574 (abstract).
12. Goodenough, D. J. (1976): Assessment of image quality of diagnostic imaging systems. In: *Medical Images: Formation, Perception and Measurements*, edited by F. A. Gray, pp. 263–277. Wiley, New York.
13. Goodenough, D. J., and Weaver, K. E. (1979): Overview of computed tomography. *IEEE Trans. Nucl. Sci.*, NS-26, No. 1.
14. Goodenough, D. J., Weaver, K. E., and Davis, D. O. (1975): Potential artifacts associated with the scanning pattern of the EMI scanner. *Radiology*, 117:615–619.
15. Goodenough, D. J., Weaver, K. E., and Davis, D. O. (1977): Physical measurements of the EMI imaging system. In: *Reconstruction Tomography in Diagnostic Radiology and Nuclear Medicine*, edited by M. M. Ter-Pogossian et al., pp. 245–266. University Park Press, Baltimore.
16. Gordon, R., Herman, G. T., and Johnson, S. A. (1975): Image reconstruction from projections. *Sci. Am.*, October:56–58.
17. Hoffman, E. J., Phelps, M. E., and Ter-Pogossian, M. M. (1975): Attenuation coefficients of various body tissues, fluids and lesions at photon energies of 18 to 136. *Radiology*, 115:43–46.

18. Hounsfield, G. N. (1973): Computerized transverse axial scanning (tomography). I. Description of system. *Br. J. Radiol.*, 46:1016–1022.
18a. Kuhl, D. E., and Edwards, R. Q. (1963): Image separation radioisotope scanning. *Radiology*, 80:653–661.
19. Oldendorf, W. H. (1961): Isolated flying spot detection of radiodensity discontinuities displaying the internal structural pattern of a complex object. *IRE Trans. Biomed. Elect. BME*, 8:68–72.
20. Radon, J. (1917): On the determination of functions from their integrals along certain manifolds. *Ber. Saech. Akad. Wiss. Leipzig Math. Phys. Kl*, 60:262–277.
21. Robb, R. A., Greenleaf, J. F., Ritman, E. L., Johnson, S. A., Sjostrand, J. D., Herman, G. T., and Wood, E. H. (1974): Three dimensional visualization of the intact thorax and contents: a technique for cross sectional reconstruction from multi-planar x-ray views. *Comput. Biomed. Res.*, 7:395–419.
22. Rossmann, K. (1963): Spatial fluctuations of x-ray quanta and recording of radiographic mottle. *Am. J. Roentgenol.*, 90:864.
23. Rossmann, K. (1969): Point spread function, line spread function and modulation transfer function: tools for the study of imaging systems. *Radiology*, 93:257–272.
24. Thomas, S. R., McLennan, J. E., Kereiakes, J. G., Neff, R., Chambers, A. A., and Lukin, R. R. (1979): Intracranial blood clot volume and geometric parameters determined from CT images. *Radiology*, 133:741–746.
25. Zatz, L. M. (1977): The EMI scanner: collimator design, polychromatic artifacts and selective material imaging. In: *Reconstruction Tomography in Diagnostic Radiology and Nuclear Medicine*, edited by M. M. Ter-Pogossian et al., pp. 245–266. University Park Press, Baltimore.

Computed Tomography in Radiation Therapy,
edited by C. C. Ling, C. C. Rogers, and
R. J. Morton. Raven Press, New York © 1983

Specifying a CT Scanner for Use in Radiation Therapy Planning

Edwin C. McCullough

*Division of Radiation Therapy, Department of Oncology, Mayo Clinic/Foundation,
Rochester, Minnesota 55901*

Even though it is possible (and probable) that a therapy department will use a computed tomographic (CT) scanner that was designed principally for diagnosis, there is a need to state those features of a CT scanner that facilitate its use in radiation therapy treatment planning (the specifics of which are documented elsewhere in this volume). The works of Goitein (1) and Stewart et al. (2) are particularly relevant to the topic at hand.

Desirable features of a CT scanner to be employed in radiation therapy planning can be conveniently grouped into the following six categories: mechanical features, scan parameters, x-ray system, manipulative capabilities, quantitative behavior, and data transfer. Considerations such as maintainability, parts availability, cost, space requirements, compatibility with other equipment, and expected longevity of the vender are common to CT scanners for diagnosis and are not considered here.

MECHANICAL FEATURES

CT scans used for treatment planning usually require the scans to be done with a flat table top (easily accomplished by using a piece of plywood cut to fit the usual dish-shaped couches). This usually causes the patient to be offset slightly in the CT scanner gantry aperture, but, more importantly, a larger aperture is usually required. It has been suggested (1) that a scanner gantry aperture of at least 60 cm in diameter be provided.

In addition to the use of a flat table insert, one does not wish to distort the other contours of the patient, so the use of bolus bags is to be discouraged. As it is sometimes necessary to plan treatments in planes that are not perpendicular to the long axis of the patient (e.g., the pituitary), it is convenient to have angulation of the gantry and/or an angulating head holder available.

It is generally desirable that the quality of the CT scans used in therapy planning be comparable to that accepted for diagnostic scanning, so that scan times on the order of breath holding times are important. Until the argument of whether there is a significant difference in scans done at 3 sec versus 10 sec is resolved, it appears that most of the scanners currently available provide satisfactory scan times.

A perennial problem when utilizing CT scans in radiation therapy is having some correlation of scan plane location on a "plain film" view, as therapy planning is done integrating both transverse and plane film images (until the time that true three-dimensional imaging and planning is available). The recent availability of digital radiographic capabilities on most current scanners has alleviated this problem, even though we have found it difficult to convince our diagnostic colleagues to do this on every patient with suspected cancer.

SCAN PARAMETERS

"Scan parameters" include such considerations as: (a) spatial resolution; (b) contrast resolution; (c) scan slice thickness; (d) reconstruction diameter; and (e) sequential scan rate. High-contrast spatial resolutions of 1 to 2 mm are routinely achieved on all current scanners, and I have yet to hear convincing arguments that better spatial resolutions are needed. In fact, there are some alternate systems utilizing simulators that will probably achieve 2- to 5-mm resolutions at best. In this discussion of needed spatial resolutions, one must keep in mind at least three very relevant points: (a) most therapy beams do not have well-defined edges; (b) we cannot expect CT to show microscopic extension, and we will be obliged to use margins of 1 cm or more; and (c) computed treatment plans are usually done on a coarse grid with a generous amount of interpolation.

Low-contrast resolution requirements for a CT scanner used for therapy localization have yet to be defined. The principal argument for doing the best you can is that one may wish to delineate tumor/soft tissue boundaries in situations where very little attenuation coefficient difference is present. Whether this argument is particularly valid remains to be proved. Slice thicknesses on the order of 5 mm (or smaller) are probably needed to obtain reasonable axial resolution, a point that is particularly relevant to a later discussion on reformatting.

Maximum reconstruction diameters in the range of 45 to 50 cm should be available so the outer contours of "queen- and king-sized" patients are included when on a flat table top. Larger scan diameters, of necessity, decrease spatial resolution for a fixed pixel number. Scanners with options for 256 or 512 pixel diameter reconstructions may offer some advantages as far as achieving better spatial resolutions for larger scan diameters, but at the expense of low-contrast response.

In a situation where one is going to do a true volumetric reconstruction and/or treatment plan, it may be necessary to do thirty to forty 5 mm thick slices to cover the entire vertical extent of the field. For this situation, it is highly desirable to do the scanning as rapidly as possible (e.g., in less than 15 min). To facilitate this, the CT scanner should be able to defer processing. Also, accurate table indexing (± 1 mm) is a feature of interest. With these capabilities the ultimate limitation on scan sequence rate becomes tube loading considerations.

X-RAY SYSTEM

The oil-cooled, fixed-anode x-ray tubes used on the rotate-translate CT scanners were able to operate continuously, albeit at a dose rate that made them less than attractive for sub-10-sec scanning. The newer rotary motion CT scanners utilize rotating anode tubes that provide high instantaneous dose rates but suffer from cooling rate limitations. A CT scanner for radiation therapy should have as high an anode cooling rate as possible and/or the ability to lower the milliamperage so that higher throughput is achieved.

MANIPULATIVE CAPABILITIES

The availability of a series of contiguous transverse CT scans leads naturally to the idea of reformatting in order to produce sagittal, coronal, and/or oblique views. Indeed, most of the currently available CT scanners routinely provide these capabilities. In fact, one can usually reconstruct these reformatted images with varying pixel thicknesses, and if one uses all the pixels across the transverse plane one can simulate a plain film. In fact, with a little imagination (and some software development by the CT scanner manufacturers), one can envision the reformation of any therapy portal, providing adequate CT scan information has been obtained. Whether this would be cost-effective in view of the availability of simulators and their high-quality films is a topic for discussion.

QUANTITATIVE BEHAVIOR

There appears to be reasonable interest in utilizing the CT numbers from a CT scan (following appropriate conversions) to permit corrections of dose distributions to be done on a patient-by-patient basis. This use puts some requirements on the accuracy of numbers obtained *in vivo*, and the potential user of such information must establish the inaccuracies expected in patient scan geometries. The potential errors are not insignificant.

Artifact behavior is another factor that may compromise use of CT numbers. In particular, scans of the head and neck areas are obviously compromised by unaccounted for beam hardening effects. A CT scanner whose data are to be used for dose corrections should have some ability to correct for polychromatic effects and remove streaks caused by metallic clips. These software packages are available from most CT scanner manufacturers, but they usually take a fair amount of time to execute and, in the world of diagnosis where time is money, their use has been discouraged.

DATA TRANSFER

CT scan images are available to the therapy planning team in at least three forms: (a) magnetic storage on a floppy disc (usually 8 or 16 images per disc); (b) magnetic storage on a computer tape (the Philips scanner at one time was using standard compact cassettes); and (c) hard copy. Unfortunately, the use of magnetic media transfer (which is mandatory for use of the actual CT numbers) is thwarted by the incompatibility of storage formats and readers from one manufacturer to another and even between scanner models from the same manufacturer. Fortunately, many of the vendors of "turn-key" treatment planning systems can read magnetic media stored CT scans from a variety of CT scanners.

If one utilizes "hard copy" CT scans in treatment planning, there is a need to have distance indications available. It is also helpful to have a grid pattern to allow for a rough assessment of monitor/camera-introduced distortions. Only a few CT scanners provide a distance-marked horizontal and vertical grid display. Unfortunately, it is even more difficult to get our diagnostic colleagues to provide this along with all scans (and a digital radiograph) of any patient suspected of having a cancer.

SUMMARY

Even though one may never need to have a CT scanner built just for use in radiation therapy planning, there are certain unique requirements that must be kept in mind when considering this application of CT scanning. Many of the more obvious ones have been detailed above, and as the field matures we can expect to see further definition and expansion of the requirements.

REFERENCES

1. Goitein, M. (1979): Computed tomography in planning radiation therapy. *Int. J. Radiat. Oncol. Biol. Phys.*, 5:445–447.
2. Stewart, J. R., Hicks, J. A., Boone, M. L. M., and Simpson, L. D. (1978): Computed tomography in radiation therapy. *Int. J. Radiat. Oncol. Phys. Biol.*, 4:313–324.

Computed Tomography in Radiation Therapy,
edited by C. C. Ling, C. C. Rogers, and
R. J. Morton. Raven Press, New York © 1983

Patient Position During CT Scanning

Michael Goitein

*Division of Radiation Biophysics, Department of Radiation Medicine, Massachusetts
General Hospital, Boston, Massachusetts 02114, and Harvard Medical School*

Stable and reproducible positioning of the patient—at the time of treatment simulation, from simulation to first treatment, and from one treatment session to another—is a long-standing problem in radiation therapy. Over the years a variety of solutions have evolved, so that with sufficient care and attention to detail quite satisfactory patient positioning is usually possible. To a large extent, the computed tomographic (CT) scanner can fit quite readily into the existing techniques so that the problem reduces to adapting existing methods to the new technology. However, the CT scanner does introduce a number of new aspects into the problem. Among these are:

1. The fact that the CT scanner is often located in a distant department, controlled by radiologists rather than radiation therapists, and staffed by technologists unfamiliar with the special problems of radiation therapy.

2. Patients are often scanned before their diagnosis is established, certainly before radiation therapy is decided on for at least a portion of their therapy, and without consultation with a radiation therapist.

3. Inadequate time may be allocated to the generally time-consuming tasks unique to radiation therapy patient setup.

4. Interference with the CT gantry tunnel may make it impossible to scan the patient in the position which would be best for treatment.

5. All support devices must be reasonably radiolucent, and skin marks and, ideally, surgical clips should be "radio-gray."

6. Alignment lights can generally not be situated in the scan plane.

7. The scanner couch readout may be inaccurate.

8. An insufficient number of scans may be taken, and the documentation of the couch position and other conditions may be inadequate.

9. There are also several other problems: the phase of the respiratory cycle during which CT scans are performed, the use of contrast agents, the use of bolus material,

---

This chapter is based in part on Section 7 of "Applications of computed tomography in radiotherapy treatment planning" in *Progress in Medical Radiation Physics*, Vol. 1, edited by C. Orton, pp. 195–293. Plenum Press, New York, 1982.

the accuracy of CT numbers, and the occasional diagnostically derived need for scanning under conditions other than those of therapy.

None of these pose difficult technical problems. To identify any one is to suggest its solution. However, the implementation and conduct of a comprehensive "system" which can assure adequate control over patient positioning is not easy. It depends on meticulous attention to, and control of, a large number of small details. If there is any single "simple solution" to this task, it is to ensure the interest and appropriate training of the CT technician and the understanding and cooperation of the diagnostic radiologist. Without the active cooperation of the CT staff, it is impossible to realize the full benefits of CT scanning. It would be highly desirable that either: (a) the technicians have a background as radiation therapy technicians; (b) a radiation therapy technician assist in studies of patients who are likely to receive radiation therapy; or (c) at least the CT technician be exposed in a serious way to the techniques used for patient alignment in radiation therapy treatments.

LOGISTICS

There are substantial problems of communication and logistics in most hospitals. Often the CT scan is performed early in the course of the patient's workup and before a decision has been made to institute radiation therapy—often before a radiation therapist is involved in the patient's management. Thus even though a malignancy may be suspected, the scans are often not thought of as potentially contributing to the planning of radiation therapy treatments. Under such circumstances, even though attention may customarily be paid to the problems of patient positioning for known candidates for radiation therapy, the proper steps will not be taken. This has a number of possible consequences. The scan may be of diminished value, or none at all, for purposes of planning the radiation therapy field, or it may be necessary to rescan the patient under the appropriate conditions with the attendant increase in cost and unnecessary use of a valuable and limited resource. Attention needs to be given to this problem, both by those who administer the use of CT scanners within the hospital and by regulatory agencies. There is no reason that the possibility of radiation therapy treatments cannot be anticipated for the majority of patients being assessed for malignant disease and the need for accurate and reproducible patient alignment satisfied.

Therapy scans are often time-consuming as they require attention to setup details and, often, a large number of slices. Also, much more time after the scan must be devoted to interpretation and "marking-up" the scans in consultation between therapist and diagnostician. There is no sense in ignoring this. To do so can only lead to frustration.

PATIENT POSITION

The use of the anatomic information provided by CT for the design of radiation treatments depends on the patient being as nearly as possible in the same position for scanning as for treatment (or vice versa). The importance of this varies from patient to patient. In some situations it is possible to relate the CT scan findings to stable anatomic landmarks (e.g., bony structures) and, when devising the treatment, to work from these fixed landmarks. This, for example, is the case in the brain where the stability of the structures and the presence of good landmarks make it often possible to use information obtained from scans taken under quite different conditions from those of treatment. However, for the majority of situations encountered in body scanning, such a translation significantly degrades the information obtained in the CT scan. It is therefore important that attention be given to making sure that scans are performed under known and appropriate conditions of patient position and alignment. A number of details are of importance in this respect, and these are now briefly discussed.

Choice of Position

The proper choice of position can importantly contribute to the patient's therapy by assuring stability and reproducibility, as well as permitting improved normal tissue sparing. These are matters of judgment and experience. CT has much to contribute with regard to learning the influence of position on the disposition of tissues, both for whole classes of treatment problems and for the individual patient. Repeat scans with the patient in different positions may well be indicated in special cases. In any event, the patient's position for therapy should be considered *before* scanning. General policies should be established for common categories of disease. Not only need the question of prone, supine, or other position be considered, but details of arm, leg, and head position and support must be determined. Adequate documentation is important—an instant camera would be a valuable addition to the scanner room.

Despite the best intentions, it is not always possible to achieve the desired patient position on the CT scanner. This happens, for example, when the normal treatment policy is to have the arms outstretched in some manner (akimbo, clasped over the head, or out to the side as is done in some chest wall radiation). Although this is sometimes unavoidable, necessitating careful analysis of the relative motion likely between the scanning and treatment situations, it is worth considering a modification in the treatment position. Due to the generally modest diameter of the scanner tunnel, the CT scanner imposes more severe restraints than the therapy machine. It may therefore be preferable to adopt a position which is compatible with the CT scanner than to accept different positions in treatment and scanning situations.

Immobilizing Devices

CT-compatible immobilization casts can be helpful, particularly for treatments of the head and neck area and the extremities. We have used a perforated thermoplastic (Perforated Aquaplast; AliMed, Inc., Boston, MA) which can be softened by immersion in 65°C water, then stretched over and formed to the patient's skin surface. It hardens within a few minutes. This material can be secured to a plywood board (covered with the mattress material mentioned below) which can be used both in the CT scanner and on the therapy machine. In fact, we have several such boards, one of which is kept permanently at the CT scanner and the others at the appropriate treatment units. The advantage of perforated material is that the patient's skin surface can be seen through it so that the correct registration of the patient and the mask can be verified, skin marks can be seen, some skin sparing is possible, and the patient can breath and perspire freely (both during cast fabrication and subsequently). However, the periodicity of the perforations can give rise to artifacts in some types of scanner. In those situations a nonperforated thermoplastic can be used.

Table Top

Flat table tops are in almost uniform use in radiation therapy. It is not clear if the use of a flat table top achieves more stable patient positioning—probably not. However, it seems to offer greater reproducibility of patient position from one treatment to the next. Whatever the reason, the fact that the patient will be treated under these conditions makes it mandatory to use a flat surface for the support of the patient in the CT scanner. Ideally, not only should the patient surface be flat, but it should have the same width as the treatment table top and should use the same covering material. In this connection, we have had very good results with the use of a thin vinyl-covered foam mattress (crinkled "Vy-foam" mattress; AliMed Inc., Boston, MA). This mattress is thin enough (6 mm) to ensure stability of the patient and thick enough to be reasonably comfortable; it has a washable nonslippery surface and is radiolucent.

Alignment Marks

Most treatments are set up with the aid of superficial marks, or landmarks, on the patient. These may be ink outlines of the treatment field or, more commonly, fiducial marks used to align the patient in the scanner coordinate system (usually there are three of these). If these marks were already established before the CT scan, they have only to be overlaid by a "radio-gray" material which is dense enough to be visible in the CT scan but not so opaque as to produce artifacts. We use narrow-gauge (about No. 5) radiopaque plastic catheter tubing. A thin bead of barium paste or thin steel wire also works.

More often, the CT scan is performed before skin marks are established. Two alternatives are then available: Skin marks can be more or less arbitrarily chosen in sensible locations once the patient is satisfactorily positioned. These would ideally be placed with the aid of pencil light beams forming an orthogonal reference coordinate system (see below). Often such marks can be used for treatment positioning, especially if irregular fields are used. If the setup strategy requires a shift of these marks, or additional skin marks, these can be established at a subsequent session using the therapy simulator. Schemes for transferring information derived from CT data onto skin marks have been developed for a commercial scanner (Pfizer

Medical Systems, New York, NY) and in a prototype optical scanner. These schemes suffer from the problem that such a transfer is possible only after extensive analysis of the CT data, which is generally not completed before the patient leaves the scanner couch.

In some cases it may well be that the target volume and relevant normal structures are most directly and accurately related to internal bony landmarks. In this case these can be identified and, subsequent to the CT scan, radiographically identified, usually using a radiotherapy simulator, and "transferred" to skin marks. That is, skin marks appropriate for setup can be put on the patient's skin in a well-defined relationship to the bony landmarks, so that the CT-defined anatomy can then be referenced to these *ex post facto* marks. Even with this strategy it may be useful to have skin marks put on the skin before the scan in order to define the patient alignment at the time of the scan so as to reproduce it when the bony landmarks are related to new skin marks. The old marks can then be dispensed with.

Alignment Lights

Two opposed horizontal pencil beams and one vertical one, all lying in the same plane, are needed for alignment. Lasers are convenient but surely not necessary for this purpose. It is difficult and not necessarily desirable (because of the difficulty of observing the patient) to have the alignment beams in the scan plane. It is sufficient that it be a *known* distance from the scan plane and that the couch position readout be accurate and not prone to slippage.

Breathing

The question of what to do about breathing depends to a large extent on the speed of the CT scan. Machines whose scan time is in excess of a reasonable breathhold offer no practical alternative other than to have the patient breathe as shallowly as possible during the course of the scan. Machines whose scan time is of the order of 15 to 20 sec have only two realistic choices: Either the patient is asked to maintain deep inspiration throughout the course of a scan, or the patient can maintain shallow respiration. Fast scans, of the order of 10 sec or less, can be performed in any phase of suspended respiration but are prone to artifact if scans are taken with continuous breathing.

The extent to which breathing represents a serious problem depends, of course, on the anatomic site. Clearly the thorax is likely to be significantly affected by respiration, as is the abdomen where diaphragmatic motion can cause significant distortion of organs. It is probably a lesser problem in the pelvis and relatively insignificant in the head, neck, and extremities.

If one is in a situation, as with a fast scanner, to be able to scan under any desired condition of respiration, what would be the best respiratory condition to employ when scanning the patient? If it is possible to take scans under only one condition, one would pick the condition which would result in the best possible quality of scan, i.e., a state of suspended respiration. With a fast scanner this should probably be with lung filling of the order of what is obtained in shallow respiration. With a 15- to 20-sec scanner one is obliged to work with deep inspiration. Usually, if attention is being paid to these matters, it should be possible to repeat at least a few critical sections in another state of respiration to assess the extent to which respiration causes significant change in the anatomic relationships. In such cases, in what phase of respiration should the second scan be taken? It is commonly suggested that the second scans should be repeated with the patient breathing normally. I find myself in some disagreement with this position, which is primarily based on some notion of using "average" absorption coefficients for purposes of dose evaluation. I think it more valuable to perform the second scan also in suspended respiration, in a phase of the respiratory cycle taken so that the pair of scans bracket the expected treatment situation. This is because one is really interested less in the average position of organs than in their extreme excursions. That is, if the tumor mass is to be included in the treatment field, its margin should be within the field during all phases of respiration, and so knowing that some average position is encompassed is of little value. Thus if organ and tissue localization are of primary concern, one is better served by scanning once in inspiration and once in expiration, thereby defining the limits of possible motion.

Of course, very often, and particularly with fast scanners, these issues are academic and it is only occasionally that a significant effort is necessary to monitor the degree of motion during respiration. However, it is important to recognize that respiration can give rise to problems and so to be prepared to make an analysis when necessary.

Bolus Material

Bolus distorts. This is the only circumstance in which I would advocate some degradation of the diagnostic capabilities for purposes of treatment planning applications. In part this is because the diagnostic quality of scans is often very good even when bolus is omitted. As the dynamic range of scanner detectors increases in the more modern machines, bolus is likely to become increasingly unnecessary.

Contrast Media

Another ingredient of the CT recipe is the use of contrast media. Oral contrast medium for intestinal delineation, intravenous contrast medium for kidney and bladder delineation, gas contrast medium for vaginal and bladder delineation, and various surgical clips for correlation with surgical findings are all routinely used. It is sometimes proposed that treatment planning scans be taken in the absence, where possible, of such contrast agents. This notion, of course, arises from the desire to use the CT scan for dose calculation purposes. However, the delineation of tissues is, as repeatedly emphasized, extremely important for the design of the treatment field and should receive the highest priority in treatment planning scans. It is relatively easy to take care of contrast media in the dose calculation process. Emphasis should be placed on making the treatment planning program capable of this rather than denying these enormously useful techniques when obtaining scans for treatment planning purposes.

Unavoidable Changes

There are circumstances in which one cannot avoid very significant differences in patient condition between the therapeutic situation and that needed for the best diagnostic evaluation. An example might be treatment of bladder carcinoma, where some centers prefer to treat with an empty bladder in order to maximize normal tissue sparing, whereas evaluation of the tumor may require a full bladder. Under such circumstances two sets of scans should be made.

Relating Scans to Other Studies

I strongly advocate the use of a large number of finely spaced CT scans to guide the planning of radiation therapy. This results in improved definition of the target volume in all directions and facilitates the interpretation of scans by establishing contiguity of structures in adjacent sections. The consequent availability of sagittal and coronal (and oblique) reconstructions provides an additional tool for interpretation of the CT data.

The provision of digital radiographic capability on the scanner is extremely helpful in referencing the CT data to other studies taken in anteroposterior or lateral positions, or to a subsequent simulation procedure. This is true even though the data are taken from a different, indeed peculiar, perspective. If a large number of CT scans have been made, a computer reconstruction of any projection view with full perspective correction is feasible. I have implemented this capability in a treatment planning program, and it has proved very helpful in the use of the CT data.

"TREATMENT PLANNING" VERSUS "DIAGNOSTIC" SCANS

A dichotomy has frequently been drawn between scans taken for diagnostic purposes and those needed for planning radiation therapy. In its extreme, but widely espoused form this division boils down to the philosophy: "Let the diagnostic radiologists do whatever they need to do (it is too hard or impossible to influence them at that stage), then perform a repeat scan for treatment planning under controlled conditions, usually taking a reduced number of slices."

I do not like this strategy for two main reasons: (a) It is wasteful of the CT scanner time, which is a precious and expensive resource; and (b) it tends to result in planning the treatment using inferior data.

Rather, I prefer that the necessary effort and planning go into making the first scan adequate for *all* functions associated with diagnosing and staging the disease and planning its therapy. Only in rare instances is it likely that a properly performed initial study would not provide all the information needed. The advantage of this approach is that it draws the diagnostic and therapeutic aspects of the patient's evaluation closer together, probably to the benefit of both.

Computed Tomography in Radiation Therapy,
edited by C. C. Ling, C. C. Rogers, and
R. J. Morton. Raven Press, New York © 1983

Three-Dimensional Reconstruction of CT Images for Treatment Planning in Carcinoma of the Lung

*†L. E. Reinstein, *†D. L. McShan, †‡R. E. Land, and
*†A. S. Glicksman

*Department of Radiation Oncology, Rhode Island Hospital,
Providence, Rhode Island 02902; †Section on Radiation Medicine, Brown University,
Providence, Rhode Island 02912; and ‡Department of Radiology, St. Joseph Hospital,
Providence, Rhode Island 02907*

The process of radiotherapy treatment planning for radiation therapy involves the selection and design of radiation beams tailored to deliver a uniformly high dose to the volume at risk while minimizing the dose to the surrounding healthy tissues. For many years the RT simulator has played an important role in providing diagnostic images which aid in the choice of beam parameters and the design of irregularly shaped fields. Although the simulator can be extremely useful in certain situations, it suffers from the limitation of all conventional x-ray units: Its images lack sufficient density discrimination to distinguish soft tissue structures. Thus with the simulator, most treatment planning is performed on the basis of bony landmarks, surgical clips (when available), and radiopaque dyes.

At institutions where computed tomographic (CT) scans have been routinely available for radiotherapy, it has been repeatedly observed that the use of conventional simulator images (combined with the presumption of "standard anatomy") do not necessarily result in the optimum treatment (1,2,6). For this reason an increasing number of institutions are relying on multiplane CT images to provide the soft tissue information needed to adequately determine the tumor volume. With the current state of CT technology, it is now possible to acquire a large number of CT images within a reasonable amount of time. These images can be used to determine the target contour for each plane.

This multiplane approach is insufficient, however, for treatment planning situations where the tumor and surrounding anatomical structures change rapidly throughout the volume, and a means for visualizing in three-dimensional (3-D) perspective the spatial interrelationship between the radiation beam, the external contour, and the internal structures is essential. Several of the new CT treatment planning systems which feature (so-called) 3-D planning options superimpose a two-dimensional planar display of anatomical contours and overlaying isodoses onto each CT image.

155

Unfortunately, none is capable of displaying these data as an interpretable 3-D image for use in treatment planning. Therefore the actual field design remains the task of the conventional simulator.

A fresh approach to the problem of 3-D treatment planning and simulation was initiated at Rhode Island Hospital (RIH) in 1977, and the system which was developed is currently in clinical use (3,5,7). The method involves the creation of multicolor video images of the relevant internal patient anatomy in 3-D perspective. These anatomical surface features are mathematically reconstructed by the DEC PDP 11/45 computer using data from multiple CT scans and can be viewed by the radiotherapy planner in any spatial orientation.

One of the most useful features of the RIH 3-D treatment planning system is the "computer-simulation" or "side view" mode. In this mode, the images can be interactively manipulated and viewed as if along the central axis of the radiation beam; the beam parameters (gantry angle, collimator angle, and field size) can be chosen, and the field shaping block can be designed in a real-time computer simulation session using only the color video monitor, four push buttons, and a "joystick." The computer algorithms used for automatic contour recognition from CT data and for 3-D surface generation are discussed in detail in a separate paper (4). The clinical application of this system to radiotherapy for carcinoma of the lung is described here.

EXAMPLE

Consider the case of a patient who was sent to our Radiation Oncology Department for treatment of carcinoma of the right lung; the lesion was situated in the right hilum and extended from the carina to halfway into the lung parenchyma, approximately from T_3 to T_6. As indicated in Fig. 1, CT scans of this patient were taken at 20 levels spaced 1 cm apart. The patient was lying supine on a flat table during this procedure in an attempt to replicate the usual treatment position. A triangulation reference system was established using skin marks and radiopaque barium paste to ensure the accurate setup of the patient according to the resulting treatment plan. Although more data were available, the computer was able to reconstruct the surfaces of the relevant anatomical structures using only nine of the cross-sectional images. At each of these levels, it "semi-automatically" tracked the boundaries of the relevant internal structures, which were identified (4). The contour of the target volume was outlined by the radiotherapist interactively using the joystick with the video display (Fig. 2).

For this patient, the target contours were drawn to include the entire visible extent of the tumor, as well as the mediastinum. The therapist noticed that on levels 7 and 8 the tumor approached close to the anterior chest wall. This fact had not been appreciated from the diagnostic x-rays prior to the CT examination, and the proposed target volume was adjusted accordingly. An anteroposterior (AP) reconstruction of the relevant anatomical surfaces is shown in Fig. 3 These include the right and left lungs, a section of the sternum, the spinal cord, and the posterior half of the external surface. These surfaces are seen here in gray tones; the display on the video monitor

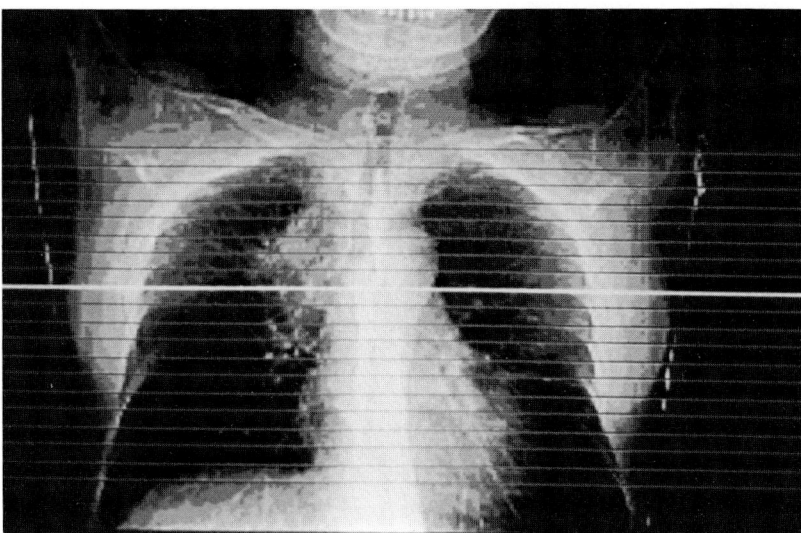

FIG. 1. Scout view of thorax reconstructed from CT scans of the patient discussed in this example.

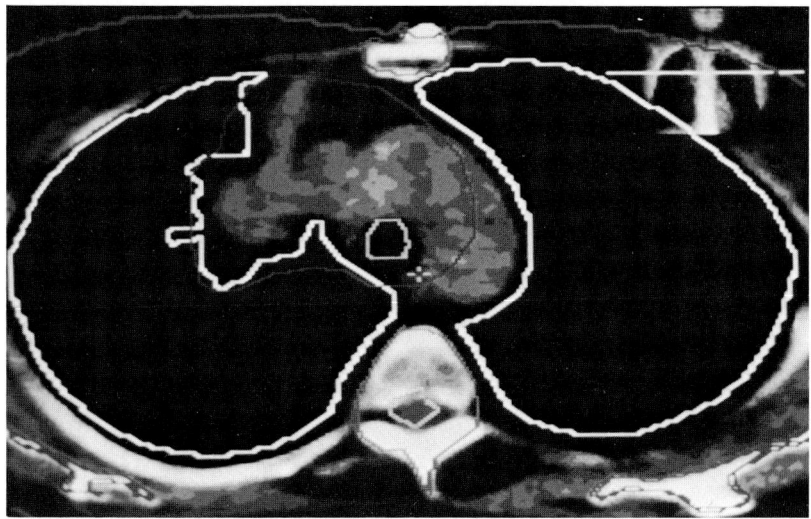

FIG. 2. A magnified CT section through the center of the target volume. Contour boundaries of lungs, spinal cord, sternum, and trachea were tracked semiautomatically by the computer, while the target contour was outlined interactively by the radiotherapist.

is actually in multiple colors, which render the various surfaces highly distinguishable.

The entire image can be rotated to any desired viewing angle, creating a clearer understanding of the tumor's three-dimensional extent and its placement with respect to the adjacent organs. In Fig. 4, an anterior oblique view, the tumor is seen to

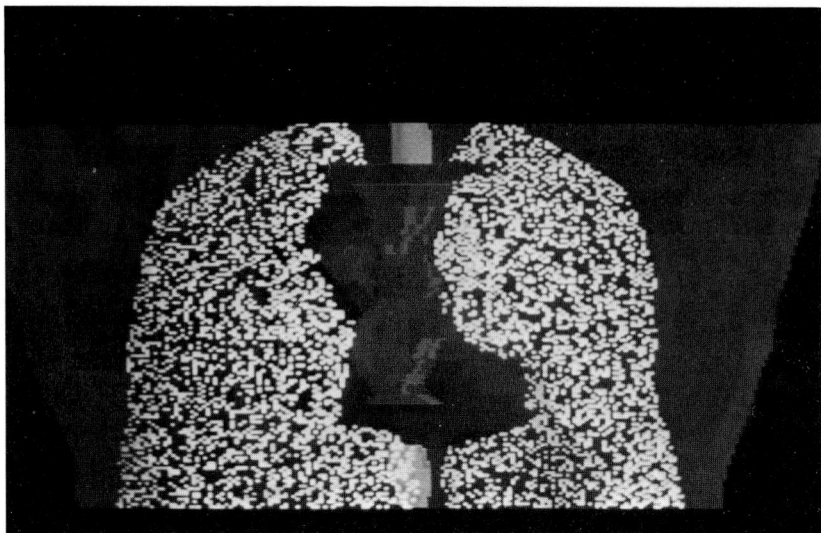

FIG. 3. AP reconstruction of relevant internal surfaces by the computer. The actual video monitor display is in multiple colors, which render the surfaces of the lungs, sternum, target volume, and spinal cord as well as the posterior external surface highly distinguishable.

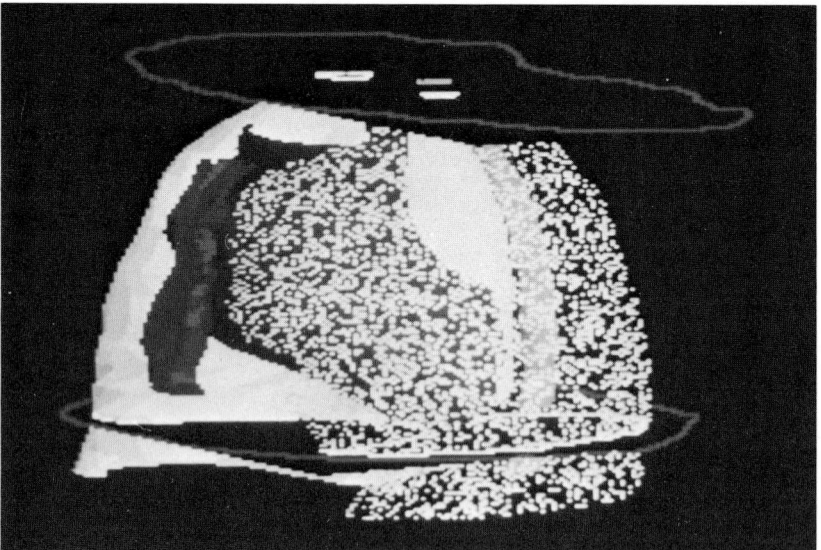

FIG. 4. An anterior oblique view of the reconstructed internal anatomical surfaces. The left lung is shaded in a "see-through" mode (only random pixels are plotted) to reveal the underlying structures. The actual video monitor display here is in multiple colors, which renders the surfaces of the lungs, sternum, target volume, and spinal cord highly distinguishable; applies to Figs. 5–12 also.

project anteriorly at the upper levels and to approach close to the spinal cord as it descends. Note that the left lung is shaded in a "see through" mode to reveal the underlying structures. Based on the information gained from these 3-D images, the decision was made to irradiate the tumor through two anterior oblique portals and a single posterior portal; it was hoped that the dose delivered to uninvolved lung tissue and the spinal cord could be minimized by proper design of gantry angle, collimator angle, and custom shaped blocks.

Although the display and rotation of "full-surface" images are helpful in attaining insight into the planning problem as a whole, it is at present too slow (on the order of 2 to 4 min) and therefore impractical as a tool for interactive beam design. It is for this reason that the "side view" or "portal beam simulation" mode was developed. In this mode, the computer graphics are simplified and visual completeness is exchanged for high speed. The result is a responsive, highly interactive display which retains a sufficient amount of anatomical structure to be useful for detailed treatment planning.

A "side view" display for this patient is seen in Fig. 5. The contour of a single transverse plane appears in the upper left hand corner of Fig. 5 to indicate the placement of the proposed radiation beams. The rectangular outline represents the field borders of the radiation beam, whose central axis is actually parallel to the transverse planes. The projections of the nine transverse planes are shown relative to the incoming beam (for clarity, the computer displays only the target and spinal cord contours in this mode). The contours, which from this "side view" angle appear only as horizontal lines, are connected to reveal the shapes and the relative positions of these volumes. As the image is reconstructed using the perspective of the x-ray

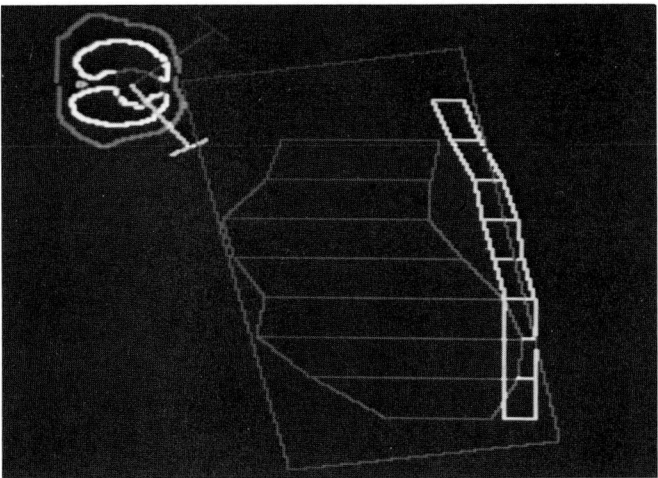

FIG. 5. "Side view" display for interactive beam simulation. Note that a portion of the spinal cord as well as the target volume is included in the radiation field (*rectangular outline*) at its gantry angle. The single transverse plane in the upper left aids in orientation of the proposed beam placement.

target (i.e., the anatomy is seen from a "beam's eye view"), it is geometrically analogous to a portal or simulator film.

If the anterior oblique beam (seen in Fig. 5, 45° to the lateral direction) were used, it is clear that there would be no way to include the entire tumor in the radiation field without overlapping with the spinal cord. Although shifting to a completely lateral field would create a "separation" between the target volume and the spinal cord, it would also result in excessive irradiation of the uninvolved lung tissue. As the beam direction can be instantaneously rotated by adjusting a potentiometer on the control console, it is a relatively easy task for the planner to find the optimal projection which eliminates the target-volume/spinal cord overlap while minimizing the high-dose irradiation of the lung. These goals are met using a more laterally oriented oblique beam (Fig. 6).

The central axis placement, collimator, orientation, and field size as seen in Fig. 6 are also easily and interactively controlled. The geometrical beam parameters which are selected (central axis coordinates, collimator angle, field width and height, respectively) are immediately displayed and stored for use by the isodose calculation routines. Note that even at this optimized gantry angle (Fig. 6) with a 10° collimator tilt the beam would still "nick" the cord at the superior and inferior field corners, without incorporating some form of beam blocking into the plan.

The design of customized beam shaping blocks can be accomplished by using this computerized simulation. The interactive joy-stick is used to superimpose the required block outline on the simulated portal image (Fig. 7). Extensive, highly tailored blocking can be designed to reduce unnecessary lung irradiation; once

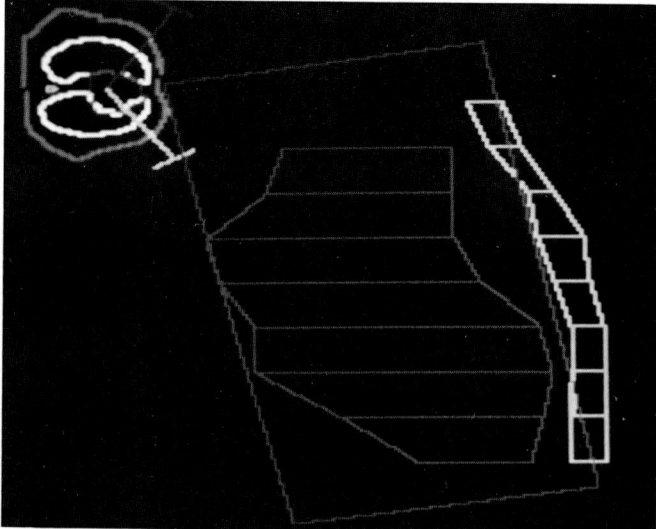

FIG. 6. The "side view" display viewed from a more lateral gantry angle. Although there is separation between the projection of the spinal cord and the target volume at this angle, beam blocking is still needed to avoid irradiating small portions of the cord.

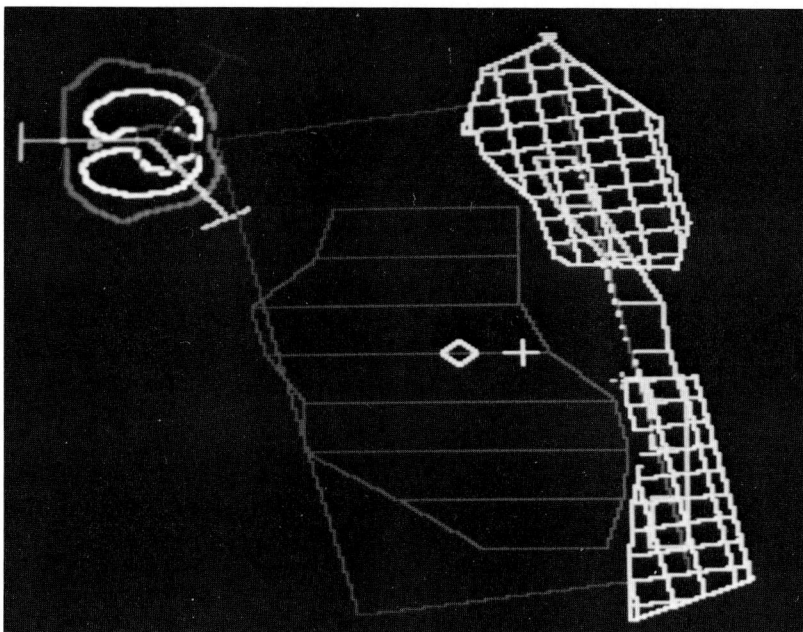

FIG. 7. Side view display at the selected gantry angle after the beam block outlines have been interactively drawn in on the video monitor.

designed, the resulting field shape is displayed in the full surface format seen in Fig. 8. A hard-copy printout of the block design (at the proper magnification) is generated as a pattern for cutting a shaped styrofoam mold on the "hot-wire" block cutter.

The final step in the treatment planning process is the calculation, display, and evaluation throughout the treatment volume of the absorbed dose distribution. The calculation routine used is a version of Cunningham's CBEAM program. Several methods have been devised for displaying the results. These include 3-D isodose surface display, anatomical surface dose display, continuous color-to-dose mapping (single or multiplane), and interactive color bands (3). The last of these, which allows the planner to define and display dose ranges as discrete color bands, has been found to be most useful in assessing the quality of an external beam plan.

Several color bands are created by adjusting the console potentiometers to set the lower dose limit and the width of one (or more) bands of uniform color. The result (Fig. 9) shows the dose distribution in the central ($z = 0$) plane for the three-beam treatment plan just described. Four distinct color bands were created to help locate "hot spots," define uniform areas of high dose, and determine the dose to the spinal cord and uninvolved lung. The homogeneity of the dose distribution was judged to be acceptable (95 to 105% within the target contour) despite a small "hot spot" of 106 to 111%. An alternative display format (color-to-dose mapping) is seen in Fig. 10. Note that this display includes a graphic representation of the field

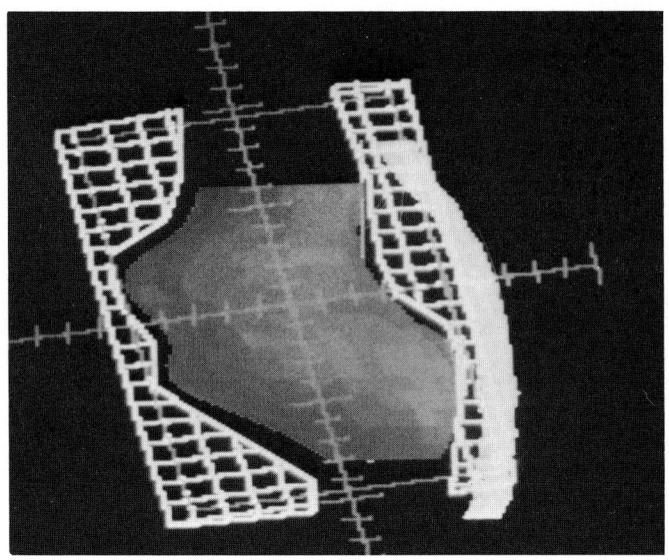

FIG. 8. A full surface image of the target volume and spinal cord, displayed at the chosen treatment angle. Note the 10° collimator rotation and the customized field shaping blocks used for this treatment plan.

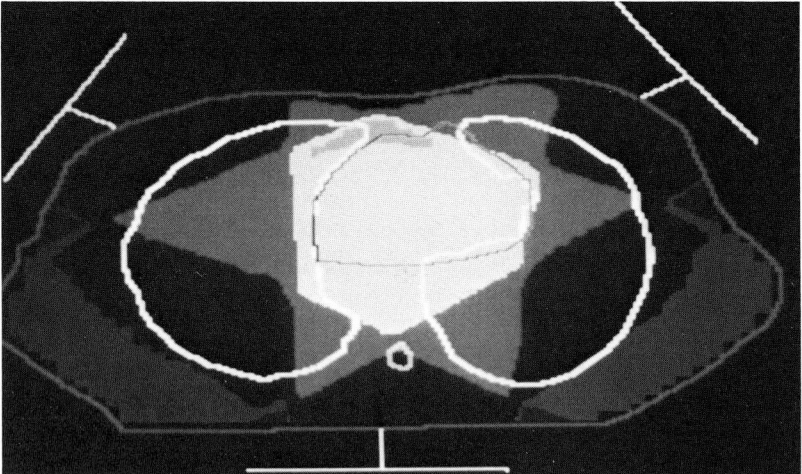

FIG. 9. Dose distribution in the central plane of the target volume. Bands of uniform color represent four separate dose ranges on the video monitor. The assignment of color to a specific dose range is interactive, and the resulting color key is seen at the upper right.

shaping blocks and illustrates the "point-dose" feature, which allows an instant readout of the relative dose at any point on the plane where the "cursor" is located.

An appreciation of the variation in relative dose throughout the treatment volume can be gained by simultaneous multiplane dose display (Fig. 11) or by sequential display of the individual planes of interest. The color band dose display for this

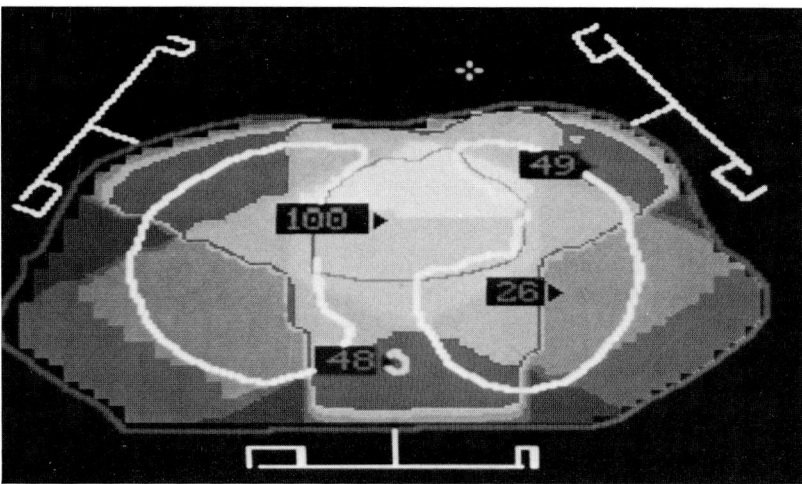

FIG. 10. Alternative display of calculated dose distribution in central plane. In this format, a pixel-by-pixel mapping of dose to color is displayed. Also shown is the capability of interactively displaying the relative dose at points in the plane which are selected by movement of the cursor. Note the representation of the planar cross sections of the beam shaping blocks.

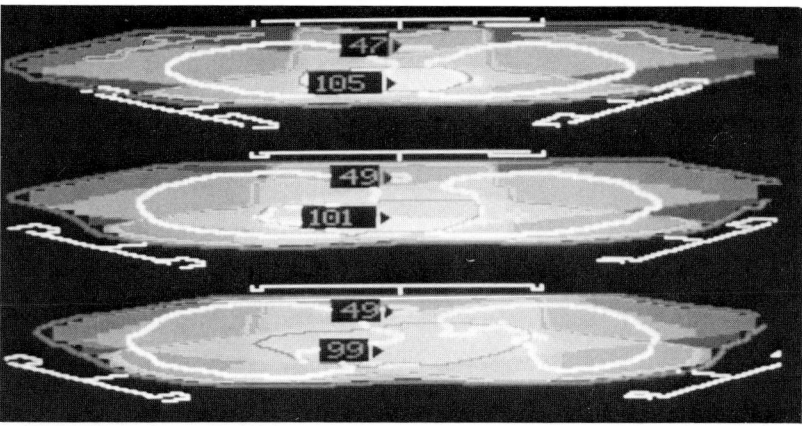

FIG. 11. Multiplane dose display. The dose distributions in several of the planes can be viewed simultaneously to gain insight into the variation of dose throughout the treatment volume.

same plane, at a level 6 cm inferior to the central plane, is shown in Fig. 12. Note that the collimator tilt (10°) successfully projects the 95 to 105% color band toward the patient's posterior to completely encompass the target volume as drawn.

DISCUSSION

In conventional two-dimensional (2-D) treatment planning and isodose calculations, the central plane is considered to represent the entire volume, and the relationship of the tumor to the normal surrounding tissues is perceived solely in this

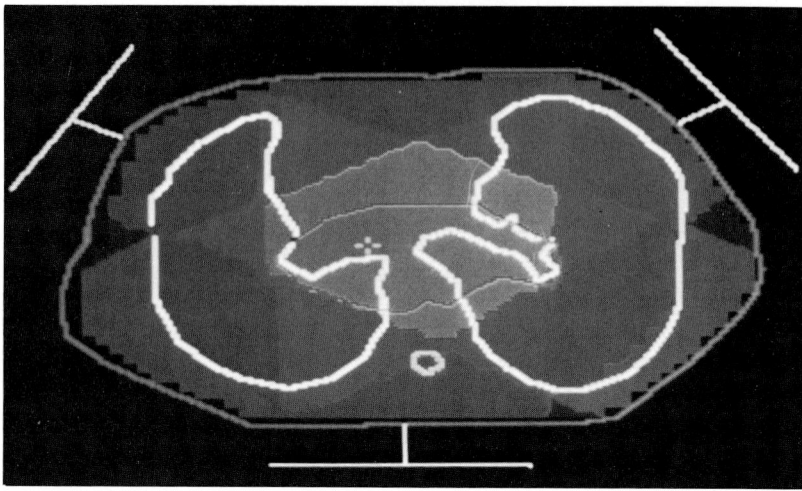

FIG. 12. Color band dose display is seen at a level located 6 cm inferior to the central plane. The collimator tilt successfully projects the uniform high dose region toward the posterior surface to encompass the target volume.

plane. The RT simulator used in conjunction with this single plane approach can aid in the perception of the 3-D perspective *only* with respect to structures which are easily seen using standard radiography. The important soft tissue features, which may be invisible to the RT simulator, can, however, often be located with state-of-the-art CT scans. Although allowing one to visualize these features from plane to plane, the CT scans do not by themselves create an integrated 3-D picture. This need has been satisfied through the development of a 3-D treatment planning system, which mathematically manipulates the multiplane CT data to construct a rotatable 3-D image.

Using this system, the treatment planner perceives the spatial relationships between the soft tissue features, bony structure, and target volume with respect to the borders of the proposed treatment field for any combinations of gantry angle, collimator angle, and field dimensions. As the patient's presence is not required during the process of "computerized simulation," the derivation of the ideal beam parameters and the careful design of individualized field shaping blocks can now be performed without the time pressure inherent in a lengthy and uncomfortable session on the simulator table.

REFERENCES

1. Goitein, M., Wittenberg, J., Mendiondo, M., Doucette, J., Friedberg, C., Ferrucci, J., Gunderson, L., Linggood, R., Shipley, W., and Fineberg, H. (1979): The value of CT scanning in radiation therapy treatment planning: a prospective study. *Int. J. Radiat. Oncol. Biol. Phys.*, 5:1787–1798.
2. Hobday, P., Hodson, N., Husband, J., Parker, R., and MacDonald, J. (1979): Computed tomography applied to radiotherapy treatment planning: techniques and results. *Radiology*, 133:477–482.

3. McShan, D., Haumann, D., Reinstein, L. E., and Glicksman, A. S. (1979): An interactive three-dimensional radiation treatment planning system. *Br. J. Radiol. [Suppl.]*, 15:144–146.
4. McShan, D., Reinstein, L. E., Land, R. E., and Glicksman, A. S. Auto-contour recognition in three-dimensional treatment planning. This volume.
5. McShan, D., Silverman, A., Lanza, D., Reinstein, L. E., and Glicksman, A. S. A computerized three-dimensional treatment planning system utilizing interactive color graphics. *Br. J. Radiol.*, 52:478–481.
6. Munzenrider, J., Pilepich, M., Rene-Ferrero, J., Tchakarova, I., and Carter, B. (1977): Use of body scanner in radiotherapy treatment planning. *Cancer*, 40:170–179.
7. Reinstein, L. E., McShan, D., Webber, B, and Glicksman, A. S. (1978): A computer-assisted three-dimensional treatment planning system. *Radiology*, 127:259–264.

Computed Tomography in Radiation Therapy,
edited by C. C. Ling, C. C. Rogers, and
R. J. Morton. Raven Press, New York © 1983

Automatic Contour Recognition in Three-Dimensional Treatment Planning

*†D. L. McShan, *†L. E. Reinstein, †‡R. E. Land, and
*†A. S. Glicksman

*Department of Radiation Oncology, Rhode Island Hospital,
Providence, Rhode Island 02902; †Section on Radiation Medicine, Brown University,
Providence, Rhode Island 02912; and ‡Department of Radiology, St. Joseph Hospital,
Providence, Rhode Island 02907*

For the past several years, we have been involved in developing a three-dimensional (3-D) radiation treatment planning system (4–6,8). The system that has evolved provides computer-generated graphics which assist the treatment planner in visualizing and appreciating the extent of the tumor and its relationship to the surrounding anatomy. The system provides simulation and interactive selection of beam portals and provides displays to help visualize resulting dose distributions in relation to the target volume and surrounding anatomy.

One of the difficulties in using our 3-D system in the past has been the requirement to manually enter cross-sectional outlines. Conventional transverse tomographic images were commonly used and lacked the precision and detail now available with computed tomographic (CT) data. Work was therefore begun on developing automatic-contouring techniques for abstracting outline information from CT scans as well as techniques for identifying the data for use in our 3-D treatment planning system.

The hardware used in our system consists of a DEC PDP11/45 computer with floating point hardware and 112k bytes of core memory (although the actual programs are limited to less than 16k). The image display device used is a 256×256 pixels (12 bits each) raster color graphic system. An interactive console with potentiometers, a joystick, and pushbuttons are used for interaction with the display software. CT data are transferred via magnetic tape and are stored on disc for rapid retrieval. The CT data used in this presentation were obtained on a GE/CT 8800 scanner which has scout film imaging capabilities.

The case presented here concerns the thoracic region (details of the tumor and target volumes are discussed elsewhere in this volume). For this case, 20 slices spaced 1 cm apart were obtained. Figure 1 shows a scout image with the positions of the slices indicated.

In order to present a 3-D view of the anatomy, our system requires that serial cross-sectional contours be obtained for each structure to be displayed. In general

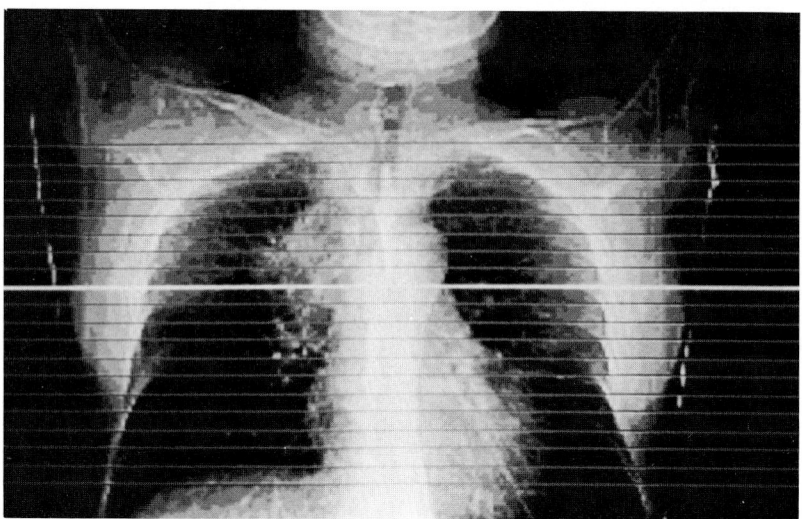

FIG. 1.   AP scout image with position of CT slices indicated (spaced 1 cm apart).

we are concerned with extracting the target volume and the location and extent of neighboring anatomy, which may be structures to which we wish to minimize dose or which may serve as landmarks to help visualize the anatomy. In almost all situations the target volume must be entered manually by the therapist or treatment planner; but most of the remaining anatomy can be identified with automatic contouring techniques.

Our approach to automatic contouring has been to use a fairly simple boundary detection algorithm coupled with *a priori* information based on standard anatomical data. The boundary detection algorithm is similar to others reported in the literature (3,7). In brief, the region to be outlined is "windowed" using upper and lower thresholds on the CT data.

A binary image map is generated with ones, set for those pixels within the region. The region thus defined is outlined using an edge or boundary tracking routine. The outline data are chain coded with an eight-way coding scheme and stored in a random access file that has been set up with a tree-structure directory, which allows grouping and rapid retrieval of the contour data. The contour data thus defined can then be connected to form a 3-D surface that can be displayed using computer-generated graphics.

To proceed with automatic contouring using our technique, it is necessary to first define the *a priori* information for standard anatomy. This process consists of defining threshold values, expected locations, shape classifiers, and other identifying information for each structure which might be of interest. Once defined, this information remains fixed from patient to patient, with some variations based on patient positioning, sex, age, or other physiological classifications. For CT data input, the identification process is based on cross-sectional data; therefore the *a priori* information is organized as cross-sectional information. A cross-sectional anatomy book (1) was used to obtain representative cross-sectional data (1,2). Specified at approximately 2-cm spacings, the data are abstracted by first defining a normalized coordinate system based on the size of the external contour. The relative location and shape are specified for each structure.

Table 1 shows a representative data file. The file begins with a list of thresholds. Because (with our computer system) rapid random access to the CT data is not possible, the program first scans the data and defines the binary image maps based on the threshold data. Up to eight of these maps can be generated on one pass

TABLE 1. *Representative data file*

SECTION 24: Thoracic anatomy
Thresholds
$1 − 350 to 250   external boundary and internal tissue and bone
$2 − 880 to − 420 lungs and esophagus
$3 − 30 to 20   spinal cord
$$ End of thresholds
Contour specifications
  Format (starts with line starting with '$')
    Line 1: $N NAME
          Where: N = threshold map number
                  Name = name of structure
    Line 2: ITYPE, ICOLOR, IFLAG
          Where: ITYPE = contour type number (unique)
                  ICOLOR = contour color
                  IFLAG = 1 IF target, @- display in side view option
    Line 3: XC,YC,DIRX,DIRY
          Where: XC = expected center x-value (starting point)
                  YC = expected center y-value (starting point)
                  DIRX = x-direction for boundary search (− 1,0, + 1)
                  DIRY = y-direction for boundary search (− 1,0, + 1)
    Line 4: MAX-X, MIN-X, MAX-Y, MIN-Y, DEV-YC, MAX-AREA,MIN-AREA
          Where: MAX-X = maximum height
                  MIN-X = minimum height
                  MAX-Y = maximum width
                  DEV-XC = maximum deviation of center from specified center
                  DEV-YC = same for y dimension
                  MAX-AREA = maximum area
                  MIN-AREA = minimum area
1$ External
1,3840,0 3840 = blue
  Start scan at − 16.0,0 scan right (1,0)
  50.,10.,50.,10.,50.,50.,2500.,100.
  The following dimensions are relative to center or external contour
2$ Lungs/left lung
  4,4095,1 495 = white
  Start scan at .4,0. scan right (1,0)
  1.,0.24,2.,12,0.2,0.2,2.0,0.2
2$ lungs/right lung
  14,1095,1
  Start scan at − 4.0 scan right (1,0)
  1.,0.25,2.,1.,0.2,00.2,2.0,0.2
2$ Esophagus

through the data (approximately 4 sec). The maps are bit-oriented and a 256×256 image can be reduced to 16 physical disc-resident records, allowing rapid retrieval for the second phase of boundary detection. The choice of threshold values were obtained using either a histogram or a cross-cut profile taken from representative CT scans.

Figure 2 shows an example of the latter. The diagonal line shows the position of the cut, and the profile of CT numbers is plotted at the bottom of the image. The horizontal band represents a threshold window, and the upper and lower limits can be interactively adjusted. In general, the limits are selected to include the characteristic CT numbers of the desired region. The limits are set at approximately the midpoint of the transition between the interior and exterior density values. Typically, only the upper or lower limit is important when defining the region boundary; in some cases, however, both are necessary, e.g., when the region borders both higher- and lower-density regions. Figure 3 illustrates the binary map (uniformly shaded areas) generated for the thresholds defined in Fig. 2.

With the binary threshold maps defined, the program then continues reading the *a priori* data (Table 1). For each structure to be identified, there are four lines of data. The first line specifies the name of the structure (must be unique) and the corresponding threshold map to be used. The second line contains information regarding the type of structure and display color for the structure. The third line contains the expected center of the structure (used as a starting point for the boundary searching routine) and the direction to scan for the initial boundary determination. At this point, the program proceeds with the edge detection process. Starting at the expected center, the program scans in the direction specified looking for the first perimeter pixel (pixel within the region) (ones) with one or more neighboring pixels outside of the region (zeros). The program then tracks the perimeter with a preferred

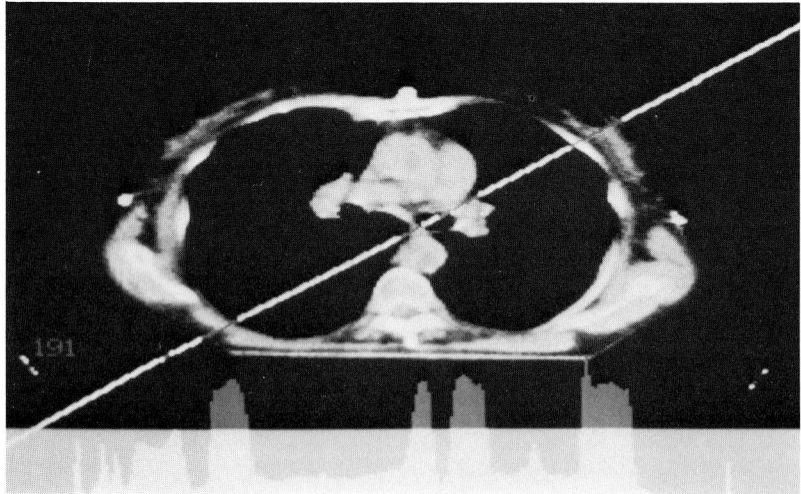

FIG. 2. Cross-cut profile with threshold region (*solid bond*) used to delineate lungs and thorax.

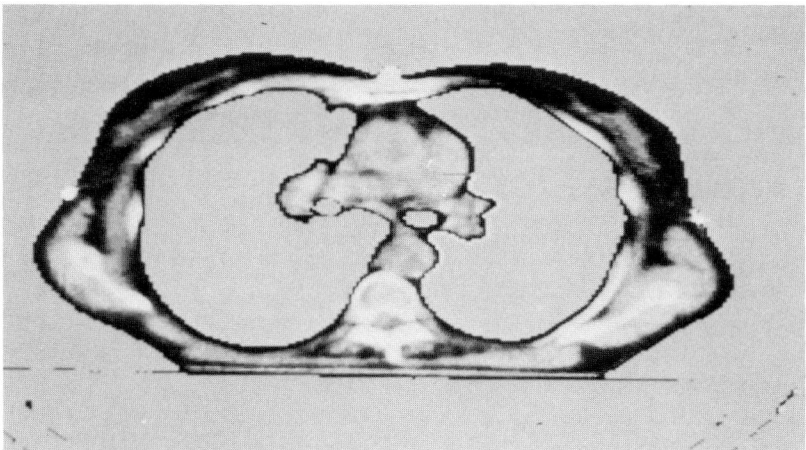

FIG. 3. Binary image map (*solid shaded regions*) generated using thresholds defined in Fig. 2.

"left-hand-on-the-wall" direction. The resulting contour is then checked for appropriateness. Using the fourth line from the standard anatomy data file, the shape of the detected contour is checked for size (maximum and minimum height and width), location, and area. A mismatch in any of these classifiers will cause the contour to be rejected. Rejects may occur either because of localized "holes" in the threshold region (interiorly located nonregion pixels) or because of normal (or abnormal) deviations from the standard anatomy. To handle these situations, the program can operate in two modes, automatic and semiautomatic. In the semiautomatic mode, the program will stop and allow the user to either accept the identified contour, skip the identification, or try again (with the user defining a new starting point). In the automatic mode, the program will shift the starting point slightly and try again twice. If still unacceptable, the last try will be stored but flagged as questionable, and the contour recognition will continue for the remaining structures. (The times involved for automatic contouring are under a minute per slice.) Questionable contours can then be checked and either accepted, edited, or deleted.

Once the necessary contours have been identified, the program can then construct surfaces by aligning and interpolating between levels to form a grid of 3-D coordinates. A spline interpolation algorithm is used to allow reasonable looking surfaces even when only a few widely spaced slices are involved. This is useful, as in many cases the variation from slice to slice is small, and a smaller sampling of slices can be used. Generation of surface grids takes about a minute per structure.

The identification and reconstruction of surfaces can be checked by projecting them onto a scout image, as shown in Fig. 4. This image also serves to relate the extent of the manually identified target volume to an image with which the therapist is more familiar.

Satisfied, the user can then request a full surface anatomical display (Fig. 5). Structures are shown as solid shaded surfaces. Individual surfaces can be added or

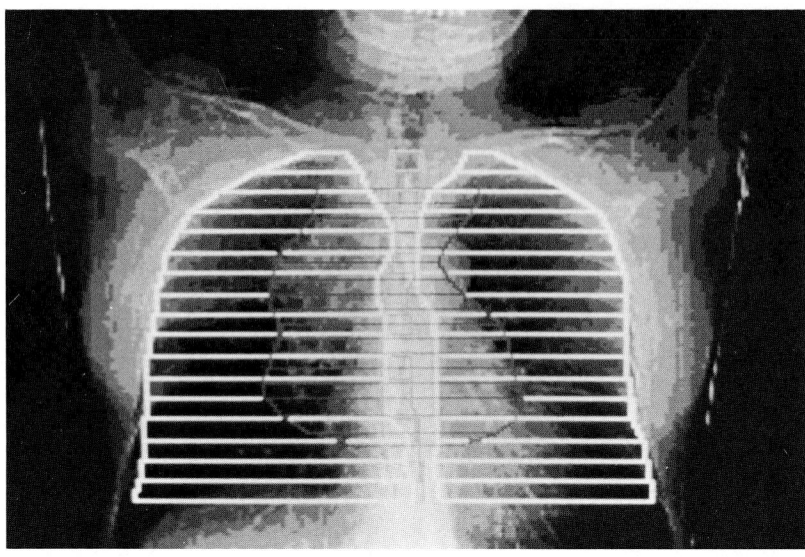

FIG. 4.   AP scout image with projection of abstracted lung, spinal cord, and target boundaries.

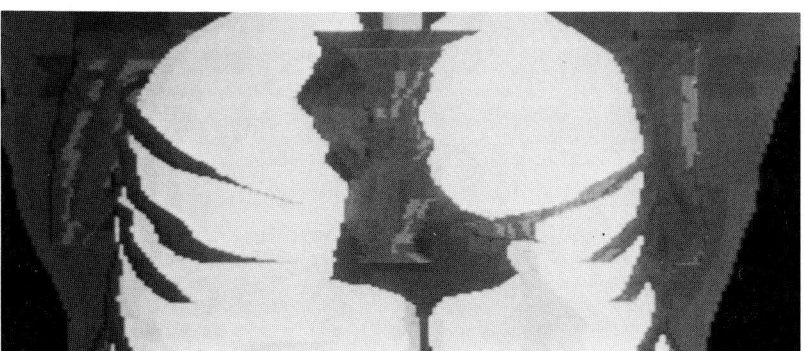

FIG. 5.   AP reconstructed surface image.

removed. Figure 6 shows the image rotated 45° to give a left lateral view. The left lung has been placed in a see-through mode. These types of images are useful for appreciating the full extent of the target volume and its relationship to the neighboring anatomy. Projection of this anatomical data as viewed by a proposed beam portal is useful for quickly planning optimal beam parameters and for designing beam shaping blocks.

Figures 5 and 6 also show an attempt at reconstructing and displaying a portion of the skeletal system, i.e., the lower ribs and scapula. The ribs are difficult to identify on the cross-sectional scans due to the thickness of the slices and the oblique incidence of the bone. Therefore the images of these structures are somewhat crude. Nevertheless, the relative positioning of the structures is accurate. Although not

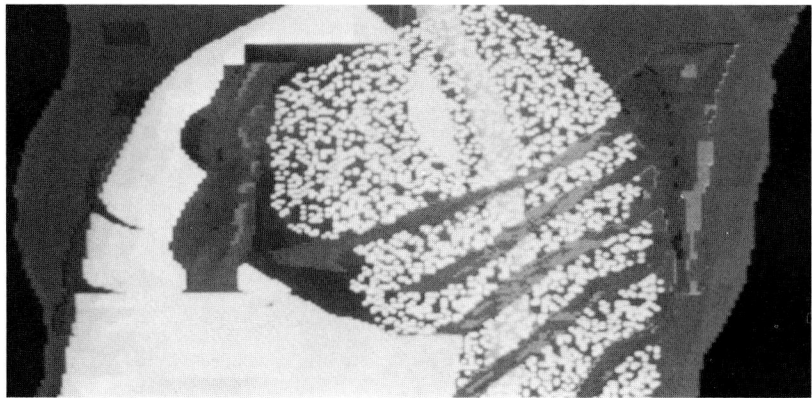

FIG. 6. Left lateral (45° from AP) view of surfaces (left lung in see-through mode).

particularly useful for planning in this case, it is anticipated that reconstruction of bony structures will be useful for correlating computer-generated portal images with verification films taken at therapeutic beam energies where the bony landmarks are often the only or the best alignment guides.

CONCLUSIONS

The rapid abstraction of anatomical contours from CT data is a useful and perhaps necessary component for 3-D treatment planning. The need to visualize adequate irradiation to the full 3-D extent of treatment volume can be fulfilled with a display of reconstructed surfaces. The ability to do this on a routine basis calls for, as much as possible, automatic contouring techniques. The approach taken at our institution thus far appears to achieve this end.

REFERENCES

1. Carter, B. L., Morehead, J., Wolpert, S. M., Hammerschlag, S. B., and Griffiths, H. J. (1977): *Cross-sectional Anatomy/Computed Tomography and Ultrasound Correlation*. Appleton-Century-Crofts, New York.
2. Eycleshymer, A. C., and Schoemaker, D. M. (1970): *A Cross-Section Anatomy*. Appleton-Century-Crofts, New York.
3. Keller, J. M., Edwards, F. M., and Rundle, R. (1981): Automatic outlining of regions on CT scans. *J. Comput. Assist. Tomogr.*, 5:240–245.
4. McShan, D. L., and Glicksman, A. S. (1979): An interactive three-dimensional radiation treatment planning system. A motion picture. Rhode Island Hospital.
5. McShan, D. L., Haumann, D. R., Reinstein, L. E., and Glicksman, A. S. (1979): An interactive three-dimensional radiation treatment planning system. *Brit. J. Radiol. [Suppl.]*, 15:144–146.
6. McShan, D. L., Silverman, A., Lanza, D. M., Reinstein, L. E., and Glicksman, A. S. (1979): A computerized three-dimensional treatment planning system utilizing interactive colour graphics. *Br. J. Radiol.*, 52:478–481.
7. Neighborhood coding of binary images for fast contour following and general binary array processing. Irwin Sobel Computer Graphics and Image Processing, Vol. 8, pp. 127–135, 1978.
8. Reinstein, L. E., McShan, D. L., Webber, B. M., and Glicksman, A. S. (1978): A computerized three-dimensional treatment planning system. *Radiology*, 127:259–264.

Computed Tomography in Radiation Therapy,
edited by C. C. Ling, C. C. Rogers, and
R. J. Morton. Raven Press, New York © 1983

A Multidimensional Treatment Planning System

*Michael Goitein, *Mark Abrams, **Derek Rowell,
**Helen Pollari, and **Judy Wiles

*Division of Radiation Biophysics, Department of Radiation Medicine, Massachusetts General Hospital and Harvard Medical School, Boston, Massachusetts 02114; and **Department of Mechanical Engineering, Massachusetts Institute of Technology, Cambridge, Massachusetts 02138

Three recent technical developments are likely to change the way in which radiation therapy is planned: computed tomography (CT), interactive raster-scan computer graphics, and the lowering cost of memory and associated development of 32-bit virtual memory minicomputers. We present features of a program being developed around these capabilities and oriented toward assisting the therapist to decide which organs and tissues should be included in the radiation fields and which can be excluded from some or all fields.

The general features we have developed or plan to provide are:

1. *Interactive display of CT (and other) data.* The full capabilities for interactive display, which have become routine for CT scanners, should be made available and enhanced to facilitate appreciation of the three-dimensional relationships among anatomic features.

2. *Means for identifying structures of interest.* Facilities for "marking up" the CT data should be as easy to use as a grease pencil; in particular, the marks should be easy to alter and add to.

3. *Synthesis of all the diagnostic information available.* Much vital data come from diagnostic information other than CT. The availability of CT data must not lead to a failure to take full advantage of such data, which can include: radiographic studies, e.g., plane films or special studies (small bowel series, angiograms, etc.); conventional laminograms or polytomes; xerograms; ultrasonograms; radioisotope scintigrams; and findings from the history, the physical examination, and surgical exploration. It is also important that the program can be used in the absence of CT data.

4. *Assistance in choosing an external beam approach and field shape from any available direction.* The goal of encompassing the target volume and avoiding, as much as possible, adjacent normal tissues is a three-dimensional task and is not well solved by viewing only one or a few selected transverse planes. A beam's-

eye view of the structures of interest, in which the planner is shown the structures as though looking along the central axis of a radiation beam with an eye placed at the radiation source, is particularly helpful. From this stance the relative disposition of all identified structures is readily appreciated, and a field-shaping aperture or collimator setting can be very naturally designed.

Any motion of the treatment beam or patient support device which can be achieved in practice should be emulated by the program. Thus there is no requirement that external beams be coplanar, and fully "three-dimensional" treatments should result.

5. *Provide output of direct use in treatment design and implementation.* The program should generate such information as: (a) the outline of the field shaping aperture; (b) treatment machine parameters necessary for patient setup; (c) alignment film simulations to verify the treatment accuracy; (d) design parameters for compensating filters (e.g., life-size tracings for lead sheets to be used in a sandwich); and (e) parameters necessary for dynamic therapy.

6. *Provide calculation and display of dose at any point or points, taking into account inhomogeneities, for any available radiation modality.* The estimated dose throughout the irradiated volume must be displayed and its relationship to the anatomy established. The dose from several components of therapy must be capable of being shown, both separately and in sum.

7. *Compare rival treatment plans.* Conventionally, two or more plans are compared by showing the plans side by side. With fully three-dimensional dose distributions and beam angulations not restricted to lie in a single plane, more versatile presentations of the data are mandatory.

8. *Be interactive and easy to use.* The program features should be easy to summon up and rapid in execution; changes should be readily incorporated.

We call programs which provide these or similar capabilities "multidimensional," rather than the more usual term "three-dimensional," in order to emphasize the need to present to the planner numerous types or dimensions of information. In addition to the three spatial dimensions, one may wish to display anatomical information such as CT number, data from one or more diagnostic studies, a dose distribution, a rival dose distribution, and annotations. At a minimum, one should be able to display six dimensions simultaneously, a requirement which poses a formidable challenge.

ACKNOWLEDGMENTS

Supported in part by grant CA-21239 from the National Cancer Institute, a grant from the Whitaker Foundation, and a Research Career Development Award CA-00251 from the National Cancer Institute (M.G.).

Computed Tomography in Radiation Therapy,
edited by C. C. Ling, C. C. Rogers, and
R. J. Morton. Raven Press, New York © 1983

Current Industrial Developments in the Application of Computed Tomography to Radiotherapy Planning

N. Suntharalingam

Thomas Jefferson University, Philadelphia, Pennsylvania 19107

"Computerized axial tomography scanners have proved themselves as diagnostic tools. They are here to stay. I am convinced it makes sense for any hospital to have at least a head scanner" (4). So said the head of Iowa's Health Facilities Council, as his council gave what amounted to routine approval for the purchase of two computed tomographic (CT) scanners by two Des Moines hospitals. Certainly such views from a state health planning head would have been unheard of a year ago, and they appear to reflect a changing environment across the United States. This change signifies the acceptance of CT as a conventional medical procedure and not as an experimental technique. By the end of 1979 there were 1,254 CT scanners in the United States. One manufacturer alone sold about 400 new scanners in 1980 and hopes to reach the 1,000 mark by the end of 1981. Industry experts expect the number of scanners sold in 1981 to double the 1980 sales.

In this context, it might be useful to look at some data on the practice of radiation therapy in the United States with special attention on the type of facilities and equipment in current use. These data have been collected in an on-going study (3). Table 1 shows a comparison of the data collected for the years 1977 and 1980. Even though the data for 1980 are not complete, they show that there are more than 1,500 megavoltage treatment machines in current use, with a trend to move toward high-energy accelerators as the preferred unit. Simulators have not been widely accepted in the past, but the new data show that about 40% of the megavoltage facilities do perform simulation on a dedicated simulator. This is an indication of the current direction of the radiotherapy community in obtaining accurate information for the management of patients. Unfortunately, questions relating to use of CT and computerized treatment planning were not included in the last survey but will be included in the survey for 1982.

If industrial developments are to be initiated to meet the needs of the radiation therapy community, it would be useful to have some information on the patient population in the United States. It is estimated that the total number of cancer patients who receive some form of radiation treatment is close to 360,000 per year,

TABLE 1. *Practice of radiation therapy in the United States*

Type of facility	1977	1980[a]
Megavoltage facilities	1,068	993
Megavoltage machines	1,479	1,509
Cobalt-60 units	881	748
Accelerators	598	761
Simulators	268	409
With fluoroscopy	159	250
Radiographic only	109	159
Facilities		
>1,100 New patients	17	24
350 to 1,100 New patients	367	364
<350 New patients	684	605

Data from ref. 3.
[a]1980 Data incomplete.

and about 45% of these patients are treated with curative intent. It should also be of interest to note that a large proportion of the patients are treated at hospital-based facilities and not at university-type or free-standing facilities. About 24 facilities treat over 1,100 new patients a year, whereas about 600 facilities treat fewer than 350 new patients a year. Thus it is not difficult to see that radiation therapy is a small patient volume discipline with the need for high-cost sophisticated equipment.

NEEDS IN RADIATION THERAPY

Certain modern trends in radiation therapy were recognized and documented in 1976 (1). Two trends selected from this list are: (a) the digital computer is widely and increasingly used as a means of calculating dose distributions; and (b) considerable stress is now placed on the acquisition of accurate data concerning the patient's anatomy and delineation of the target volume. The gradual utilization of the simulator—an apparatus incorporating a diagnostic x-ray tube constructed so as to simulate a radiation treatment unit in respect of its geometrical, mechanical, and optical properties—partly established the need for accurate data. In fact, in the same report (1) the simulator functions were defined as: (a) to assist in localizing tumor and internal organs in one of several views, to make the projections of points of interest on the skin, and hence to construct accurate cross-sectional diagrams of the patient; and (b) to check the suitability of the proposed beams and to facilitate small adjustments.

Anticipating the future impact of CT scanning on the practice of radiation therapy, the Committee on Radiation Oncology Studies prepared a report (5) in 1978 defining and emphasizing the importance of local-regional control to ultimate survival and decreased morbidity of cancer. It was recognized that CT scanning coupled with computerized treatment planning and dosimetry offer a great potential for improving outcome of radiation treatments through accurate localization of tumor and critical normal structures and by utilizing the tissue density and attenuation coefficients to increase the accuracy of dose calculations. In view of the fact that there are already hundreds of CT scanners installed for diagnostic use, some basic additional requirements that such units should satisfy to meet the particular requirements of radiation therapy were suggested and are given in Table 2. It was the opinion of the Committee that none of the specifications requested would lead to substantial modification of existing units, nor would they detract from their use as a diagnostic scanner.

Of course, the ideal situation would be to have CT scanners dedicated for use in a radiation therapy department. Some might question the cost justification for such a unit, but it certainly would not be difficult to show how valuable such a device would be at least in some of the large facilities. A dedicated scanner would be particularly useful for addressing relevant clinical research questions, particularly in the areas of tumor localization, tumor staging, treatment planning, and dose-response studies. The CROS report has presented design criteria for a dedicated scanner, and these are given in Table 3. These requirements are in addition to those mentioned for diagnostic scanners. A similar list of required features of a CT scanner for dedicated use in radiation therapy has been proposed by Goitein (2), and these are given in Table 4. All these requirements are quite realistic, both technically and economically, and most CT manufacturers should be in a position to satisfy the desires of the radiation therapy community.

TABLE 2. *Diagnostic CT scanner with therapy options*

1. Ability to transfer accurate position information from CT scanner to therapy treatment machine.
2. Data format and data transfer to dose calculation computer.
3. Derivation of information in three dimensions. Sagittal/coronal reconstruction as well as simulation of a portal view.
4. Good reproducibility of scans.

From ref. 5.

TABLE 3. *Dedicated CT scanner for radiotherapy*

1. High-contrast spatial resolution 2 mm with 256 × 256 matrix covering 50 cm.
2. Attenuation coefficients at treatment energies.
3. Variable kVp and filter combination.
4. Multiple scans to be made in less than 15 min.
5. Storage capability for up to 100 slices per patient.
6. Variable scan times.
7. Life-size hard copy of scan image.
8. Presentation of CT data in any plane.

From ref. 5.

TABLE 4. *Required features of a CT scanner used in radiation therapy*

1. Excellent spatial and absorption coefficient resolution.
2. Capability of continous scanning of a large number of thin sections at one per 10 sec.
3. High anode and x-ray tube housing cooling rates.
4. High geometric and photon conversion efficiencies of detectors.
5. Large patient aperture and large diameter of reconstruction.
6. Scan without bolus material.
7. Generate AP and lateral "plain films."
8. Display sagittal and coronal views.

From ref. 2.

TABLE 5. *Manufacturers' recommended scanners for radiation therapy*

Manufacturer	CT scanner	CT and radiation therapy planning
Pfizer	0200 FS	PZ-SIM (TP-11 software)
General Electric	CT/T 8800	RT/Plan (stand-alone) (Royal Marsden software)
		RTP software (with scanner)
Picker	Synerview	SYNERPLAN (independent/shared) (TP-11 software)
Technicare	Deltascan 200 HR	Deltaplan II (stand-alone or add-on) (Memorial/Sloan-Kettering software)
Siemens	Somatom 2	EVADOS with EVALUSKOP (independent)
		SOMADOS (with scanner) (Uppsala SI-DOS U-2 software)
Philips	Tomoscan 310	GEMINITPS (stand-alone)

CURRENT DEVELOPMENTS

When attempting to obtain information on current developments in CT for radiation therapy, a simple, short questionnaire was mailed to various manufacturers known to be involved with CT scanners and CT-based radiation treatment planning computer systems. Most manufacturers recommended, as seen in Table 5, their top-of-the-line diagnostic CT scanners for use in radiation therapy. Pfizer is the only group that has developed and is marketing a scanner dedicated for radiotherapy. (It has now become known that Elsinct has purchased Pfizer Medical Systems.) Although most of the CT scanners currently recommended are third- or fourth-generation scanners and are priced in the range of $800K to $950K, Pfizer chose to develop their second-generation 0200 FS scanner as a dedicated unit for radiation therapy with software packages for both "simulation" and dose calculations for a total package price of about $400K. This special unit is called the PZ-SIM, and it is intended to integrate three therapy processes usually performed separately, i.e., CT scanning for localization, dose calculation, and treatment planning and simulation. All of the scanning and image manipulation functions of the 0200 FS are preserved in PZ-SIM. A fully CT-interfaced treatment planning system using the AECL TP-11 software is provided for dose distribution calculations, with the ability to display dose distributions superimposed on the CT images. Treatment plans are "simulated" by illuminating on the patient's skin for marking the user-defined regular or irregular beam portals. The total planning process will thus require a rather long time with the patient remaining on the CT scanner table while all three processes are completed. At this early stage it is somewhat difficult to predict the overall acceptability of such an integrated device. There are a total of six units, either already installed or awaiting delivery, and it should be of interest to hear about the experiences and acceptance in the field. The CT-interfaced treatment planning software package is always available as an option on all Pfizer CT scanners for a price of about $37K. Several facilities have made this feature available on their Pfizer diagnostic scanners.

The General Electric CT/T 8800 scanner is today the most widely used body scanner in the United States. The high spatial and contrast resolution with the choice of 4.8-sec. or 9.6-sec. scanning time has made this scanner very acceptable for therapy patients as well. General Electric has two products classified as CT/treatment planning packages, the GE RT/Plan and the RTP software. The GE RT/Plan is a stand-alone radiation treatment planning computer system with high-quality CT image display and real-time dose matrix calculations and display of isodose contours. This requires the transfer of CT scan data from the scanner to the independent system, which is housed in the radiation therapy department. The important feature is the ability to manipulate and display the CT scan image without any degradation of the quality. Additionally, the interactive capabilities and the speed of dose calculations are very good, these being achieved by improved software techniques. The RT/Plan dose calculation software was originally developed by the physics group at the Royal Marsden Hospital in England. There are eight such systems installed in various departments of widely different patient population size, and it is somewhat early to comment on their acceptability. This stand-alone system is priced at about $235K. The RTP system is simply a software package that runs in the CT hardware configuration or in the independent physician's diagnostic console. This software is limited to only external beam calculations and is available on all GE scanners at no additional cost. Eleven radiation therapy facilities are currently using this software for their treatment planning dose calculations.

Picker International has developed a CT/treatment planning package for use with their SYNERVIEW fourth-generation CT scanners. The treatment planning system, called SYNERPLAN, uses the AECL TP-11 software and has been extended to include three-dimensional scatter correction capability utilizing information from multiple CT slices. The SYNERPLAN is available as a shared system with the CT scanner for an extra $35K. It is also available as an independent CT-based treatment planning system for about $167K.

Technicare, in collaboration with the Memorial/Sloan-Kettering medical physics group, has developed a CT-based treatment planning system for use with their

Deltascan 2000 series CT scanners. The Deltaplan II system is available as a stand-alone system and has all of the display and image manipulation capabilities similar to those available on the Delta-2000 scanners. CT images need to be transferred from any Delta scanner via magnetic tape or floppy discs. The dose computational software represents the latest in programs developed at Memorial/Sloan-Kettering over the past 25 years. The stand-alone system is now available for a cost of $180K. The treatment planning software is available as an optional add-on configuration for a cost of $20K.

The two large European manufacturers of radiology equipment, Siemens and Philips, have both developed CT-based treatment planning systems. The Siemens system is an updated version of the original planning system developed at Uppsala. The EVADOS system is quite elaborate and uses an auxiliary operating console called the EVALUSKOP, which permits full handling and interpretation of the CT scans away from the scanner. The EVADOS system is priced at about $280K, and even though a large number of such systems have been sold in Europe they are yet to be installed in the United States. A slightly less sophisticated version called SOMADOS is also available but as an add-on to the CT scanner. Philips recently announced the availability of a stand-alone CT-based treatment planning system called GEMINI in the price range of about $200K. Very little additional information is available at this time except that it is an extension of the algorithms developed by Van de Geijn for the Philips treatment planning computer system.

The second category of industrial developments in the use of CT in radiation therapy is in the incorporation of CT scan information into treatment planning computer systems. Table 6 lists the manufacturers and the treatment planning systems offered by each of them. AECL, a pioneer in treatment planning computer systems with about 145 of their TP-11 systems in current use, has announced the availability of Theraplan, which allows display of and interaction with CT images for treatment planning purposes. The new system integrates all the existing software features and dose calculation programs of the TP-11 together with an expanded inhomogeneity correction algorithm based on the equivalent TAR method. Theraplan is a universal CT planning system which has been designed to accept CT scan information from most major CT scanners in use today. Theraplan requires CT scan information to be transferred via magnetic tape and offers color-enhanced visual display of isodose distributions superimposed on the gray scale CT image.

TABLE 6. *Radiation therapy planning systems with CT*

Manufacturer	Treatment planning system
AECL	Theraplan (magnetic tape)
ADAC Laboratories	CT connection (magnetic tape/floppy disc), also integrated digitizer/back-projector
ATC	RAD Plan
Capintec	CTS series
CMS	Modulex

The stand-alone Theraplan system is priced at $133K, and about 18 systems have now been installed. Also, TP-11 users can upgrade their system to a full Theraplan system with the needed hardware and software modifications for about $70K.

ADAC Laboratories have an interactive computer-based system for treatment planning using a unique back-projection system to utilize contour information from CT scans or echograms. The system features the full complement of external beam and intracavitary dose calculation software developed in collaboration with the Northwest Medical Physics Center. This complete system is priced at $79K. More recently ADAC have also made available an optional CT connection. This allows the direct use of digital CT scan data, transferred via magnetic tape or floppy discs, in the treatment planning process. Patient scans may be displayed on the treatment planning system console together with superimposition of isodose distributions. This total system with the CT connection is priced at $99K. There are about 60 ADAC systems in use, and about half of them are using some CT scan information in their planning process.

Three other treatment planning systems in current use have also incorporated the use of CT information; they are the ATC RAD Plan (old Rad-8 system), the Capintec CTS Series 8 systems, and CMS Modulex systems. These systems are all priced in the range of $70K to $95K.

DISCUSSION

It is quite clear that little if anything is happening in the CT industry toward the development of a CT scanner dedicated to radiation therapy. This is not surprising, as there is considerable concern whether the radiation therapy community as a whole is ready to have dedicated CT scanners for their exclusive use in patient treatment planning and management. Although certain large departments would prefer to have their own scanners and probably could easily justify their use from a cost-benefit point of view, several facilities believe they could handle their needs on diagnostic scanners already available in their hospitals. Certainly CT scanning activities and primarily body scanning are bringing together once again the diagnostic radiologist and the radiation oncologist. If an improved working relationship could be established, there is no doubt that currently available diagnostic scanners could be put to good use in also satisfying the needs of radiation therapy. This does not mean that further improvements or modifications on diagnostic CT scanners are not required. Some of the special requirements addressed earlier are needed. There is some evidence of progress toward meeting some of these requirements, and new developments in this regard are to be announced toward the end of the year.

The primary development of use of CT in radiation therapy has no doubt been in the area of treatment planning dose computations. While physicists have been addressing problems relating to dose distribution calculations in the presence of tissue heterogeneities for both photon and electron beams, the manufacturers have been busy with developing improved software for interactive and display purposes. An important question that needs to be addressed soon is the adequacy of the quantitative nature of the electron density data for automatic entry into dose computation systems. What corrections, if any, should be considered for beam hardening, frequency response of reconstruction algorithms, motion artifacts, alignment difficulties, and statistical variations of CT numbers? Another area of concern has been the method of transfer of digital CT scan information from scanner to independent dose computation systems. Should the transfer be via magnetic tape, floppy discs, or hard copy? What are the advantages and disadvantages of each approach? Answers to these questions are badly needed, and industry needs to get together with the user to arrive at an optimal selection of hardware.

While CT manufacturers have moved toward developing high-priced, elaborate, and sophisticated stand-alone treatment planning systems primarily for use with their own CT scanners, treatment planning computer systems manufacturers have expanded into the area of using CT scan information for both dose calculation and display. These developments and their rapid acceptance by the radiation therapy community will certainly impact on the overall outcome of radiation therapy treatments. An important question in the minds of several potential users of these systems is: What is one getting that is different and worth about $100K extra from the independent CT-based treatment planning systems? Some obvious factors are speed, interactive capabilities, on-line changes in treatment plans and subsequent display of dose distributions, diagnostic quality of CT image displayed, and last but not least the accuracy of the dose calculation algorithms. At this stage there is some difficulty in identifying the advantages of one system over the other, but it is obvious that there are certain trade-offs and compromises to keep the cost down. The true answers will have to come from the users themselves.

Finally, it is worth emphasizing that when one considers the use of CT in radiation therapy one is looking at the whole process of radiation therapy and not just radiation dose calculations. It is rather unfortunate that our community has accepted the terminology "treatment planning" as being interchangeable with "dose calculations." It may be more useful to refer to the whole process of the management of the patient as "planning of treatment," which then includes a sequence of processes beginning with diagnosis, tumor staging, localization, selection of treatment technique, dose calculation, simulation, implementation of intended treatment, and finally ending with follow-up during and after treatment. It is toward this whole process that one should consider the impact of CT. The need for a close collaboration between the CT industry and the radiation therapy community then becomes clear.

ACKNOWLEDGMENTS

The help provided by several individuals from industry on their respective systems is acknowledged. In particular, Joseph Ting (General Electric), Brian Heidtman (Pfizer), John Rhodda (Technicare), Tom Morgan (Philips), Larry Windedahl (ADAC), and David Hall (AECL) were also helpful in participating in the round-table discussion during the symposium.

REFERENCES

1. Determination of absorbed dose in a patient irradiated by beams of x- or gamma rays in radiotherapy procedures. ICRU Report No. 24, 1976.
2. Goitein, M. (1979): Computed tomography in planning radiation therapy. *Int. J. Radiat. Oncol. Biol. Phys.*, 5:445 (editorial).
3. Kramer, S. (principal investigator): *Patterns of Care in Radiation Therapy*. American College of Radiology, Philadelphia.
4. Special report: Scanning the CAT scene. *Cost Containment Newsletter*, 1981.
5. Stewart, J. R., et al. (1978): Computed tomography in radiation therapy (CROS report). *Int. J. Radiat. Oncol. Biol. Phys.*, 4:313.

Computed Tomography in Radiation Therapy,
edited by C. C. Ling, C. C. Rogers, and
R. J. Morton. Raven Press, New York © 1983

Current Methods and Algorithms in Radiation Absorbed Dose Calculation and the Role of Computed Tomography: A Review

James A. Purdy and Satish C. Prasad

Physics Section, Mallinckrodt Institute of Radiology, Washington University School of Medicine, St. Louis, Missouri 63110

Since the introduction of computer treatment planning in radiation therapy during the mid-1950s, the development of dose computational algorithms has principally been directed toward external photon beam and interstitial and intracavitary treatment techniques. However, the increased availability of high-energy linear accelerators capable of multienergy electron beams and the complexity of treatment techniques currently in use has spurred interest in the development of electron beam dose computational algorithms in recent years.

In general, the presently available methods of absorbed dose calculation for an irregular field and for a heterogeneous medium are only approximate, and therefore their use for radiation therapy treatment planning is limited. The dose distribution in a patient is usually computed using central axis depth dose data in conjunction with dose profiles measured at several depths over a range of field sizes. The radiation beam data refer in one way or another to measurements in a homogeneous water phantom under reference conditions, i.e., beams of square cross section, symmetrical energy fluence, and standard distance to and normal incidence on a flat surface. Tissues which differ from water in composition (in terms of electron density), e.g., lung, bone, and fat, perturb the dose at a point in a patient by modifying the primary radiation as well as the scatter component of the radiation beam. The various algorithms that have been developed to correct for these effects all suffer in some degree in not being a three-dimensional computation which can take into account the composition, size, and shape of the inhomogeneity.

The development of computed tomography (CT) has generated new enthusiasm in treatment planning by providing detailed geometric and physical data for tumor and normal tissue localization. As CT numbers are related to the linear attenuation coefficients for x-rays of diagnostic energies, they may be correlated with the electron density of the corresponding tissues. For the x-ray energies used in radiation therapy, Compton scatter is the dominant mode of interaction, and thus the absorption and scattering of photons in tissue depends primarily on the electron density. In fact, several treatment planning systems which utilize CT data directly are already commercially available. In these systems the emphasis has been on CT data transfer and display capabilities. However, the most important component in a treatment planning system is the dose calculation in a specified medium at a specified point under specified geometric and physical conditions of beam and medium. Much work is still needed in the development of true three-dimensional dose computation algorithms if CT is to realize its true potential in radiation therapy treatment planning.

This chapter presents an overview of the various algorithms which have been used to compute the absorbed dose within a heterogeneous medium for photon and electron beams. This material is to serve as the foundation for the subsequent discussion on the specific details of the physics of the inhomogeneity problem and the current and future developments in clinical dosimetry as a result of CT application in radiation therapy.

EXTERNAL PHOTON BEAM DOSE COMPUTATION

At the present time, most radiotherapy treatment plans consist of two-dimensional dose distribution in transverse planes of a patient. The dose computations performed on the commercially available digital computers are based on algorithms developed over the last 15 years. Among the methods most commonly used are those developed by Cunningham et al. (6), Milan and Bentley (13), and van de Geijn (19). A brief discussion of each method follows.

Cunningham's Method

In the Cunningham method the dose at any point in an irradiated volume is separated into a primary component and a scatter component. The primary and scatter components are calculated separately, and the total dose at any point is obtained by summing the two. This method uses experimentally determined quantities, e.g., the tissue/air ratio (TAR) and the scatter/air ratio (SAR).

The dose ($D_{primary}$) at depth d in a phantom due to a primary beam is given by

$$D_{primary} = D_A(d) \cdot TAR(d,0) \cdot f(x,y)$$

where $D_A(d)$ is the dose in air along the central axis at the depth of calculation, $TAR(d,0)$ is the zero area TAR at the depth of calculation, and $f(x,y)$ is a factor describing the radiation beam intensity in air at the point in a plane perpendicular to the central axis. The function $f(x,y)$ depends on three parameters: the diameter of the radiation source, the slope of the beam intensity profile in air at the point where the intensity falls to 50%, and the collimator transmission factor. These parameters are determined by fitting the mathematical expression for the intensity function with experimentally determined intensity profiles. The scatter dose at the point of interest is determined by summation of the SAR using Clarkson's method (4).

For routine treatment planning, beams are generated on a computer for a given source-skin distance (SSD), field size, and beam quality. These beams are generated assuming a homogeneous water medium and flat surface. The beam data usually consist of dose matrix points at the intersection of lines called fan lines and depth lines. One of the most common commercial treatment planning systems, the Artronix PC-12, uses 19 fan lines and 11 depth lines or 209 matrix points. Some of the more recent and larger systems have greatly increased these numbers (e.g., 41 fan lines and 31 depth lines on the CMS Modulex system). In the presence of the curvature of the body surface and internal homogeneities, appropriate corrections are required. For air gaps due to the body curvature, corrections based on methods similar to the "effective SSD method" are typically applied to the doses at appropriate points in a beam (9). One of the advantages of Cunningham's method is that it is general enough to handle irregular fields and blocked beams.

Milan and Bentley Method

The Milan and Bentley method relies heavily on beam data generated experimentally and stored in a computer for dose calculations. The data measured and stored consist of central axis depth dose tables (CAX data) and beam profile tables (off-axis ratios, OAR). The CAX data usually consist of percent depth dose (%DD) values at several depths (e.g., the RAD-8 uses 17 depths) for square field ranging from the smallest to the largest field size in steps of 2 cm for a given SSD. CAX data for an intermediate field is generated by interpolation. Rectangular fields are taken into account by using the data for the corresponding equivalent square field sizes. Profile data are measured and stored for several off-axis points (e.g., the RAD-8 uses 47 off-axis points at five depths ranging from d_{max} to the deepest CAX value). These 47 off-axis ratios lie on fan lines, 23 to left, 23 to right, and 1 on the central axis. Dose profile measurements are recommended for a square field in steps of 1 cm.

Again, note that the measured beam data stored in the computer are for a homogeneous water phantom and normal incidence. Therefore appropriate corrections similar to those used with Cunningham's method are needed to take into account body curvatures with inhomogeneities. A shortcoming of this method is that it is not readily applicable to irregular fields.

van de Geijn Method

In the van de Geijn method, the dose at any point is calculated from a knowledge of central axis percent depth dose, off-axis ratios, and TARs. For the purpose of dose calculations, four functions are stored in the computer or calculated from fits to the data: central axis percent depth dose, off-axis ratios in two principal plans of the beam, and TARs. A computer program based on these functions was described by van de Geijn (19). The interested reader should consult the original paper.

EXTERNAL PHOTON BEAM INHOMOGENEITY CORRECTION

The improved spatial and density description of tissue inhomogeneities provided by CT has produced renewed emphasis on the development of more accurate inhomogeneity correction algorithms for external photon beams. As indicated previously, the usual procedure for most inhomogeneity correction methods is to first assume that the irradiated medium is homogeneous and water-equivalent, and then obtain a correction factor to account for the presence of the inhomogeneity. Generally it is necessary to determine the water-equivalent path length between the point of calculation and the beam entrance point along a ray within the patient. These correction methods include the "effective attenuation method," the "isodose shift method," the "effective SSD method," the "TAR method", and the "power law TAR method" (9). All of these methods have inherent shortcomings associated with them, which will be discussed in detail in subsequent presentations.

For the purpose of overview and background, the algorithms for the most common methods are presented. The "effective attenuation method" correction factor (CF) is given by

$$CF = e^{\,\bar{\mu}\,(d - d_{\text{eff}})},$$

where $\bar{\mu}$ is the effective linear attenuation coefficient, which is empirically determined; d is the actual thickness; and d_{eff} is the water-equivalent thickness. A serious shortcoming of the method is that values of μ for different photon energies have not been sufficiently determined.

The "isodose shift method" was originally used to correct depth dose values for the curvature of the patient's skin surface and later applied to internal inhomogeneity considerations. Isodose lines are shifted by an amount equal to a constant $\times$ the thickness of the inhomogeneity as measured along a line parallel to the central axis and passing through the calculation point. The isodose curves are shifted away from the surface for lung and air cavities and toward the surface for bone. Values for the shift constant are empirically determined. This method suffers in that values for the shift parameters for the various beam qualities are not well determined.

The "effective SSD method," used by several of the commercial computer treatment planning systems, corrects the percent depth dose at a point behind a heterogeneity by calculating the water-equivalent depth based on the relative electron density. Thus for a point at depth (d) located behind a heterogeneity of thickness t, with a relative electron density of ρ_e (with respect to water), the percent depth dose is replaced by the percent depth dose at $d - t(1 - \rho_e)$ multiplied by an inverse square correction term:

$$[(\text{SSD} + d - t \cdot (1 - \rho_e))/(\text{SSD} + d)]^2$$

The "TAR method" correction factor (CF) is simply the ratio of two TARs in which the numerator is the TAR for the water-equivalent thickness (d_{eff}) and the denominator is the TAR for the actual thickness (d) of tissue along a ray from the surface of the phantom to the point of calculation. W_d is the width of the beam at the depth of calculation

$$CF = \frac{TAR(d_{eff}, W_d)}{TAR\ (d, W_d)}$$

The "power law TAR method" is a more sophisticated method originally proposed by Batho (2) and generalized by Young and Gaylord (20). This method accounts for the composition of the inhomogeneity and its position relative to the point of calculation. However, the extent or shape of the inhomogeneity is not taken into account. The correction factor (CF) for a point (P) beyond the inhomogeneity is given by

$$CF = \left(\frac{TAR(d_2, W_d)}{TAR(d_1, W_d)}\right)^{(\rho_e - 1)}$$

where d_1 and d_2 refer to the distances from point P to the near and far side of the non-water-equivalent material, respectively; W_d is the beam dimension at the depth of P; and ρ_e is the relative electron density of the inhomogeneity with respect to water.

The "equivalent TAR method" recently proposed by Sontag and Cunningham (16) makes direct use of CT scan slices for dose computation. The correction factor is based on the assumption that a quantity, analogous to a TAR, may be determined for nonhomogeneous medium by scaling the depth and field size in an appropriate manner. The scaling requires a knowledge of the relative electron densities over small volume elements. The correction factor (CF) is given by the ratio of two TARs

$$CF = \frac{TAR(d', \tilde{r})}{TAR(d, r)}$$

where d is the depth of calculation and r is the field radius at depth; d' and $\tilde{r}$ are the scaled values of these quantities. TAR $(d', \tilde{r})$ is determined by separating it into zero area TAR and SAR terms. The scaled quantities d' and $\tilde{r}$ are related to d and r, respectively by

$$d' = \frac{d}{n} \cdot \sum_{j=1}^{n} \rho_j \ \text{ and } \ \tilde{r} = r \cdot \tilde{\rho}$$

The summation over j is taken along the primary photon ray where there are n discrete inhomogeneity elements with relative electron density ρ_j. The term $\bar{\rho}$ is effective density which is a weighted average of relative density over the entire irradiated volume. Determination of $\bar{\rho}$ is crucial in this method.

The method has been tested in simple geometries, and good agreement (within 3.5%) has been found between measurements and calculation. This method reduces computational requirements by assuming that the scattered dose reaching the point of calculation in an irradiated volume can be adequately described by a single equivalent plane with appropriately scaled parameters. It has recently been adopted by one of the commerical systems.

The "delta volume method" is probably the more sophisticated inhomogeneity correction method being considered today. It was first proposed by Cunningham and Beaudoin (5) and later extended by Prasad et al. (10,15). In this method, the absorbed dose at each point is separated into primary and scatter components. The scatter component is obtained by summing contributions from small-volume elements (delta volume) of the entire irradiated body. TAR and SAR data are appropriately modified to account for the structural inhomogeneities in the irradiated volume. Multiple-slice CT data are required to characterize the irradiated volume in terms of electron density.

The scatter component can be cast into a summation over differential SAR terms $(\Delta^3 S_{water})$, which describe the scatter contributions from small volume elements (ΔV) in the irradiated volume. In the presence of inhomogeneities, $\Delta^3 S_{water}$ must be appropriately modified. Thus the scatter, $\Delta^3 S_{inhomo}$, coming from the volume element ΔV to a point P in the presence of inhomogeneities can be written as

$$\Delta^3 S_{inhomo} = \Delta^3 S_{water} \, N(x', y', z) \, f_1(x', y', z) \times f_2(x', y', z),$$

where $N(x', y', z)$ is the ratio of electron densities in volume element ΔV to that in water; $f_1(x', y', z)$ is a factor describing the attenuation of the beam (relative to water) due to inhomogeneities between the source and the volume element ΔV; and $f_2(x', y', z)$ is a factor describing the attenuation of scatter radiation (relative to water) due to the path inhomogeneities between ΔV and the calculation point. The function $f_2(x', y', z)$ can be obtained from a knowledge of electron densities along the path and the average energy of the scattered radiation. The average energy of the scattered beam can be calculated from the angle of scattering and the energy of the incident beam. The total SAR at the point P can be obtained by summing $\Delta^3 S_{inhomo}$ over the whole irradiated volume.

The primary component of the beam at point P can be calculated by correcting for the attenuation of the beam (relative to water) from a knowledge of the electron density along the beam path between the source and point P. The dose at P can thus be calculated from the scatter component, the primary component, and the dose in air at point P.

Agreement between computed values and experimental measurements in both simple and complex geometries have been found to be on the order of 2 to 3%. This method, however, suffers from the large computational effort required to obtain a full dose distribution in routine treatment planning. It is expected though that dedicated high-speed digital hardware may render this method practical in the not too distant future.

ELECTRON BEAM DOSE COMPUTATIONAL ALGORITHMS

As indicated previously, the increased availability of high-energy linear accelerators capable of multienergy electron beams and the complexity of treatment techniques currently in use has led to increased activity in this area of dose computation development. In addition, electron beam arc therapy is now being studied at several universities and appears to be a viable treatment technique which will require sophisticated treatment planning capability if it is to reach its potential.

An excellent discussion of the various algorithms proposed for quantitatively describing an electron beam dose distribution within a patient may be found in the review article by Sternick (18). Again, for purposes of background information, several of the more common electron beam dose computation algorithms are described here in general terms.

The "absorption coefficient method" (7) makes use of the fact that electron beam depth dose data show an empirical relationship with any medium, which can be expressed by a simple exponential

$$I(d) = 110 - 10 \exp (\mu d),$$

where $I(d)$ is the relative percent ionization, d is the distance beyond the depth at which depth $I(d)$ is 100%, and μ is an empirically determined coefficient for heterogeneous media, e.g., bone and lung.

The "coefficient of equivalent thickness (CET) method" (3) is based on empirical measurements either in a suitable phantom or *in vivo* in order to define a CET value which can be used to determine the dose distribution in a heterogeneous medium. The method may be illustrated as follows. The absorbed dose distribution data measured in a unit density medium are used as the reference. The depth doses are corrected along a ray by assuming that the attenuation of the electron beam by a thickness (t) of an inhomogeneity is equivalent to the attenuation by a thickness (t) multiplied by the appropriate CET value. The isodoses are shifted toward the entry surface if the CET value is greater than one and toward greater depth if the CET value is less than one.

The "absorption equivalent thickness (AET) method" (11) is similar to the CET method. Appropriate AET values based on empirical measurements are used to shift the unit density measured depth dose curves toward or away from the surface depending on the density of the inhomogeneity.

The "modified absorption coefficient (MAC) method" (1) extends the techniques described above to make additional corrections for the polarization effect, the deviation of the central axis percent depth dose from relationship $I(d) = 100 - 10 \exp(\mu d)$ for energies above 20 MeV, and the variation in densities of internal organs for a specific patient. The interested reader should consult the original paper (1).

The "age diffusion equation method" (17) is one of the more recent electron beam dose computation methods developed. The method significantly reduces the amount of data required for an accurate characterization of an electron beam. The method is based on the general age diffusion equation and has been successfully implemented for both a betatron and a linear accelerator. The development of this equation leads to

$$D(x,y,z,\tau) = \frac{D_0}{2}\left[\text{erf}\left(\frac{x_0(z) - x}{2(k\tau)^{1/2}}\right) + \text{erf}\left(\frac{x_0 + x}{2(k\tau)^{1/2}}\right)\right]$$

$$\times \left[\text{erf}\left(\frac{y_0(z) - y}{2(k\tau)^{1/2}}\right) + \text{erf}\left(\frac{y_0 + y}{2(k\tau)^{1/2}}\right)\right]$$

$$\times \cos\left[G_1(z/R_p)^2 + G_2(z/R_p) + G_3\right] \cdot \left[F/(F + z)\right]^2$$

$$\times \exp\left[-(2\pi/3R_p)\cdot(k\tau)^{1/2}\right]^2$$

where

$$
\begin{aligned}
D(x,y,z,\tau) &= \text{dose at depth } z \\
(k\tau)^{1/2} &= (C_z/R_P + P)^N \\
F &= \text{source-skin distance} \\
x_0 &= \tfrac{1}{2}(\text{width} + K_e)\cdot[(F + z)/F] \\
y_0 &= \tfrac{1}{2}(\text{length} + K_e)\cdot[(F + z)/F] \\
R_p &= \text{practical range}
\end{aligned}
$$

$$
\left.
\begin{aligned}
&G_1 \\
&G_2 \\
&G_3 \\
&C \\
&N \\
&P
\end{aligned}
\right\} \quad \text{constants for a given energy}
$$

$$
\begin{aligned}
K_e &= \text{field size correction for edge effects} \\
k\tau &= \text{age diffusion parameter}
\end{aligned}
$$

The error function factors account for the percent depth dose variation with field size. The shape parameter P characterizes the beam diffuseness at the surface, C characterizes the increase in the diffuseness with depth, and N is the overall shape-changing parameter. G_1, G_2, and G_3 are parameters calculated from measured central axis depth dose data, N and P. In practice, the parameters are determined at each energy for a single field size. The algorithm can then be used to predict the dose distribution for the other field sizes. Modifications of the generated dose distributions to account for the presence of inhomogeneities can be made using any of the ray methods previously discussed.

The "pencil beam approximation method" (8,12) is based on the hypothesis that the dose distribution in a broad, parallel electron beam entering a uniform phantom can be constructed from a series of narrow pencil beams. The narrow beam dose distribution in a plane at a right angle to the beam axis must be either measured or calculated. The broad beam dose distribution in a plane is then calculated by summing the narrow beam profiles at appropriate spacings. This method has great potential to be able to account for the presence of even very small inhomogeneities.

ROLE OF CT IN BRACHYTHERAPY DOSE CALCULATIONS WITH INHOMOGENEITY CORRECTION

Among the various sources of errors in brachytherapy dose calculations are the uncertainty in localization of sources within the patient, uncertainty in the calibration of the source strength, the limitation of the computational algorithm, and dose perturbations due to the presence of inhomogeneities. CT scans will play an increasingly important role in eliminating some of the sources of uncertainties associated with brachytherapy calculations. Multiple CT scans with coronal and sagittal reconstruction should be able to localize sources more accurately within the patient. The thin linear sources and radioactive seeds used in brachytherapy do not appear to pose a significant problem to good CT image quality, and therefore hard-copy images of the CT scans can be used for precise localization of the sources. Even in the presence of metallic materials (e.g., a tandom), reasonably good CT scan images can be obtained. However, ovoids, which contain a large amount of metallic material, still pose a problem.

CT will surely help in developing computational algorithms by which tissue inhomogeneities can be taken into account. Prasad et al. (14) recently proposed a method in which a correction factor to the dose in unit density tissue is determined by suitably modifying the attenuation of the primary dose and the changes in scatter buildup factor in the presence of inhomogeneities. The water-equivalent path length between the source and the point of calculation is determined from a knowledge of the electron densities of the intervening tissue (which can be determined from CT scans). Then for a given gamma ray energy, the attenuation of the primary is calculated and the changes in scatter dose determined using the buildup factor for the water-equivalent path length. The dose from a finite linear source is obtained by summing doses from small elemental lengths.

CONCLUSIONS

In radiation therapy the accurate computation of absorbed dose to many anatomical sites within a patient is complicated by the presence of dose-perturbing inhomogeneities, e.g., bone and lung tissue. The location and absorption properties of these inhomogeneities must be precisely known in order to accurately account for the dose-perturbation effects. The absorption properties of tissues irradiated using beam modalities common to radiotherapy are determined primarily by the electron densities of the tissues. It is now well established that the CT numbers, which are proportional to the linear attenuation coefficient at diagnostic energies, can be related to the electron density of the various tissues. This capability of providing detailed geometric and physical data for tumor and normal structure specifications has generated considerable interest in the development of treatment planning algorithms which utilize CT scan data. Several commercial CT-based treatment planning systems are now available in which two-dimensional dose distributions can be overlaid on CT scans. In these systems the CT scan data are transferred to the treatment planning computer via magnetic tape or floppy disc. The CT number of each pixel is converted to an electron density by an empirically determined curve correlating CT numbers with electron density. The absorbed dose is then computed in two dimensions using algorithms developed prior to CT, with the exception that the difference in electron density of an individual pixel element relative to water is now taken into account.

The dose computational algorithms presently being used do not adequately account for the dose in transition regions, e.g., the buildup region at the patient's surface or near heterogeneous tissue interfaces within the body: nor do they account for the three-dimensional nature of the problem. For photon dose computation, the inhomogeneity correction for lung is the most significant. For electron beams, the inhomogeneity problem is even more serious because of the finite range and scattering properties peculiar to electrons. It is now clear that the CT scan can provide the detailed information concerning tissue localization and tissue composition that is required to greatly improve the patient model used in the dose computation algorithm. Thus the dose computation algorithm itself must now also be improved if it is not to be the limiting factor in determination of the dose within a patient.

SUMMARY

In radiotherapy the determination of the absorbed dose distribution within a patient is based on measurements in a homogeneous water phantom. Numerous corrections to such data are needed to compute the dose distribution within a patient. The accuracy of the computed dose distribution depends on a precise knowledge of the patient's contour as well as the size, location, and composition of the internal structures. The development of CT has given a new level of precision in internal structure localization and tissue characterization which has motivated new approaches to dose computations.

Techniques by which the quantitative anatomical data inherent in a CT scan can be directly used in radiation therapy dose calculations are reviewed herein. Emphasis is placed on the newly developed inhomogeneity correction algorithms which make direct use of three-dimensional arrays of CT numbers after they have been converted into electron densities. In addition, a review of our recent efforts in the development of a three-dimensional dose computation method using the differential scatter/air ratio (delta volume) approach is presented.

REFERENCES

1. Bagne, F. (1976): Electron beam treatment planning system. *Med. Phys.*, 3:31–38.
2. Batho, H. F. (1964): Lung corrections in cobalt 60 beam therapy. *J. Can. Assoc. Radiol.*, 15:79–83.

3. Boone, M. L. M., Almond, P. R., and Wright, A. E. (1969): High energy electron dose perturbations in regions of tissue heterogeneity. *Ann. N.Y. Acad. Sci.*, 161:214–232.
4. Clarkson, J. R. (1941): A note on depth doses in fields of irregular shape. *Br. J. Radiol.*, 14:265.
5. Cunningham, J. R., and Beaudoin, L. (1973): Calculations for tissue inhomogeneities with experimental verification. In: *Proceedings of the XIII International Congress of Radiology*, Madrid.
6. Cunningham, J. R., Shrivastava, P. N., and Wilkinson, J. M. (1972): Program IRREG—calculation of dose from irregularly shaped radiation beams. *Comp. Prog. Biomed.*, 2:192.
7. Dahler, A., Baker, A. S., and Laughlin, J. S. (1969): Comprehensive electron-beam treatment planning. *Ann. N.Y. Acad. Sci.*, 161:198–213.
8. Hogstrom, K. R., Mills, M. D., Cundiff, J. H., and Almond, P. R. (1981): Clinical evaluation of an electron beam algorithm. *Med. Phys.*, 8:577.
9. *ICRU Report 24* (1976): Determination of absorbed dose in a patient irradiated by beams of x or gamma rays in radiotherapy procedures. ICRU, Washington, D.C.
10. Larson, K. B., and Prasad, S. C. (1978): Absorbed-dose computations for inhomogeneous media in radiation-treatment planning using differential scatter-air ratios. In: *Proceedings of the Second Annual Symposium on Computer Application in Medical Care*, Washington, D.C.
11. Laughlin, J. S. (1965): High energy electron treatment planning for inhomogeneities. *Br. J. Radiol.*, 38:143–147.
12. Lillicap, S. C., Wilson, P., and Boag, J. W. (1976): Dose distributions in high energy electron beams: production of broad beam distributions from narrow beam data. *Phys. Med. Biol.*, 20:30–38.
13. Milan, J., and Bentley, R. E. (1974): The storage and manipulation of radiation dose data in a small digital computer. *Br. J. Radiol.*, 47:115–121.
14. Prasad, S. C., Bello, J., and Abrath, F. G. (1981): Tissue inhomogeneity corrections in implant radiotherapy. Presented at the 23rd Annual Meeting of the American Association of Physicists in Medicine, Boston.
15. Prasad, S. C., Purdy, J. A., Chen, W., and Larson, K. B. (1981): Experimental tests of three-dimensional dose calculations using differential scatter-air ratios. *Med. Phys.*, 8:559–560.
16. Sontag, M. R., and Cunningham, J. R. (1978): The equivalent tissue-air ratio method for making absorbed dose calculations in a heterogeneous medium. *Radiology*, 129:787–794.
17. Steben, J. D., Ayyangar, K., and Suntharalingam, N. (1979): Betatron electron beam characterization for dosimetry calculations. *Phys. Med. Biol.*, 24:299–309.
18. Sternick, E. S. (1978): Algorithms for computerized treatment planning. *Med. Phys. Monogr.*, 2:52–69.
19. van de Geijn, J. (1972): Revised and expanded version of the EXTDOS: a program for treatment planning in external beam therapy. *Comp. Prog. Biomed.*, 2:169.
20. Young, M. E. J., and Gaylord, J. A. (1970): Experimental tests of corrections for tissue inhomogeneities in radiotherapy. *Br. J. Radiol.*, 43:349–355.

Computed Tomography in Radiation Therapy,
edited by C. C. Ling, C. C. Rogers, and
R. J. Morton. Raven Press, New York © 1983

Physics of the Inhomogeneity Problem and the Present Status of Clinical Dosimetry

R. Mark Henkelman and John W. Wong

Ontario Cancer Institute and Department of Medical Biophysics, University of Toronto, Toronto, Ontario M4X 1K9, Canada

Considerable effort has been expended by clinical physicists on adapting the idealized physical measurements of dose in regular phantoms to the unique and irregular actualities of a cancer patient. Whatever the academic interest in precision or absolute dosimetry, clinical radiation therapy needs to know the amount of radiation delivered to an actual tumor within a given living patient.

Computed tomography (CT) has made us visually aware of the potentially large discrepancy between our physical dosimetry in phantoms and the highly irregular patient. Figure 1 illustrates the inhomogeneity problem by depicting a two-dimensional section through the real three-dimensional situation. The question to be addressed then is the following: Knowing the dose at a point P in a homogeneous

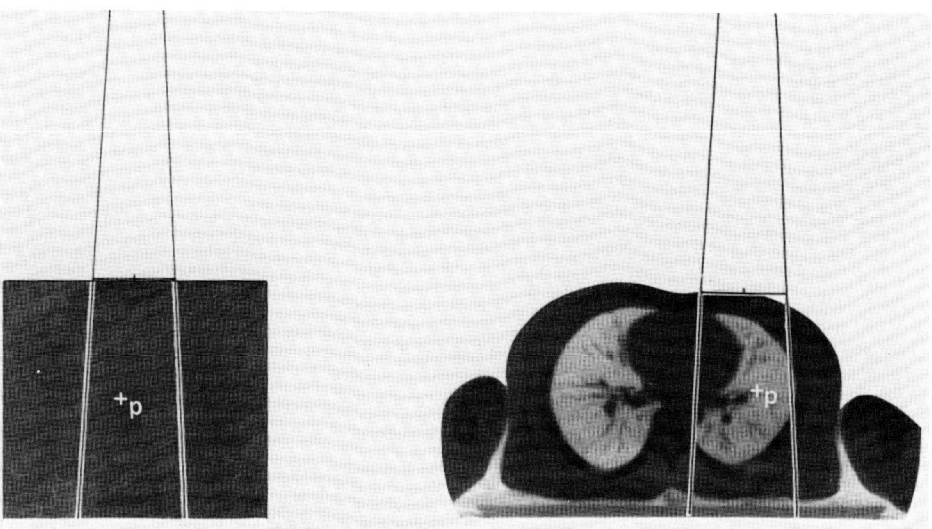

FIG. 1. The inhomogeneity problem. What is the relationship between the dose at a point P in a homogeneous phantom and the dose at a corresponding point P within the patient?

rectangular phantom (probably of unit density), what is the dose that will be delivered by the same radiation beam to a corresponding point P within the patient, taking into account the surface shape, density variation, and anatomical geometry of the individual? In showing us the range of anatomical variabilities among patients (e.g., marked left-right asymmetries in regions usually thought to be symmetrical, lung densities ranging from 0 to 0.5 g/ml rather than conforming to a literature specification of 0.35 g/ml, a transverse section that bears little quantitative correspondence to a standard anatomical atlas), CT has forced us to recognize that the inhomogeneity problem cannot be solved for a couple of textbook examples and then applied to all patients. Rather, it needs to be solved for at least a certain percentage of cases on an individual basis.

Figure 1 poses the inhomogeneity problem appropriately as a perturbation problem. The broad features of the exceedingly complex scattering processes that contribute to the dose in the phantom are generally preserved in the more complex patient anatomy. Therefore, at least for photons, only calculations of the change in dose should be attempted, as this is usually more efficient than calculating the absolute dose itself.

BASIC PHYSICS FACTORS

The important physical processes that need to be considered in solutions to the photon inhomogeneity problem are summarized in Fig. 2. A high-energy photon

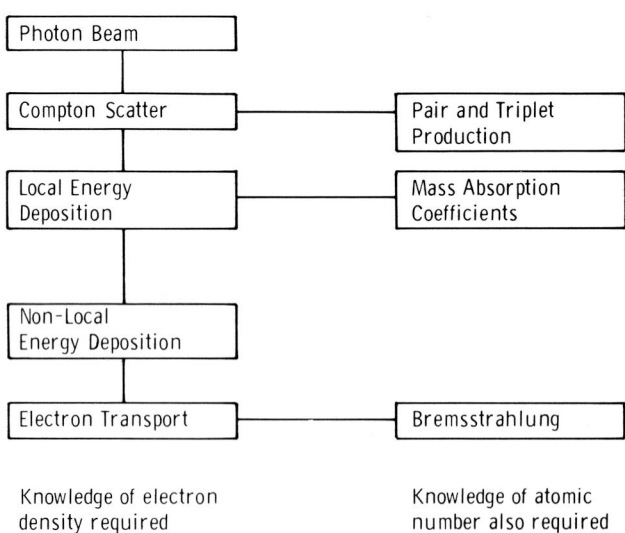

FIG. 2. Factors that need to be considered when arriving at solutions to the photon inhomogeneity problem.

beam interacts primarily through Compton scattering and pair or triplet production. Because in carbon at a photon energy as high as 10 MeV pair and triplet production amounts to only 20% of the interaction probability and falls to 3% at 3 MeV, Compton scatter is the only primary process that needs to be considered in inhomogeneity perturbation calculations.

In a photon radiation field, energy is not deposited by photons but rather by recoil electrons either from Compton scattering or from atomic photoelectric absorption. This energy absorption can be divided, for our purposes, into local and nonlocal energy deposition, depending on whether the range of the electrons exceeds the distances in which we are interested. Local energy deposition can be characterized by the mass energy absorption coefficient under conditions of charged-particle equilibrium. Nonlocal energy deposition results from energetic Compton electrons whose subsequent transport must be followed, including the possibility that they will convert kinetic energy to photons through *bremsstrahlung*. Although nonlocal energy deposition is affected significantly by inhomogeneities and increases in importance with primary photon energy, it is not considered further in this chapter. Instead, energy deposition will be assumed to be local and characterized by the mass absorption coefficient. Nonlocal energy deposition in the region of inhomogeneities (or, as it is frequently designated in the literature, the interface problem) has not yet been adequately studied and deserves more research, particularly as higher photon energies are becoming popular for therapy.

Figure 2 has been arranged into two columns. The factors in the left-hand column require a knowledge of only the electron density of the scattering medium (variations in electron stopping power due to differing atomic numbers of different tissues are not large and are not important for clinical inhomogeneity problem). The factors in the right-hand column would require information about the atomic number of the medium as well. CT measures the x-ray attenuation coefficient of tissue at a photon energy of around 100 KeV, which depends in a complex way on both the tissue electron density and the atomic number. However, adequate empirical relationships between CT number and electron density have been derived (2,12), particularly in light of the demonstration by Geise and McCullough (8) that a 4% error in electron density produces an error in dose of less than 2%. We assume, therefore, for the remainder of this work that an adequate conversion between CT numbers and electron density exists. Inhomogeneity calculations that depend on atomic number as well would require some form of dual energy CT scanning to provide the input parameters (1,5,13).

METHODS OF CALCULATING THE INHOMOGENEITY PROBLEM

Several distinct mathematical approaches to calculating the inhomogeneity problem have been considered: analytical, Monte Carlo, and, failing these, approximate.

Heroic attempts have been made by a number of researchers to find analytical solutions to the photon transport problem. Although much of this work has been motivated by a need to understand the physics of radiation shielding, it is still germane to radiation therapy. A good summary of available analytical methods and approaches is contained in an article by Fano et al. (6). Considerable progress can be achieved in calculating the photon transport in situations with simple boundary conditions, e.g., infinite fields, parallel beams in homogeneous infinite media. However, in geometrics with boundary conditions as restrictive as finite field size and finite depth, the integrals rapidly become intractable, leading to the conclusion that in the tortuous geometry of a heterogeneous patient little could be achieved along the lines of analytical solutions. The situation does not seem to have changed in the past 15 years, so that a conclusion drawn in 1967 still adequately summarizes the present situation: "At the present time, no generally acceptable method of handling the problem [of scatter dose in multiple layers] is available" (7).

At the other extreme, the increasing speed and capacity of electronic computers are making Monte Carlo calculations of photon transport possible. This approach has no problem with boundary conditions, except for the proviso that the speed of calculation decreases rapidly as the complexity of the geometry increases. However, Monte Carlo calculations are orders of magnitude too slow to be considered realistic clinical solutions to the inhomogeneity problem. Webb and Parker (16) have shown that to achieve 2% precision for a 20×20 cm^2 ^{60}Co field, 1.8×10^7 photon histories were required, taking 350 min on a CDC 7600 computer. From such figures it can be estimated that to achieve 2% accuracy by Monte Carlo calculation in a patient using a PDP 11/70 (a sizable computer by radiotherapy standards) would require about 10^5 min. The exact number is unimportant. What is important is that Monte Carlo calculations are orders of magnitude too slow for clinical use. This conclusion is not affected by the possibly faster hardware, array processors, or clever algorithms in the future. What does not yet seem to have been considered is a perturbational Monte Carlo calculation in which the change in dose from the homogeneous phantom due to changed scatter fluences is accounted for, instead of the customary calculation of total scatter dose from all photon histories. Such a perturbational Monte Carlo approach would need to follow photons through fewer orders of scatter and might achieve satisfactory accuracy within a reasonable length of time.

Due to the failure of analytical and Monte Carlo approaches, clinical algorithms for calculating the inhomogeneity problem are all approximate. It is quite appropriate to be using approximate corrections, as dosimetric accuracy of better than 2% is clinically irrelevant. However, with any approximate dose calculation method, it is essential to know what has been neglected and hence to be aware of the strengths of the approximation and also to be aware of the situations in which the method will give poorer results. Approximate corrections cannot be evaluated solely by testing a few sample cases. Instead, the inherent physical assumptions must be understood to allow one assurance of the range of validity of the approximation.

Approximations in the calculation of dose in an inhomogeneous medium need only to be made for the scattered component of the dose. The correction to the primary dose (or unscattered photons) due to inhomogeneities can easily be handled explicitly. This is true of each of the familiar correction methods, summarized by

Cunningham (4): the radiological path length method, the power law or Batho correction, the equivalent tissue/air ratio (TAR) method, and the differential scatter/air ratio method (dSAR). Any correction method that does not handle the primary dose without approximation is not worthy of consideration. The scatter component of the dose, however, will need to be approximated.

CONDITIONS TO BE SATISFIED BY APPROXIMATE CALCULATIONS OF THE SCATTER DOSE

Approximate solutions to the inhomogeneity correction problem will not yield rigorously correct answers for situations of arbitrary geometry. There are, however, a couple of specific geometries that we believe should be well approximated by any inhomogeneity correction method purported to be of general usefulness. These specific geometries are: (a) the small void in unit density material and (b) the homogeneous, non-unit density medium. Consideration of these two conditions gives some general insight into the necessary form of a correction algorithm.

Extensive experimental measurements have been made of the change in dose in water when a small void is introduced into the medium. Figure 3 shows the results of such experiments, the details of which are described elsewhere (17). As expected, a small void is most effective in changing the dose at the point of measurement (*P*) when it is introduced in the region above *P*. More surprising, however, is the observation that such removal of scattering material can result in increased scatter to *P*, as shown by the positive contours in Fig. 3. Such positive change is readily understood when attempts are made to calculate the effects seen in the experiment. Removal of scattering material from a region not only decreases the scatter fluence originating from the region but also increases the fluence of all photons passing through the region. When a cavity is introduced above the point *P*, it is the loss of attenuation of primary and scattered photons that contributes to the net increase in scatter dose to *P*. Figure 4 shows that calculations which follow perturbations of photon fluences up to second-order scattering satisfactorily account for the experimental measurements. First-order scattering alone is inadequate.

Such experiments provide a "benchmark" for proposed inhomogeneity correction methods. Any method designed to calculate the change in dose in an arbitrary complex geometry, we believe, should be able to give a good approximation to the much simpler problem of a single small inhomogeneity in a unit density phantom. In particular, any correction algorithm should predict an increased scatter dose when a small void is introduced in the region above the point of measurement, as shown in Fig. 3.

The other geometry in which we believe dose should be satisfactorily approximated is that of a homogeneous, non-unit density medium. Fortunately, the actual dose in a non-unit density medium is known if the dose in unit density has been fully characterized as a function of depth and field size due to an elegant theorem first stated by O'Connor (11). The theorem, illustrated in Fig. 5, can be stated as follows: The TAR at depth d in a medium of density ρ irradiated by a field of

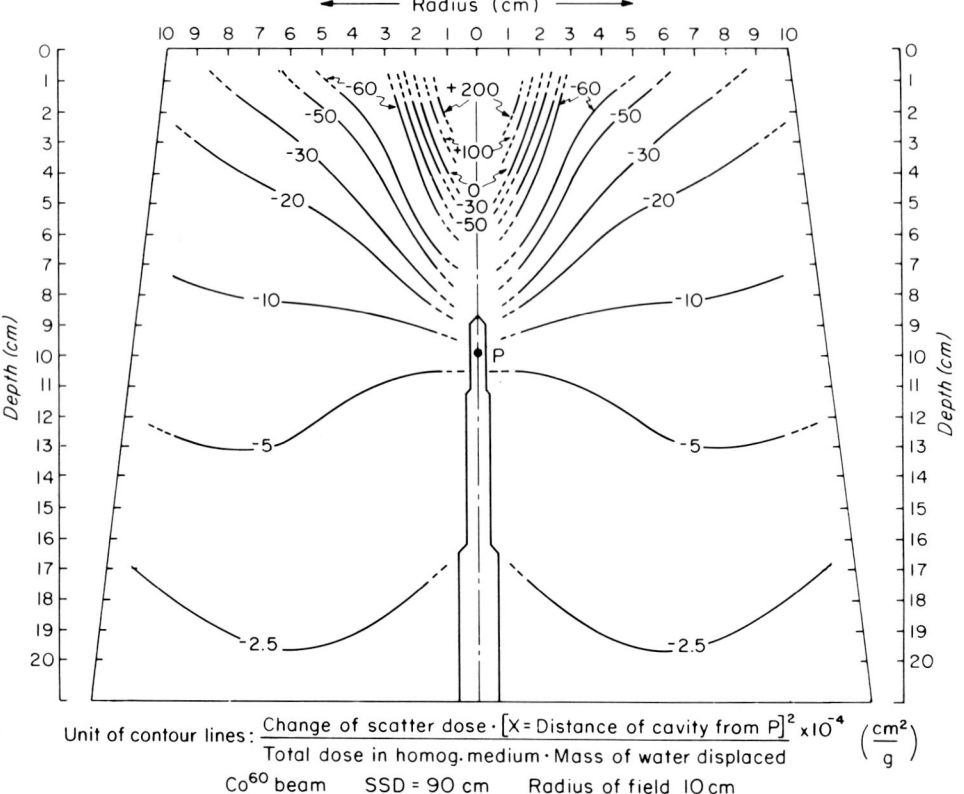

Radius (cm)

FIG. 3. Isoeffect contour plot of the measured change in dose with respect to the position of the small void in the water medium. (From ref. 17.)

radius r is equal to the TAR in a unit density medium at a depth of ρd with a field of radius ρr. This density scaling theorem can be generalized to irregularly shaped fields and phantoms but will be satisfactory for our use in the more restricted form given here. The theorem is valid under conditions in which the scatter dose all arises from Compton scattering.

The theorem can be easily proved by writing down the transport equation or by considering the conformal mapping illustrated in Fig. 5. A homogeneous, non-unit density medium is a particularly simple inhomogeneous geometry for which the true dose is known from the density scaling theorem and which should be well approximated by any correction method. In patients the most important inhomogeneity is lung, which approximates a homogeneous medium with density less than unity. The equivalent TAR correction method proposed by Sontag and Cunningham (15) was specifically designed to satisfy the constraint of this particular geometry.

Requiring a correction algorithm to satisfy both experimentally measured effects of a small void and the dose in a homogeneous, non-unit density medium teaches us something about the mathematical form of a valid solution to the inhomogeneity

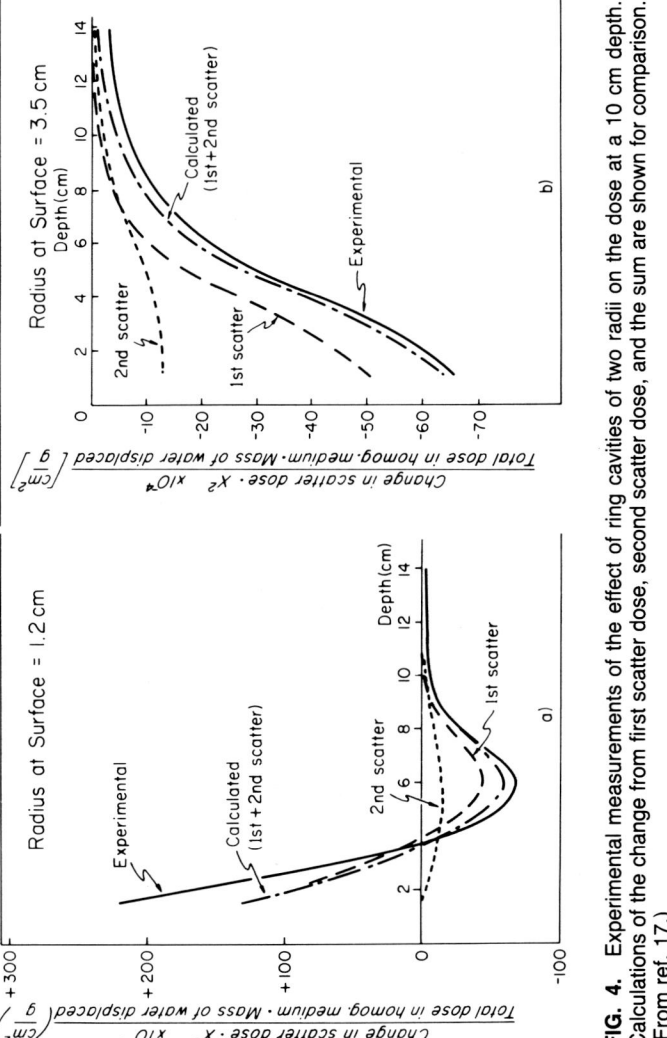

FIG. 4. Experimental measurements of the effect of ring cavities of two radii on the dose at a 10 cm depth. Calculations of the change from first scatter dose, second scatter dose, and the sum are shown for comparison. (From ref. 17.)

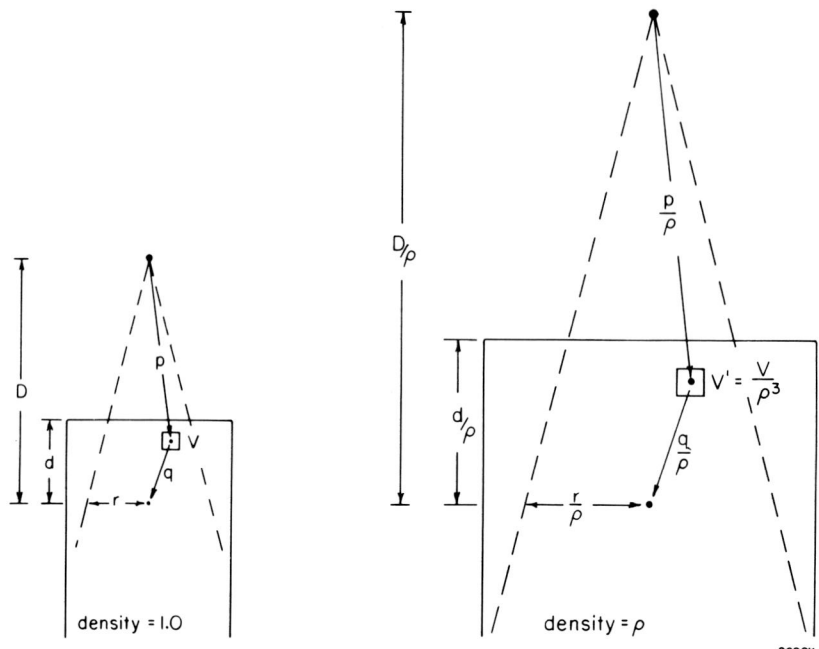

FIG. 5. Density scaling theorem that relates dose in a homogeneous unit density medium to that in a homogeneous, non-unit density medium.

problem. Consider a numerical example. In a medium $\rho = 0.5$, for a ^{60}Co field size of $r = 11$ cm at a depth of $d = 10$ cm, the TAR can be obtained from tabulated TARs in water using the density scaling theorem as TAR $(r = 5.5, d = 5) = 0.894$. Alternatively, a medium of density $\rho = 0.5$ can be thought of as consisting of many small cells of water in which half of the cells have been replaced with voids. Knowing the effect of each such void on the scatter dose as plotted in Fig. 3, and making the assumption (later to be shown invalid) that individual voids act independently (i.e., that the effects of small voids can be added), we can perform an appropriate integral over Fig. 3, from which we conclude that the change in SAR is -0.052. Therefore the TAR calculated from this alternative approach would be 0.942. Yet this answer deviates from the correct answer by more than 5% and would be even worse for the smaller densities of lung tissue. We conclude, then, that it is invalid to assume that individual inhomogeneities act independently; therefore, their effects are amenable to simple addition. Hence we conclude that any satisfactory solution to the inhomogeneity problem *must be intrinsically non-linear* in its handling of individual volume elements or pixels.

ARE PIXEL-BASED CORRECTION METHODS MORE ACCURATE THAN SIMPLER METHODS?

The increasing availability of CT-derived anatomical information for treatment planning is generating a pressure to use the great wealth of three-dimensional density data for inhomogeneity corrections. However, correction methods that account for the effects of pixels independently are of the wrong mathematical form, as was pointed out above. It is possible, therefore, for more refined pixel-based correction methods to give less accurate results than simpler methods.

Figure 6 shows a comparison of several inhomogeneity correction methods. Three pixel-based correction methods are shown as dashed lines: (a) the dSAR method developed by Beaudoin and Cunningham (3) and implemented by Larson and Prasad (9); (b) the summation of the measured effect of individual voids (Fig. 3) scaled by density, which assumes each void element acts independently; and (c) the scatter contribution from each pixel is again assumed to act independently but is assumed to be proportional to the density of the pixel, as would be the case in the method proposed by MacDonald et al. (10). As in the numerical example previously presented, we have used these methods to calculate the TAR at a depth of 10 cm in a homogeneous medium of density ρ irradiated by a ^{60}Co beam of radius 10 cm. The calculated approximate TARs are compared to the true TAR obtained from the density scaling theorem and are shown as a function of density. Each of these pixel-based methods is inferior to the simple Batho or power law correction (14). It is apparent then that "refined pixel-based correction algorithms," which use inappropriate functional forms, may be inferior to simpler bulk corrections that implicitly take into account the nonlinearity of the inhomogeneity corrections problems.

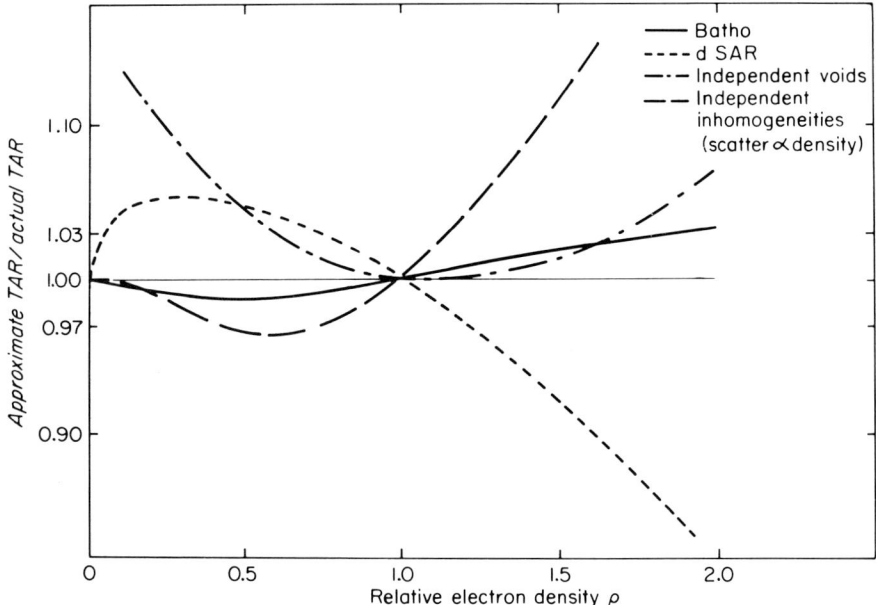

FIG. 6. Comparison of TARs calculated by approximate methods with the actual TAR obtained from the density scaling theorem in homogeneous medium of non-unit density. The differential scatter-air ratio (dSAR) method, the independent summation of the effect of individual voids, and the independent summation fo the contribution from individual volume elements that are proportional to density are all pixel-by-pixel corrections. The simpler Batho method, which treats the medium as a bulk inhomogeneity, gives superior results.

CONCLUSIONS

1. Solutions to the inhomogeneity correction problem will necessarily be approximate in any clinical implementation.

2. A knowledge of the physical assumptions of an approximation is essential to establishing its range of validity.

3. A valid solution to the inhomogeneity problem will treat the effect of individual pixels nonlinearly.

4. CT pixel-based correction methods are not guaranteed to be better than simpler methods, particularly if they treat inhomogeneities independently.

ACKNOWLEDGMENTS

This work is supported by the National Cancer Institute of Canada and the Ontario Cancer Treatment and Research Foundation. The authors have benefited immensely from discussion of this work with Drs. J. R. Cunningham and H. E. Johns, as well as other members of the staff at the Princess Margaret Hospital.

REFERENCES

1. Alvarez, R. F., and Marovski, A. (1976): Energy selective reconstructions in x-ray computerized tomography. *Phys. Med. Biol.*, 21:733–799.
2. Battista, J. J., and Bronskill, M. J. (1981): Compton scatter imaging of transverse sections: an overall appraisal and evaluation for radiotherapy planning. *Phys. Med. Biol.*, 26:81–99.
3. Beaudoin, L. (1968): M.Sc. thesis, University of Toronto.
4. Cunningham, J. R. (1981): Current and future development of clinical dosimetry with the use of CT. In: *Computed Tomography in Radiotherapy*, edited by C. Ling. Raven Press, New York.
5. Drost, D. J., and Fenster, A. (1980): Experimental dual xenon detectors for quantitative CT and spectral artifact correction. *Med. Phys.*, 7:101–107.
6. Fano, U., Spencer, L. V., and Berger, M. J. (1958): Penetration and diffusion of x-rays. In: *Handbook der Physik XXXVIII*, pp. 767–817. Springer-Verlag, Berlin.
7. Fitzgerald, J. J., Brownell, G. L., and Mahoney, F. J. (1967): *Mathematical Theory of Radiation Dosimetry*. Gordon and Breach Science Publishers, New York.
8. Geise, R. A., and McCullough, E. C. (1977): The use of CT scanners in megavoltage photon-beam therapy planning. *Radiology*, 124:133–141.
9. Larson, K. B., and Prasad, S. C. (1978): Absorbed dose computations for inhomogeneous media in radiation treatment planning using differential scatter-air ratios. In: *Proceedings of the Second Annual Symposium on Computer Applications in Medical Care*, pp. 93–99. IEEE, New York.
10. MacDonald, S. C., Keller, B. E., and Rubin, P. (1976): Method for calculating dose when lung tissue lies in the treatment field. *Med. Phys.*, 3:210–216.
11. O'Connor, J. E. (1957): The variation of scattered x-rays with density in an irradiated body. *Phys. Med. Biol.*, 1:352–369.
12. Parker, R. P., Hobday, P. A., and Cassell, K. J. (1979): The direct use of CT numbers in radiotherapy dosage calculations for inhomogeneous media. *Phys. Med. Biol.*, 24:802–809.
13. Rutt, B., and Fenster, A. (1980): Split-filter computed tomography: a simple technique for dual energy scanning. *J. Comput. Assist. Tomogr.*, 4:501–509.
14. Sontag, M. R., and Cunningham, J. R. (1977): Corrections to absorbed dose calculations for tissue inhomogeneities. *Med. Phys.*, 4:431–436.
15. Sontag, M. R., and Cunningham, J. R. (1978): The equivalent tissue-air ratio method for making absorbed dose calculations in a heterogeneous medium. *Radiology*, 129:787–794.
16. Webb, S., and Parker, R. P. (1978): A Monte Carlo study of the interaction of external beam x-radiation with inhomogeneous medium. *Phys. Med. Biol.*, 23:1043–1059.
17. Wong, J. W., Henkelman, R. M., Andrew, J. W., van Dyk, J., and Johns, H. E. (1981): Effect of small inhomogeneities on scatter dose in a cobalt-60 beam. *Med. Phys.*, 8:783–791.

Computed Tomography in Radiation Therapy,
edited by C. C. Ling, C. C. Rogers, and
R. J. Morton. Raven Press, New York © 1983

Current and Future Development of Tissue Inhomogeneity Corrections for Photon Beam Clinical Dosimetry with the Use of CT

J. R. Cunningham

Physics Division, The Ontario Cancer Institute, Toronto, Canada M4X 1K9

Henkelman et al. discussed some of the physical complexities relevant to making allowance, in dose calculations, for the presence of inhomogeneities in an irradiated medium (*this volume*). They indicated that, with the exception of Monte Carlo methods, all must be approximate. A number of methods developed for calculating dose are listed in Table 1 in order of increasing complexity and grouped according to the parameters they take into account. All of the methods, with the exception of the last two, are most easily applied in the form of a correction factor (C) determined as follows

$$C = \frac{\text{dose in heterogeneous patient}}{\text{dose at same place in homogeneous water-equivalent patient}} \qquad (1)$$

The algorithms listed in the first two groups in Table 1 were developed for hand (noncomputer) calculations and are described in an ICRU report (6). They are reviewed and compared here by applying them in turn to the situation shown in Fig. 1a. This diagram shows a beam of radiation incident on a phantom which

TABLE 1. *Algorithms for making corrections to absorbed doses in heterogeneous phantoms*

Algorithm	Method can take account of				
	Path length	Field size	Position of structure	Shape of structure	Electronic equilibrium
Linear attenuation coefficient	Yes	No	No	No	No
Ratio of TARs	Yes	Yes	No	No	No
Effective SSD	Yes	Yes	No	No	No
Isodose shift	Yes	Yes	No	No	No
Power law TAR (Batho)	Yes	Yes	Yes	No	No
Equivalent TAR	Yes	Yes	Yes	Yes	No
Volume integration of differential scatter/air ratios (Beaudoin)	Yes	Yes	Yes	Yes	No
Monte Carlo	Yes	Yes	Yes	Yes	Yes

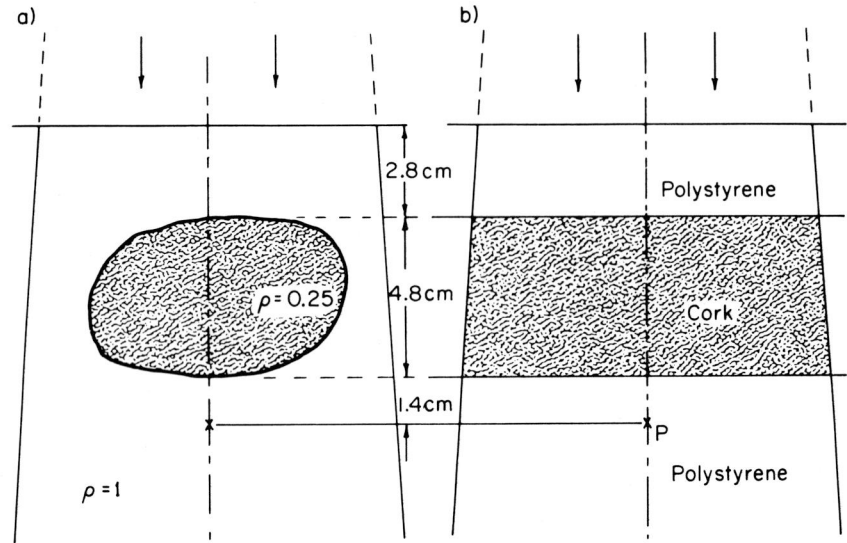

FIG. 1. (a): A phantom of relative density 1.0 containing an inhomogeneity of relative density 0.25. **(b):** Experimental arrangement for testing simple methods of making corrections to absorbed dose calculations in the phantom of **a**. The phantom is made up of layers of polystyrene (water-like) followed by layers of cork, followed by more polystyrene. Ion chamber measurements are made at points along the axis of the beam with the cork in place and then with the cork replaced by a layer of polystyrene of the same thickness.

contains a low-density region. Point P is at a depth of 9 cm below the surface along the central ray of the beam and is 1.4 cm below the lower edge of the low-density inhomogeneity. The inhomogeneity has a density of 0.25 and, along the ray to P, has a thickness of 4.8 cm.

Figure 1b shows an experimental arrangement that was used for testing calculated correction factors. The phantom consists of layers of polystyrene overlying layers of cork overlying more polystyrene. Measurements were made with a Farmer-type ionization chamber at several depths along the central ray both in the inhomogeneous phantom and with the cork replaced by polystyrene. The quotient of pairs of ion chamber readings taken at the same depth was taken as the correct value for the correction factor given in Eq 1.

ALGORITHMS BASED ON RADIOLOGICAL DEPTH

Effective Attenuation Coefficient

For the effective attenuation coefficient, the simplest algorithm of all, it is assumed that the dose is increased by a certain fraction for each centimeter of water-equivalent material that is missing. This fraction plays the role of an attenuation coefficient. Using this method the correction factor for the dose at a point such as P would be:

$$C = e^{\mu' (d - d')} \tag{2}$$

where d is the actual depth to the point and d' is the water-equivalent depth. In the example, for point P, d is 9.0 cm, $d' = 2.8 \times 1.0 + 4.8 \times 0.25 + 1.4 \times 1.0 = 5.4$ cm and, using $\mu' = 0.05$ cm^{-1}, $C = e^{0.05(9-5.4)} = 1.197$. Correction factors calculated by this method for points along the beam axis for the phantom of Fig. 1a (or Fig. 1b) are plotted as the upper dashed curve in Fig. 2. This procedure takes account of neither the field size nor the shape and position of the inhomogeneity.

Frequently the calculation is carried out as a linear rather than an exponential correction

$$C = 1.0 + \mu' (d - d')$$

This is the first term in the expansion of the exponential and is shown as the lower dashed curve in Fig. 2.

Tissue/Air Ratios

A slightly more sophisticated correction factor may be obtained by using tissue/air ratios (TARs):

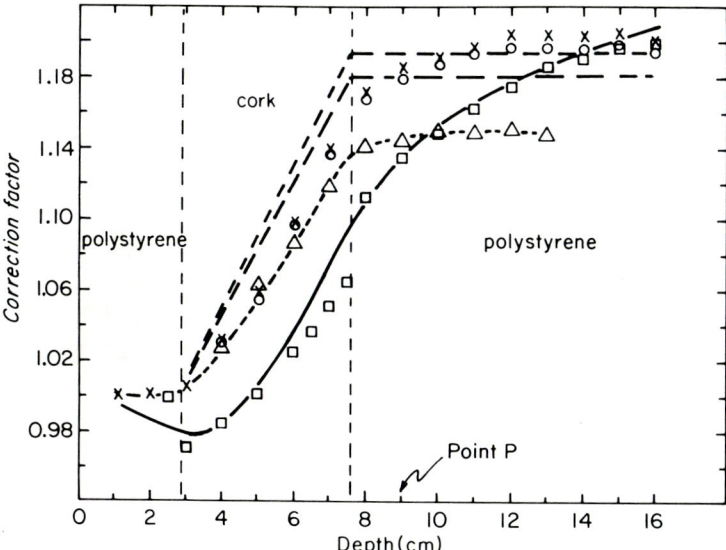

FIG. 2. Correction factors for points in the phantom of Fig. 1b when it is irradiated by a 10 × 10 cm beam from a cobalt unit. The solid line was drawn from measurements made with a Farmer-type ion chamber. The dashed lines represent results obtained from the effective linear attenuation coefficient algorithm, the crosses from ratios of TARs, the circles from the effective SSD method, the triangles from the isodose shift method, and the squares from the power law (Batho) algorithm.

$$C = [T_a(d', W_d)]/[T_a(d, W_d)] \qquad (3)$$

where d, as before, is the depth, and d' is the water-equivalent depth. W_d represents the dimensions of the cross section of the beam at depth d. For the arrangement of Fig. 1a, the beam size at point P is $10 \times (89/80) = 11.13$ cm^2. The relevant TARs for cobalt-60 radiation are T_a (5.4, 11.13) $= 0.898$ and T_a (9, 11.13) $= 0.759$ giving $C = 1.183$. Correction factors obtained by this method for different depths for the phantom of Fig. 1a are shown as crosses in Fig. 2. This algorithm takes some account of both field size and depth through the use of the experimentally determined TARs. It does not take account of either the lateral dimensions of the inhomogeneity or its position with respect to the point of calculation.

Effective Surface-Skin Distance

The effective surface-skin distance (SSD) algorithm is equivalent to that just described but makes use of percent depth dose data rather than TARs. To take account of the inhomogeneity, the isodose chart is "slid" down along a ray line so that, for example, at point P the depth of the water-equivalent depth d'. The dose is then corrected by an inverse square factor. The procedure is illustrated in Fig. 3. The mathematical statement of the correction factor is

$$C = \frac{P(d', W_0, F)}{P(d, W_0, F)}\left(\frac{F + d'}{F + d}\right)^2 \qquad (4)$$

where W_0 is the field dimension at SSD $= F$, and all other quantities are as already defined. For point P, this correction factor would be $C = (76.5/59.7) (85.4/89)^2 = 1.18$.

This procedure can be shown to be formally equivalent to the ratio of TARs method. It is the method chosen by the treatment planning systems that are the descendents of the PC (5) and Rad-8 (2) systems.

Isodose Shift Method

The isodose shift method is a simplification of the "effective SSD method." Instead of moving the isodose chart all the way down to the radiological depth and applying an inverse square correction, it is moved only part way down (for cobalt-60, only 0.67 of the way) so as to eliminate the inverse square correction.

Power Law or Batho Method

The power law or Batho method is categorized separately because it takes one more variable into account, i.e., the position of the inhomogeneity with respect to

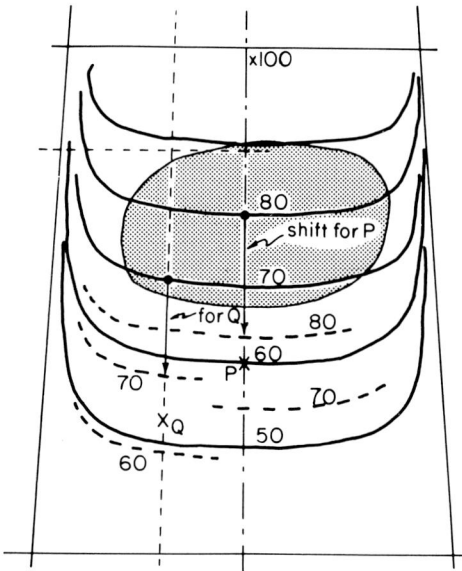

FIG. 3. Application of the effective SSD method for correcting the dose at point *P* for the presence of the low-density region above it.

the point of calculation of the inhomogeneity. The algorithm was proposed by Batho (1) for points lying below an inhomogeneity and was extended by Sontag and Cunningham (9) to include points within an inhomogeneity. The correction factor calculated by this algorithm is

$$C = \frac{T_a\,(z_1,\,W_d)^{\rho_1-\rho_2}}{T_a\,(z_2,\,W_d)^{1-\rho_2}} \tag{5}$$

where ρ_1 is the density of the material in which the point of calculation lies and z_1 is the distance from the point of calculation to the top of that material. ρ_2 is the density of the next, or overlying, material; and z_2 is the distance from the point of calculation to the top of that material. For the example point P: $\rho_1 = 1.0$, $z_1 = 1.4$, $\rho_2 = 0.25$, $z_2 = 6.2$, and therefore $C = (1.025)^{0.75}/(0.868)^{0.75} = 1.132$.

Correction factors calculated by this method for points along the axis of the beam and phantom shown in Fig. 1 are plotted as open squares in Fig. 2. This algorithm yields results which are markedly different from all of those previously discussed and produces much better agreement with the experimental data. One more variable is taken into account, i.e., the position of the inhomogeneity with respect to the point of calculation. In this restricted sense the configuration of the scattered photons are considered, and this shows up in ways that are somewhat surprising at first. For example, as seen in Fig. 2, the correction factor calculated for points in the low-density region, but just below the higher density material, are less than 1.0. All of the algorithms in group 1 predict correction factors greater than 1.0 everywhere in the low-density region. The Batho result is in agreement with the experiment. This is true because although there is an increase in the amount of primary radiation it is more than compensated for by a decrease in the local scattered radiation.

Agreement with experimental results is less good for larger field sizes. This can be seen from Fig. 4, which shows correction factors for points along the axis of the phantom of Fig. 1 when irradiated by a 20 × 20 cm beam from a cobalt unit. The open squares represent the results obtained using the Batho method, and again the experimental results are indicated by a solid curve. Agreement is good for points below the inhomogeneity but is decidely less so for points within it. For much larger field sizes (e.g., those used for half and total body irradiation) Van Dyk et al. (11) showed that errors as great as 20% may result from the use of the "generalized Batho" method within lung tissue.

The method does take the position of a structure into account but not its shape. It would not, for example, distinguish between the two configurations shown in Fig. 1.

Equivalent TAR Method

Sontag and Cunningham (10) have suggested modifying the ratio of TARs algorithm so that it takes account of the shape and position of structures as well as their composition. The procedure has been called the equivalent TAR method, and a dose correction factor may be determined as follows

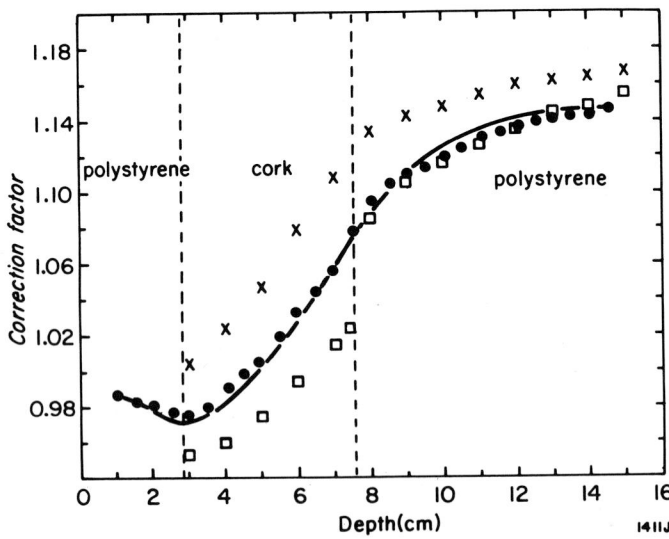

FIG. 4. Correction factors for points along the axis of the phantom of Fig. 1b when irradiated by a 20 × 20 cm beam from a cobalt unit. The crosses are obtained from the ratio of TARs algorithm, the squares from the Batho method, and the solid circles from the effective TAR method. The solid line was derived by experiment.

$$C = \frac{T_a\,(d',\hat{W}_d)}{T_a\,(d,\ W_d)} \tag{6}$$

This expression is very similar to Eq. 3, but the TAR in the numerator refers to a different field dimension $(\hat{W}_d)$, rather than W_d. The alteration of the field size is suggested by the theorem first proposed by O'Connor (8) that a beam irradiating a homogeneous but nonwater medium will produce the same dose at a point in water if all linear dimensions (e.g., depth, field size) are scaled in proportion to the relative density of the nonwater medium.

The physics of a correction procedure based on this idea is discussed at some length by Cunningham (4), and it is suggested that relative electron density rather than relative mass density should be used. The chief problem in applying the method is that of choosing the proper effective density for the nonhomogeneous patient. Sontag and Cunningham (10) suggested that primary and scattered radiation should be considered separately, so that the numerator in Eq. 6 becomes:

$$T_a\,(d',\ \hat{W}_d) = T_a(d',0) + S(d',\hat{r}) \tag{7}$$

The first term on the right is the "zero-area TAR" for the radiological depth d', and the second is the scatter/air ratio for depth d' and field size given by the radius $\hat{r}$.

Radius $\hat{r}$ is to be arrived at in two stages. First r is chosen, which is the radius of the circular field, equivalent to the field of dimensions W_d. The procedure of finding an equivalent circular field is very well established (3,7). This radius is then scaled using the relation

$$\hat{r} = r \cdot \hat{\epsilon}, \tag{8}$$

where $\hat{\epsilon}$ is "effective" relative electron density of the patient and is chosen to be a weighted average of all the relative electron densities of the structures in the irradiated volume. In this averaging procedure, regions that are close to the point where the calculation is to be made must count more heavily than regions far away from it, and regions in front of the point are more important than regions behind it.

The procedure lends itself particularly well to the use of CT images, and Sontag and Cunningham (10) chose the following procedure for determining the effective relative electron density

$$\hat{\epsilon} = \frac{\sum_i \sum_j \sum_k \epsilon_{ijk} \cdot W_{ijk}}{\sum_i \sum_j \sum_k W_{ijk}} \tag{9}$$

The CT numbers in images covering the irradiated volume are converted into relative electron densities ϵ_{ijk}, and the W_{ijk} are an assumed set of weighting factors which have the properties described above. They are intended as an expression of the relative importance of each of the ϵ_{ijk} elements in affecting the dose due to scattered radiation at the point of calculation.

There is no unique set of weighting factors for use in Eq. 9, and experience indicates that the calculated correction factor is not a strong function of the form chosen. This question is discussed at some length by Sontag and Cunningham (4,8) and is not dealt with further here.

A direct evaluation of Eq. 9 implies an integration over the entire irradiated volume for each point of dose calculation. This is not practical with present technology, and so a compromise procedure has been adopted which reduces the volume integration to one over an area. This is illustrated in Fig. 5. The left side of Fig. 5 depicts relative electron density information that could be derived from six CT images. In the example, dose calculations are to be made in the plane of image 3, which is shaded. As a first step, all the relative electron density information contained in the six images is coalesced into a single "effective" image as indicated on the right. The coalesced image consists of the weighted average of all pixels that have the same i and j indices. That is

$$\hat{\epsilon}_{ij} = \frac{\sum\limits_{k} \epsilon_{ijk} \cdot W_k}{\sum\limits_{k} W_k} \tag{10}$$

This effective image is obtained at the beginning of the calculation. It is considered to be at an effective distance, Z_{eff}, from the plane of calculation points and is used for the remaining averaging for each point

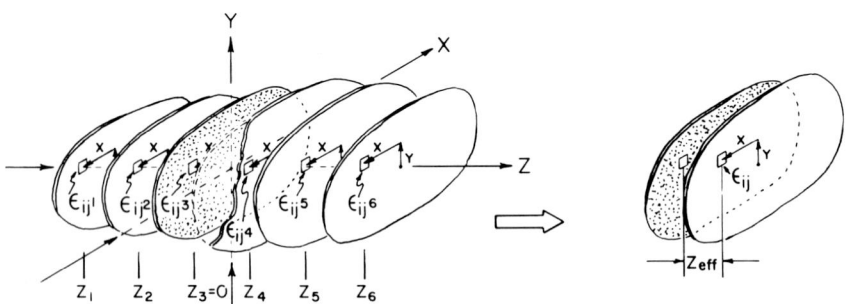

FIG. 5. Steps taken in the "equivalent TAR method" to reduce the volume integration to one over a plane. The relative electron density information contained in six CT images indicated on the left is first coalesced into a single "effective" image indicated on the right. This image is a weighted average of all six images in which regions close to the plane of calculations count more strongly. This image is formed only once, and from it a weighted average relative electron density is determined for each point of dose calculation. (From ref. 10.)

$$\hat{\epsilon} = \frac{\displaystyle\sum_i \sum_j \hat{\epsilon}_{ij} \cdot W_{ij}\,(Z_{\text{eff}})}{\displaystyle\sum_i \sum_j W_{ij}\,(Z_{\text{eff}})} \tag{11}$$

This method does, at each point, take into account the size, shape, composition, and position of all structures. It has been evaluated in a number of test phantoms and appears to be better than all of the previously mentioned algorithms. The results for a 20 × 20 cm beam of cobalt radiation irradiating the phantom of Fig. 1b are shown as solid circles in Fig. 4. The agreement can be seen to be good.

CONCLUSIONS

Algorithms for calculating dose correction factors for tissue inhomogeneities have been reviewed. They are listed in Table 1 in an order of increasing complexity. The first group, dependent only on radiological depth and field size, can all be shown to be variants of ratios of two TARs. A method due to Batho takes account of the position of inhomogeneities but not their shape. This method gives quite acceptable accuracy for small field sizes but becomes increasingly inaccurate for large fields.

Next in order of complexity is the equivalent TAR method, which takes account of the full three-dimensional structure of the irradiated body for each point of dose calculation. It is the only one reviewed which can rightly be called a "three-dimensional dose calculation method." To make it practical, however, an approximation has been introduced so that the three-dimensional integration has been reduced to a two-dimensional one. It has been tested in a variety of phantom configurations which indicate an accuracy whose standard deviation is about 3%.

Methods not discussed and considered to be more sophisticated include the volume integration of differential scatter/air ratios (discussed earlier in this volume by Purdy and Prasad) and the Monte Carlo calculations. The former is under active development and may be made practical by the use of special microprocessors. The latter is certainly the most accurate of all but will not likely be practical for routine treatment planning in the forseeable future. It will undoubtedly continue to be useful, however, in providing reference data to which results of other methods can be compared.

ACKNOWLEDGMENTS

The author wishes to acknowledge financial support from the National Cancer Institute of Canada and the Ontario Cancer Treatment and Research Foundation, and the continuing cooperation of Atomic Energy of Canada Ltd.

REFERENCES

1. Batho, H. F. (1964): Lung corrections in cobalt 60 beam therapy. *J. Can. Assoc. Radiol.*, 15:79–83.
2. Bently, R. E., and Milan, J. (1971): An interactive digital computer system for radiotherapy treatment planning. *Br. J. Radiol.*, 44:826–833.

3. Central axis depth dose data for dose in radiotherapy. *Br. J. Radiol. [Suppl. 11]*, 1972.
4. Cunningham, J. R. (1982): Tissue inhomogeneity corrections in photon beam treatment planning. In: *Progress in Medical Physics*, edited by C. E. Orton, Chap. 8. Plenum, New York (*in press*).
5. Cunningham, J. R., and Milan, J. (1969): Radiation treatment planning using a display oriented small computer. In: *Computers in Biomedical Research*, edited by R. W. Stacey and B. D. Waxman, Chap. 6. Academic Press, New York.
6. ICRU Report 24 (1976): Determination of absorbed dose in a patient irradiated by beams of x or gamma rays in radiotherapy procedures. Internal Commission on Radiation Units and Measurements, Washington, D.C.
7. Johns, H. E., and Cunningham, J. R. (1969): *The Physics of Radiology*. Charles C Thomas, Springfield, Il.
8. O'Connor, J. E. (1957): The variation of scattered x-rays with density in an irradiated body. *Phys. Med. Biol.*, 1:352–369.
9. Sontag, M. R., and Cunningham, J. R. (1977): Corrections to absorbed dose calculations for tissue inhomogeneities. *Med. Phys.*, 4:431–436.
10. Sontag, M. R., and Cunningham, J. R. (1978): The equivalent tissue-air ratio method for making absorbed dose calculatins in a heterogeneous medium. *Radiology*, 129:787–794.
11. Van Dyk, J., Battista, J. J., and Rider, W. D. (1980): Half body radiotherapy: the use of computed tomography to determined the dose to lung. *Int. J. Radiat. Oncol. Biol. Phys.*, 6:463–470.

Computed Tomography in Radiation Therapy,
edited by C. C. Ling, C. C. Rogers, and
R. J. Morton. Raven Press, New York © 1983

Cost-Benefit of Computed Tomography Application in Dosimetry Calculations

Edwin C. McCullough

Division of Radiation Therapy, Department of Oncology, Mayo Clinic/Foundation, Rochester, Minnesota 55901

The availability of computed tomographic (CT) scans brings to the therapy planning team two new dimensions: (a) the ability to accurately localize tumor sites and limiting normal structures in both two and three dimensions; and (b) the potential to use the quantitative output of a CT scanner to correct for the inhomogeneous nature of the human body.

LOCALIZATION

The benefit of having more precise localization available for treatment planning is hard to dispute *a priori*. Even though Goitein (1) presents a very penetrating analysis of the impact of this attribute on the ultimate therapeutic result, it is reasonable to assume that the localization aspect of CT scanning on isodose curve interpretations will become an important modus operandi in most careful therapy departments.

When CT is utilized for localization in connection with treatment planning, added costs may be nominal. There may be no additional costs if previously obtained CT scans can be used and if one does not require a planning system that superimposes isodoses on a gray level CT scan. However, one can easily double or triple the cost to the patient if additional "therapy" scans are needed and sophisticated hybrid hardware is purchased.

INHOMOGENEITY CORRECTIONS

The ability to incorporate CT scan measurements of tissue properties in order to provide an estimate of the effect of tissue inhomogeneities is an area of continued discussion. Even though there may be certain instances and/or modalities where single plane inhomogeneity corrected plans are of value, I suspect that those "in the know" would readily concur with the argument that it is somewhat of a compromise if one does not perform these corrections in three-dimensional geometry. This approach requires a great number of CT scans; and if an institution is to recapture this expense, the costs ($300 to $400) must be passed on to the patient.

At this time the jury is out relative to ultimate value of completely inhomogeneity corrected isodose plans for a variety of reasons, including the following:

1. Appropriate computational algorithms that can provide accurate accounting for the effect of tissue inhomogeneities on dose distributions are in various stages of development.

2. The relative merit of pixel-by-pixel versus area average needs further investigation as improved algorithms are developed.

3. The exact utilization by our clinical colleagues of the complex dose distributions that will be generated is not clear at the current time.

4. Studies documenting the *range* of doses received by target areas for uncorrected versus corrected planes have not been done to date.

On this last point, it has always been the author's contention that we will have a great deal of trouble convincing our clinical colleagues of the presumed advantage of complete inhomogeneity corrected isodose plans on the basis of being able to more accurately assign a dose value (dose values) rather than from the viewpoint that a much wider (and presumably unacceptable) range of dose values is present if we use the simple assumption of total water equivalence.

SUMMARY

The cost-benefit analysis of CT-assisted radiation therapy treatment planning is incomplete at the moment. In fact, there are those who argue that the analysis will never be completed and cite the failure to obtain comparable data relative to previous technical innovations, e.g., megavoltage radiation (especially very high energy photon beam machines), computerized treatment planning units, and simulators.

REFERENCE

1. Goitein, M. (1980): Benefits and cost of computerized tomography in radiation therapy. *J.A.M.A.*, 244:1347–1350.

Computed Tomography in Radiation Therapy,
edited by C. C. Ling, C. C. Rogers, and
R. J. Morton. Raven Press, New York 1983

Computed Tomography in High LET Radiotherapy Treatment Planning

George T. Y. Chen

*Division of Biology and Medicine, Lawrence Berkeley Laboratory,
Berkeley, California 94720*

The role of computed tomography (CT) in heavy charged particle therapy is reviewed in this chapter. Both neutral- and charged-particle therapy trials are under way in the United States and elsewhere (5). Because neutrons have depth dose characteristics similar to those of photons, treatment planning techniques similar to those used for photon beams are, to the first order, appropriate for neutron therapy. Second-order corrections and enhancements to the biologically effective dose distribution might include organ-specific radiosensitivity factors. In contrast to neutral radiations, charged particles have a well-defined range in matter and are therefore much more sensitive to variations in tissue density. It is this property of finite range which allows charged-particle dose distributions to be localized to a well-defined target volume, often sparing dose to adjacent critical tissues. The need for accurate quantitative density information as provided by CT is therefore greater with charged particles than with photons or neutrons.

Examples of highly localized dose distributions possible with charged particles are shown in Fig. 1. A two-field irradiation of the pancreas is achieved in Fig. 1, top, using an anterior and left lateral field. External compensation, shown in white, is used to conform the beam-stopping region to the distal contour of the target (broad white line). The target is uniformly irradiated to 100%, whereas liver, kidneys, and spinal cord are largely spared. The gastrointestinal tract proximal to the target volume is irradiated to approximately the 30% level. A U-shaped target has been defined in Fig. 1, bottom, which wraps around the spinal cord. Lateral and posterior fields are matched to generate a U-shaped high-dose region. The spinal cord dose is kept below tolerance, whereas the target volume is irradiated to 7,000 cobalt rad equivalent units. In both of these examples, it is clear that to successfully execute the treatment plan and spare nearby normal tissues we must be able to calculate beam penetration in the presence of substantial inhomogeneities. Inaccuracies in the calculation of the required beam penetration could lead to overdose of critical organs distal to the target or underdose of the tumor. The requirement for accurate CT values is of fundamental importance in charged-particle treatment planning.

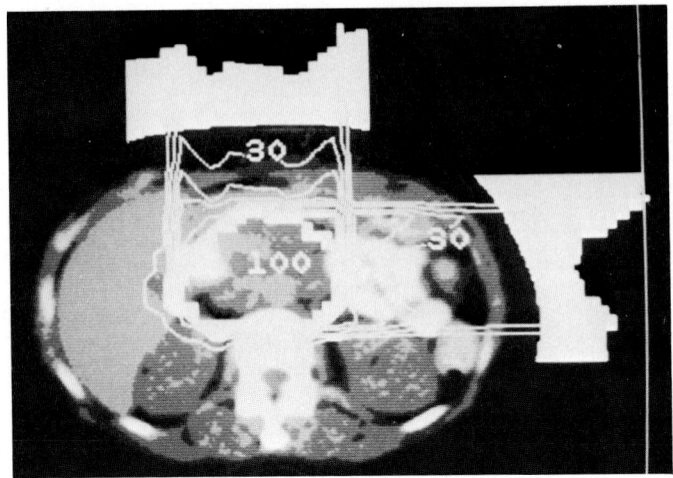

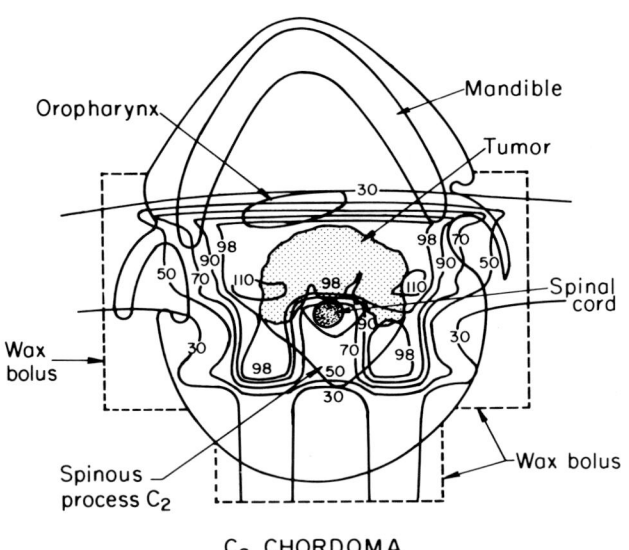

C_2 CHORDOMA

FIG. 1. Top: Isoeffective dose distribution for a pancreatic target volume treated with heavy ions. Compensation is used to conform the dose to the target volume. **Bottom:** Plan for irradiation of a chordoma at the level of C2 utilizing a helium beam. Lateral and posterior beams were abutted to produce a high-dose U-shaped region. 100% = 7,000 cobalt equivalent rads.

The approach to utilizing CT data by high linear energy transfer (LET) groups followed several general lines: (a) display axial, coronal, or sagittal CT images and define target contours on the CT data; (b) convert CT values to water-equivalent path length per pixel; (c) perform pixel-by-pixel dose calculations; (d) fabricate three-dimensional compensators to shape the high-dose region; and (e) utilize graphics based on CT contours as an aid in treatment planning.

TARGET DEFINITION

The treatment planning process for charged-particle therapy, as with conventional beams, begins with a series of sequential scans in the treatment position. The proton, helium, and heavy ion beams in the United States enter treatment rooms in a horizontal direction, leading to rather natural treatment positions of seated or standing patients. In order to scan patients in these treatment positions, both the Massachusetts General Hospital/Harvard Proton Therapy Facility and our institution have installed specially modified EMI-7070 CT scanners with this capability.

Following this initial step, target volumes on sequential scans must be defined by the radiotherapist. Ideally, this is performed interactively, with the CT scan displayed on a raster graphics unit and contours entered via trackball or joystick. As Goitein et al. have shown (3), simultaneous display of CT-based data (e.g., sagittal, coronal, and transverse planes of CT data) are often useful in this stage. Target entry must be a highly interactive process, with the ability to (a) enter, delete, or modify contours; (b) measure either water-equivalent or geometric distances; (c) annotate the presence of objects or bony landmarks; and (d) review the three-dimensional volume entered and inspect it for consistency. The target contours and CT matrix are the two basic sets of data used to calculate the shape of three-dimensional compensators which conform the charged-particle-stopping region to the distal surface of the target. The target contours are also used to define the shape of the collimator aperature. At this point, it is also useful to contour, either automatically or manually, adjacent critical structures, bony landmarks, or the external contour. These data may be used later to calculate the fractional volume of normal organ irradiated. Landmarking or denoting structures on axial slices which are also visible on anteroposterior (AP) or lateral x-rays may be used for portal alignment.

CT CALIBRATION

The quantitative information required for compensator design is the integrated path length along each beam ray from the distal edge of the target contour toward the beam source. Complementing this water-equivalent path length with the total range of the beam in water yields the amount of external absorber required for each ray. We have used a calibration curve relating CT number to water-equivalent path length/pixel obtained by scanning bone and tissue analogs (2). Data are shown in Fig. 2, for this calibration for both the EMI-5005 and the GE-7800 scanners operated at 120 kVp. The x-axis scale is in EMI units, with air nominally at -511 and bone at $+511$. A parabolic fit is made for data points between -511 and $+55$, whereas a straight line is used from $+55$ to $+511$. The relative stopping power, or water-equivalent path length per pixel, was measured in the helium ion beam and is accurate to about 2%.

The validity of this simple calibration curve has been established principally through phantom studies. Figure 3 shows a CT scan of a frozen dog cadaver. In this study a diode was placed within the brain, and the water-equivalent path from skin to diode along the indicated line was measured. Using the calibration curve

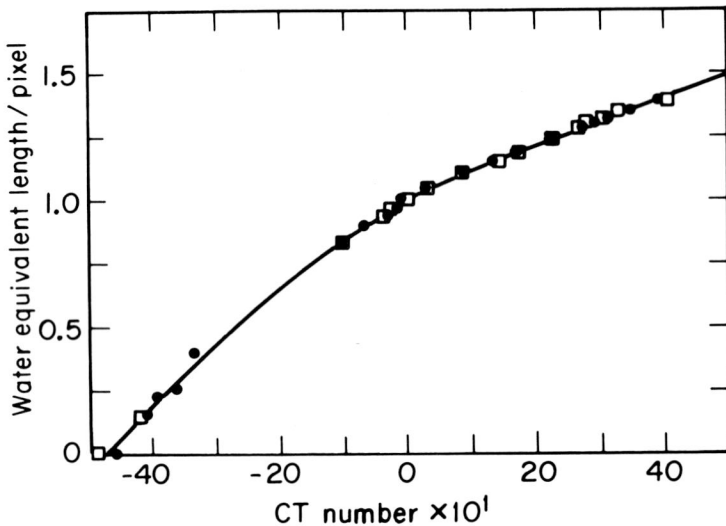

FIG. 2. Single energy calibration curve used for conversion of CT numbers to water-equivalent path length per pixel. For GE-7800 (●) and EMI-5005 (☐)scanners operated at 120 kVp.

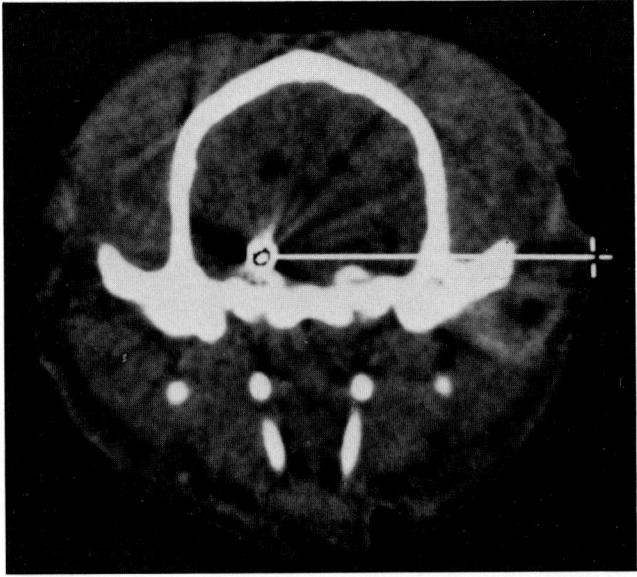

FIG. 3. CT scan of a frozen dog cadaver. A diode was implanted in the cranium and the water-equivalent path length from skin surface to diode was experimentally determined by a water column scan. Comparison with the value extracted from Fig. 2 showed agreement within 2% of the total path length.

in Fig. 2, the estimated water-equivalent path length from CT was also determined. Agreement at this site and at three other sites in the cadaver was within 2 mm, or approximately 2%. These types of data along with *in vivo* studies have led us to conclude that single energy scans are sufficiently accurate in a number of sites (abdomen, pelvis, thorax, and brain) for charged-particle treatment planning. In areas where inhomogeneities are particularly complex or where there is a very large amount of bone (e.g., the base of the skull), single energy scans may not be adequate.

Implicit in the quantitative use of CT is the assumption that the CT number of materials is independent of size or shape of the object, the presence of inhomogeneities (e.g., bone or air), and the position within the reconstruction circle. This condition is not met, to my knowledge, by current scanners. Data taken on our EMI-7070 show variation in CT number of water-equivalent plastic on the order of 5 to 7% when size and shape of phantoms are varied. However, new software on the GE-8800 at the University of California at San Francisco (1) appears to produce accurate CT values for water over a wide dynamic range of operating conditions to within ± 1%, indicating that these variations may be minimized. Research and development by scanner manufacturers in these areas is of primary importance if CT is to be used quantitatively.

Pixel-by-pixel calculations are based on CT scans taken during the tumor localization phase. It is often necessary to use oral or intravenous contrast agents to adequately define the target volume. These materials clearly affect the CT data by elevating tissue linear attenuation coefficients and often by producing streak artifacts. Furthermore, transient inhomogeneities, most commonly gas in the gastrointestinal tract, are often present. These perturbations in the scan data must be edited from the scan in order to properly design a compensating bolus which will adequately irradiate the target volume over a number of fractions spanning weeks in time. In addition, within the abdomen, daily variations in target shape and location are possible, although detailed studies documenting the magnitude are just beginning. Finally, variations in organ position due to involuntary motion (e.g., respiration) may alter target shape and position during treatment. All of these processes, which are not explicitly defined, must be considered in charged-particle treatment planning. In this sense, CT data provide a basis for computations, but techniques for folding these processes into calculations must be developed.

For instance, limits to daily patient/compensator registration must be included in the compensator design. Although immobilization techniques as described by Verhey et al. (6) indicate that patient position may be reproduced to the 2 mm level over a period of weeks for some head and neck sites, because of the steepness of gradients possible in compensators misregistration by 2 mm may produce a substantial and undesirable dose perturbation. Goitein (4) has suggested that the estimated error in alignment should be convolved with the initial compensation design to produce a bolus, which, in the event of such misregistration, will still adequately irradiate the target. In his scheme two sets of dose distributions should be calculated:

one associated with minimum beam penetration, and one with maximum penetration.

DOSE CALCULATION

The dose calculation algorithms vary among charged-particle groups and are a reflection of particle and beam optics properties. Calculations for pion treatment planning requires a fully three-dimensional approach, with contributions from scattered radiation from adjacent CT planes influencing the dose in the principle slice. With minimal scatter and forward peaked nuclear fragments, heavy ion treatment planning may proceed by calculation in each sequential scan. Dose display in planes other than the transverse (e.g., sagittal and coronal) has been implemented in several particle therapy facilities.

GRAPHICS

As stated earlier, an important part of treatment planning for charged particles is the contouring of both target and normal structures. These data may be used in two distinct ways: (a) Contours may be displayed in pseudo three dimensions as an aid in plan optimization; and (b) contours coupled with dose matrices may be used to assess the radiation dose to adjacent critical structures in an objective manner.

A series of contours representing a lesion in the brain and the cranium, as displayed on an Evans and Sutherland picture system at our institution are shown in Fig. 4. This image may be rotated, translated, magnified, and manipulated in real time by interaction with a set of knobs. Displays of this type may be used to optimize the treatment by selecting the beam direction to minimize transit through critical normal structures, by selecting a path which minimizes the complexity of compensation, and by viewing the target contours in a three-dimensional representation in order to resolve target volume inconsistencies (arising from target entry in two-dimensional images). Overall, this type of graphics assists the radiotherapist

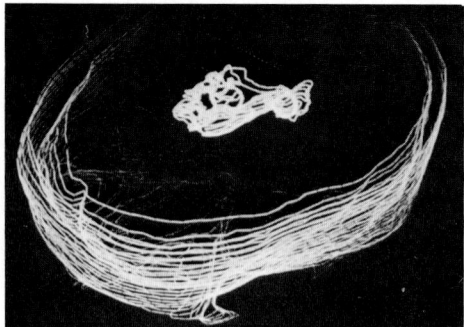

FIG. 4. Display of contours extracted from sequential CT slices and imaged on Evans and Sutherland picture system. Depth cueing is achieved through intensity variation as a function of distance from the viewer. Real time rotation and translation may be performed to optimize treatment angles.

in integrating treatment planning information from a number of sequential cuts into real space.

Contours of organs within the area of the irradiated volume and corresponding dose matrices may also be used for determining the volume of normal organ irradiated and the integral dose to such organs. These data may then be used to quantitatively compare the merits of various irradiation arrangements and, coupled with organ-specific function tests, determine the radiosensitivity of specific organs to new particle radiations.

SUMMARY

As in conventional radiotherapy, CT has been used in target localization and treatment volume definition, pixel-by-pixel dose calculations, and the evaluation of therapy by follow-up scanning. However, because of the finite range of charged-particle beams and the possibility of optimizing the irradiated volume through dose conformation, the quantitative aspects of CT are even more important in this experimental therapy modality. The technical nature of charged-particle therapy and the software tools being developed (e.g., three-dimensional graphics and manipulation and display techniques for target localization, target volume definition, and portal alignment) are equally useful in conventional therapy.

ACKNOWLEDGMENTS

Treatment planning for charged particles at Lawrence Berkeley Laboratory has evolved over the past 4 years through the contributions of S. Pitluck, R. P. Singh, J. R. Castro, J. T. Lyman, J. M. Quivey, W. Saunders, J. M. Collier, and T. Richards. The diode/dog study was developed by E. L. Alpen and A. Chatterjee. This work was supported by NCI grant 5POCA19138 and ERDA contract W-7405 ENG-48.

REFERENCES

1. Cann, C. (1981): Private communication.
2. Chen, G. T. Y., Singh, R. P., Lyman, J. T., Quivey, J. M., and Castro, J. R. (1978): Treatment planning for charged particle radiotherapy. *Int. J. Radiat. Oncol. Biol. Phys.*, 5:1809–1819.
3. Goitein, M., Abrams, M., Rowell, D., Pollari, H., and Wiles, J. (1981): A multi-dimensional treatment planning system. This volume.
4. Goitein, M. (1978): Compensation for inhomogeneities in charged particle radiotherapy using computed tomography. *Int. J. Radiat. Oncol. Biol. Phys.*, 4:499–508.
5. Thomas, R. H., and Perez-Mendez, V. (1980): *Advances in Radiation Protection and Dosimetry in Medicine.* Plenum, New York.
6. Verhey, L. J., Goitein, M., McNulty, P., Munzenrider, J. E., and Suit, H. D. (1982): Precise positioning of patients for radiotherapy. *Int. J. Radiat. Oncol. Biol. Phys.*, 8:289–294.

Computed Tomography in Radiation Therapy,
edited by C. C. Ling, C. C. Rogers, and
R. J. Morton. Raven Press, New York © 1983

Electron Beam Treatment Planning: A Review of Dose Computation Methods

Radhe Mohan, Richard Riley, and John S. Laughlin

Department of Medical Physics, Memorial Hospital, New York, New York 10021

In routine treatment planning the exact calculation of the dose distribution produced by an electron beam with the aid of techniques such as the Monte Carlo method is not practical. Such calculations require a detailed description in three dimensions of geometry and elemental composition of the patient, as well as a complete description of the incident radiation and all its interactions. These are obtainable with some difficulty, the former facilitated by use of the computed tomographic (CT) scanner. The most serious problem with the use of the Monte Carlo method, however, is the prohibitive amount of computer time required. To obtain adequate statistics, the scattering histories of a million or more electrons per beam may have to be followed. Even on the fastest computers available today, this requires several days of dedicated computer time and, for all intents and purposes, is impractical for routine work.

Therefore we must resort to approximate methods, which invariably represent a compromise between speed of computation on one hand and accuracy on the other. Quite often the approximation chosen may depend on the treatment technique and the willingness to accept a degree of error in certain regions. Different approximate methods, in general, will yield somewhat different results. In the remainder of this chapter, the work of several investigators (1–4,7,9–13) in developing such methods is reviewed.

The approximate methods of calculation can be divided into two broad categories: (a) the equivalent path length methods; and (b) the pencil beam methods.

EQUIVALENT PATH LENGTH METHOD

Typical of the equivalent path length methods is the one currently used at Memorial Sloan Kettering Cancer Center and implemented in 1979 on the Deltaplan, a CT radiation treatment planning (CT-RTP) system manufactured by Technicare Corp. This method makes direct use of the measured data as far as possible and resorts to approximations to correct for curvature and inhomogeneities. The original form of this method was developed with the electron beam represented by rays (4,8). Inhomogeneity corrections were applied using the absorption equivalent thick-

229

ness (AET) factors. These factors effectively take into account scattering and absorption of radiation, and depend not only on the density of the region of inhomogeneity but also on its depth and size. The distance dependence corrections were applied assuming an inverse square law from a "virtual source" whose position was determined empirically.

In 1979 this method was enhanced and adapted to computer calculations including pixel-by-pixel corrections for inhomogeneous structure contained in CT scans. In its current form, it employs the following expression (Fig. 1)

$$
\begin{aligned}
D_P(W,H) = D_C(W_0,H_0) \cdot G \cdot TR(Z_C,S) \\
\cdot OCR(Z_C,2x/W,\phi_W) \\
\cdot OCR(Z_C,2z/H,\phi_H),
\end{aligned}
\tag{1}
$$

$D_C(W_0 H_0)$ is the calibration dose at the calibration point C, with W_0 and H_0 being the field width and field height, respectively.

$TR(Z_C,S)$ is the tissue/air ratio (TAR), tissue/maximum ratio (TMR), or the tissue/phantom ratio (TPR) value at point P for the water-equivalent path length $Z_C = t_1 \cdot \rho_1 + t_2 \cdot \rho_2$, and S is the equivalent field size at the level of point P. Quantities ρ_1 and ρ_2 are "effective" densities of the media. Products of "effective" densities and physical path lengths are the AET factors. For the CT image, Z_C is replaced by the pixel-by-pixel summation of "effective" electron densities. There must be two sets of TR tables for different skin-surface distances (SSDs) to enable the

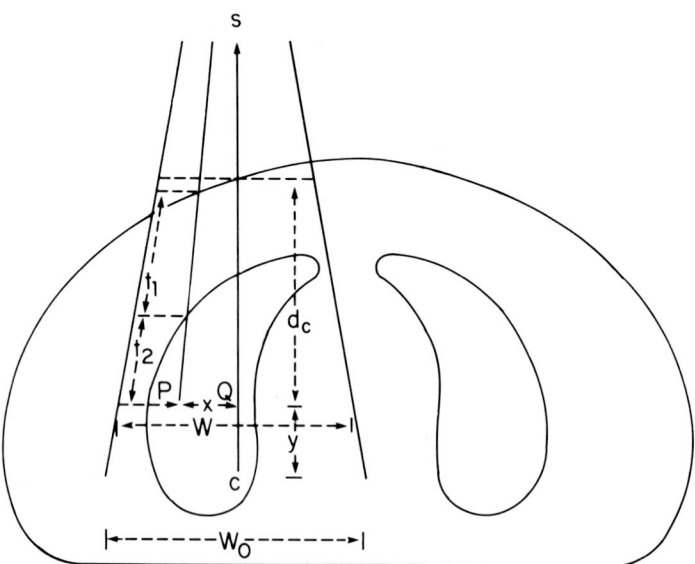

FIG. 1. The electron beam dose distribution computation model for the Deltaplan system is an example of equivalent path length methods for inhomogeneity corrections.

program to take into account the SSD variation of TPRs, TMRs, and TARs, and to apply the air gap correction.

$OCR(Z_C, 2x/W, \phi_W)$ is the off-center ratio (OCR) at P relative to point Q on the central axis, and ϕ_W is the collimator opening along the direction of width. The next term, $OCR(Z_C, 2z/H, \phi_H)$ is the off-center correction for distance z in the plane of calculation along the height axis from the central axis. The quantity ϕ_H is the collimator opening along the height. In order to apply air gap corrections, the program requires OCRs for two separate SSDs.

The distance-dependent geometric factor G for electrons is obtained from distance-dependent factors (DDFs) using the expression $G = \text{DDF}(SQ)/\text{DDF}(SC)$ (refer to Fig. 1). DDFs are obtained by measuring dose rate at the calibration depth for a series of SSDs.

The dose computation method employs the linear attenuation correction for incorporating inhomogeneities and, as such, does not take into account the changes in scatter from variations in density and the lateral diffusion of electrons in the heterogeneous medium.

The consequence of neglecting the lateral transport of electrons is illustrated in Fig. 2. The dashed curve represents the measured TMR values in cork (density =

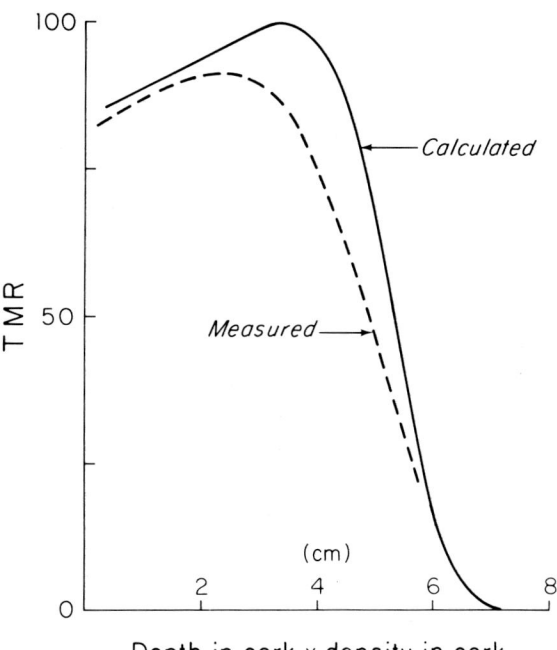

FIG. 2. Comparison between measured data and values of electron beam TMRs in cork calculated employing the equivalent path length method. A 13 MeV 10 × 10 cm² electron beam was used, and measurements were made at a fixed source to a measurement point distance of 110 cm.

0.295), and the solid curve is the corresponding values calculated using the equivalent path length method. The field size was 10 × 10 cm² at 100 cm from the source. The energy of electrons was 13 MeV. The range of these electrons is about 6.5 cm in water and approximately 22 cm in cork. The calculation using the equivalent path length method ignores the lack of scattered electrons from regions outside the beam boundary. These regions are well within the reach of the range of scattered electrons. Consequently the calculated values are much higher than the measured values. By the same reasoning, it can be shown that a 33 × 33 cm² field in cork of density 0.3 will have approximately the same central axis depth dose as a 10 × 10 cm² field in water.

PENCIL BEAM METHODS

Several investigators (1–3,10–13) have been exploring the use of electron pencil beams for calculating the dose to patients being irradiated with electron beams. In methods of this type, a broad beam of an arbitrary shape is divided into a number of narrow beams (pencils) of electrons incident on the surface of the patient. To calculate the dose at a given point in the patient, the contribution of all pencils to this point must be added. A typical beam may be divided into several hundred pencils. Although the computation time does not increase by the same proportion, it would increase on the average by two orders of magnitude compared to the equivalent path length method. There are three distinct approaches to the generation of pencil beams.

Age Diffusion Pencil Beam

Steben et al. (12) and Ayyangar et al. (1) have used a modification of the age diffusion model proposed by Kawachi (6) They used six parameters to fit beams with entrance dimensions of 0.5 × 0.5 cm such that the summation of these beams is in agreement with broad beam data. Dose computation is accomplished by the summation of such beams with corrections for surface contours and inhomogeneities being performed in essentially the same manner as the equivalent path length method.

Fermi-Eyges Pencil Beam

The approach followed by Perry and Holt (10), Hogstrom et al. (3), Werner et al. (13), and Brahme et al. (2) is based on the Fermi-Eyges solution to the Boltzmann equation applied to a narrow cylindrical beam incident on a flat homogeneous body. This theory primarily takes into account multiple coulomb scattering but ignores most other processes, e.g., secondary electron production and bremsstrahlung. This theory was originally developed to deal with beams of energy much higher (in the BeV range) than those of interest in radiation therapy. The Fermi-Eyges solution is based on the assumption of small angle scattering and does not apply well at depths greater than approximately one-third the electron range. Furthermore, the multiple scattering theory provides a solution that describes the fluence of electrons and not energy deposition.

The Fermi-Eyges multiple coulomb scattering theory shows that, for a narrow pencil of electrons incident on matter, the dose at point P (Fig. 3) is given by

$$D(x,y,z) = D_0(z) \cdot \exp \left\{ - (x^2 + y^2)/[2\sigma^2(z)]\right\} \Big/ [2\pi\sigma^2(z)] \qquad (2)$$

where $D_0(z)$ is the central axis depth dose due to an infinitely wide plane parallel electron beam incident normally on the water phantom; z is the depth of the point P along the central axis; and x and y are its lateral distances from the central axis. The quantity σ describes lateral spread of the beam and incorporates the effects of a variety of scattering processes; it can be computed from fundamental principles and published data (2,3,10).

Monte Carlo Pencil Beam

The third approach to the generation of pencil beam dose distributions makes use of the Monte Carlo method. Although not practical when used wholly and entirely for routine calculations of treatment plans, the Monte Carlo method is quite suitable and can be used successfully as a tool to generate pencil beam data. These data need be obtained only once for a given energy and can be employed in all subsequent treatment planning calculations. Riley et al. (11) used the Monte Carlo

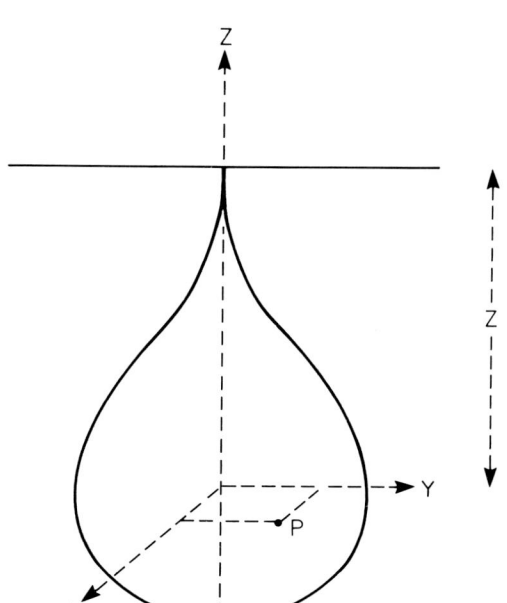

FIG. 3. Geometry of multiple coulomb scattering pencil beam expression for electron dose computation: see Eq. 2.

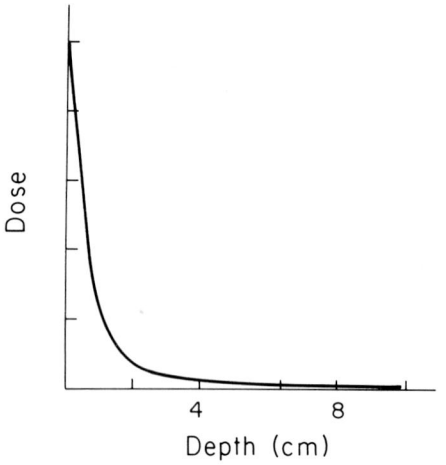

FIG. 4. Central-axis depth dose of a 20 MeV pencil beam calculated with the Monte Carlo method.

code EGS (electron gamma shower) for this purpose. This code provides for a fully three-dimensional cascade production. It includes not only multiple scattering but also secondary electron production, bremsstrahlung, and a number of other electron-scattering processes. Among its inputs, it requires scattering cross sections of the media through which the electrons traverse. Cross sections for water, tissue substitutes, bone, lead, etc. were generated using a companion code called PEGS.

Examples of pencil beam data generated with this code are shown in Figs. 4, 5, and 6. Figure 4 is the central axis depth dose curve of a pencil of 20 MeV electrons

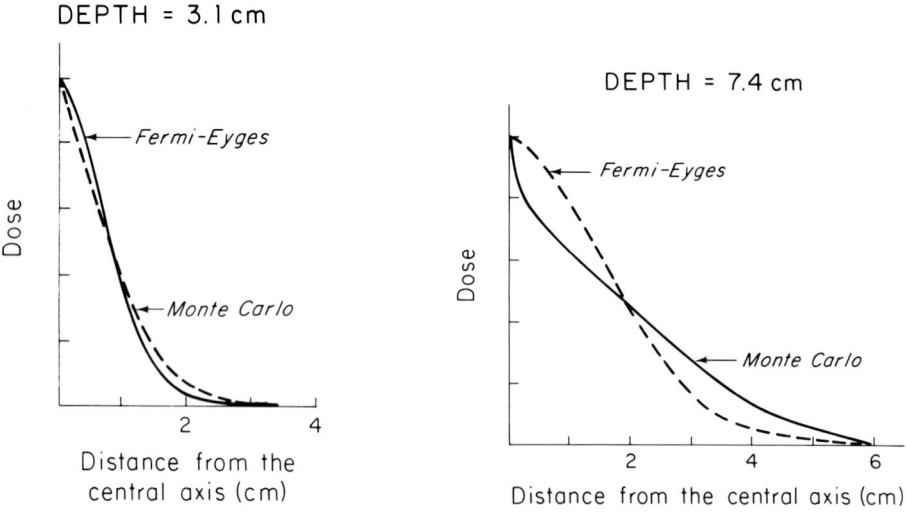

FIG. 5. Beam profiles of a 20-MeV pencil beam at depths of 3.1 and 7.4 cm. The solid curves are the results of Monte Carlo calculations; dashed curves are the gaussian shapes predicted by the Fermi-Eyges multiple coulomb scattering theory. The σ for the scattering theory was chosen to match full width at half-maximum.

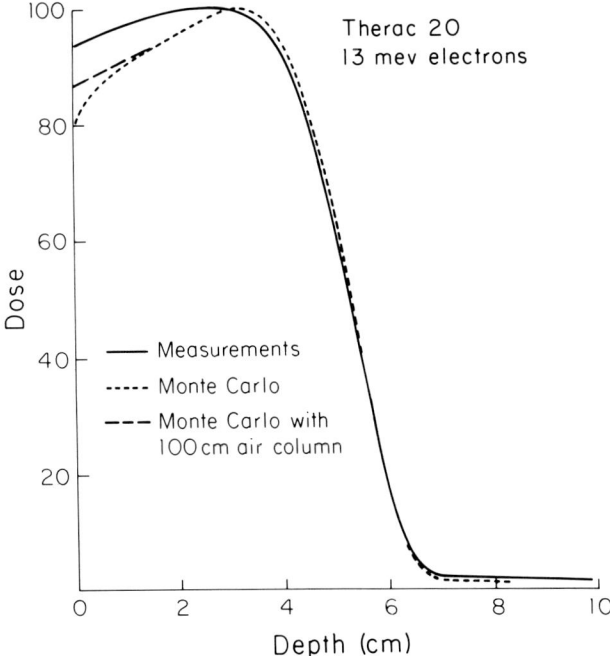

FIG. 6. Comparison of measured broad electron depth dose data (*solid curve*) with those generated by summation of Monte Carlo pencil beams. The dashed curve includes scattering from a 100 cm tall column of air between the source and the phantom surface.

in water. A notable feature is that there is no maximum at depth as for a broad beam. For the latter, the increase in dose at depth relative to entrance dose is due to lateral diffusion of electrons. Thus if pencils are added over a broad beam, they produce a central axis depth dose curve that agrees (Fig. 6) with the measured data.

Figure 5 shows the Monte Carlo generated beam profiles for 20 MeV electrons at depths of 3.1 and 7.4 cm, respectively. Comparison with the corresponding profiles from the Fermi-Eyges multiple coulomb scattering theory demonstrates that the inclusion of all major scattering phenomena makes a significant difference at depths where the lateral spread of beams is significant.

Figure 6 shows results of calculations and their comparison with experimental data from the Therac-20 linear accelerator. The calculations were done for water with a VAX-11/780 computer. The calculated data shown here are for pencils summed over a beam of infinite dimensions. For the dotted curve, a gaussian angular spread in the incident monoenergetic pencil beams was assumed, and its magnitude was adjusted to obtain the best fit with the measured data. The measured data (solid line) are for the largest (effectively infinite) electron beam obtainable. The differences in the calculated and measured values can, at least in part, be explained by the fact that the actual incident beam has a lower energy component and will give rise to a higher dose at shallow depths. For example, as illustrated by the dashed line, a 100-cm column of air between the source and the phantom surface increases the surface dose by almost 11%. Inclusion of the machine head and collimation system in the geometry should remove the remaining discrepancy. This part of the system is being refined.

In summary, Monte Carlo calculations with monoenergetic and monodirectional pencil beams give good agreement with experimental data. This agreement can be considerably improved by incorporating angular and energy spreads in the incident pencil beams.

Obtaining pencil beam dose distributions that correctly and completely incorporate most, if not all, of the important scattering processes is only a first step in the calculations of dose distributions in three dimensions in patients. The remaining steps are described below in the use of pencil beams in practical situations.

PENCIL BEAMS, SURFACE IRREGULARITIES, AND BLOCKED BEAMS

Pencil beams are ideally suited for dose calculations involving surface irregularities and blocked beams. This has been demonstrated by Perry and Holt (10). It is assumed that the pencil beams incident on an irregular surface at the time they hit the surface are identical and that they diffuse in the medium in a known and identical manner with respect to the entry point (Fig. 7). To compute the dose at an arbitrary point in the homogeneous medium, the contribution to this point due to all pencils that may have penetrated different depths is summated.

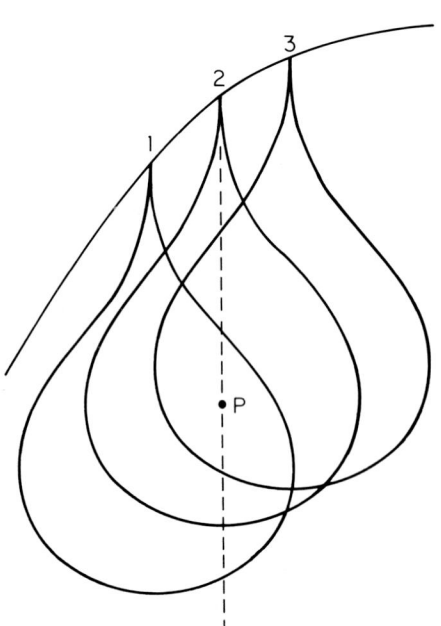

FIG. 7. Pencils of electrons propagate into a homogeneous medium in an identical manner relative to their entry point. Point P is at a different location relative to the various entry points. Contribution from each pencil is added to obtain the dose at P, thus accounting for the effect of surface irregularities.

PENCIL BEAMS AND INTERNAL INHOMOGENEITIES

The process of correcting for inhomogeneities beneath the patient's surface is considerably more complicated. This is because of the fact that by the time the pencil beam has penetrated a certain depth it is no longer monodirectional and monoenergetic, as it was at the surface. The effects of varying density and structure on such beams are complicated and difficult to compute with precision. A simple solution proposed by Hogstrom et al. (3) is to assume that each inhomogeneity lying in the path of the pencil beam is infinite in its lateral extent. The weighted path length from the surface to the depth of computation is then used to calculate the scattered contribution of each pencil to the point. This is essentially an extension of the equivalent path length method to pencil beams and should work well for an inhomogeneous structure that does not extend beyond about one-third of the range of incident electrons, i.e., in the region where the pencil beam has not yet spread out significantly. At larger depths relatively few of the electrons will still be close to the central axis of the pencil beams, and its applicability is questionable.

More work needs to be carried out in order to develop a better approach to correct for inhomogeneous structure. Two approaches we are examining are briefly described below. The first is a "pseudo Monte Carlo" method in which computation would be performed for one layer of pixels at a time. Beginning with the incident beam on the surface pixels, one could calculate, based on previously generated Monte Carlo data, the dose to these pixels and the contribution to the next layer of pixels in terms of electron energy, directions, and intensiy. For the second layer, previously generated Monte Carlo data would again be utilized and interpolated, if necessary, to determine the dose to each pixel in the second layer and the contribution to the succeeding layer.

A second approach is an extension of the ray model. Perry and Holt (10), using a multiple scattering formalism, have derived an expression for the mean (curved) path of electrons between two points in a homogeneous medium, and have shown that most particles do not deviate greatly from this (curved) path. Perhaps the mean path, determined either theoretically or by Monte Carlo methods, in homogeneous media would still be an adequately close approximation in inhomogeneous media. One would then calculate the dose to a point from a pencil beam in a manner similar to that using the equivalent path length methods by finding the effective path length along the predetermined mean (curved) path.

PENCIL BEAMS AND COLLIMATOR PERTURBATIONS

Simple summation of pencil beams cannot adequately account for the effect of a collimator system near the beam boundaries. One approach is to modulate the pencil beams by the measured primary beam intensity. Another approach, suitable for use with multiple scattering theory pencil beams, is to modify σ of Eq. 2 to take into account scattering from the collimator (3,13). We propose that the effect of collimator and housing etc. be taken into account using the following expression

$$D = [D(\text{pencil beam})/D_0(\text{pencil beam})] \cdot D_0(\text{measured}) \qquad (3)$$

where D (pencil beam) is the calculated dose using pencil beam for the patient, D_0 (pencil beam) is the calculated dose for the homogeneous phantom normal to the incident beam, and D_0 (measured) is the corresponding measured dose in the same phantom. The effects of collimator, etc. are included in the measured data. This method will require larger amounts of measured data but will be more accurate.

INCORPORATION OF CT DATA

CT numbers represent attenuation coefficients of x-rays in the diagnostic energy range and, as such, are not suitable for use in dose calculations in the therapetuc energy range. Depending on the method of electron beam dose calculation chosen, they must be transformed into a new, more appropriate set of numbers prior to their use in dose computations.

For the equivalent path length method, the dose is computed using the measured depth dose data (or TMRs) that already include the stopping power corrections. Therefore it is sufficient to transform the CT numbers into electron densities and use them to compute the equivalent path length by the addition of the electron densities of pixels lying along the path of the source-computation point ray. Several investigators (3,5,8) have designed and demonstrated techniques for determining transformation factors from CT numbers to electron densities. These factors vary from one machine to another and should be determined for each machine.

In the pencil beam technique, the pencils, if obtained by the multiple scattering theory, represent fluence of electrons and not energy deposition. Therefore a correlation between CT numbers and both the stopping powers and scattering powers must be established.

The pencil beam data generated using the Monte Carlo method are already in the form of energy deposition and are calculated using cross sections of tissue substitute materials and their densities. Therefore no transformation to electron densities or stopping power corrections are necessary. On the other hand, CT numbers must be transformed into numbers corresponding to the tissue substitute materials whose scattering cross sections are used to calculate the pencil beams.

SUMMARY AND CONCLUSION

Various methods of dose computations have been reviewed. The equivalent path length methods used to account for body curvature and internal structure are not adequate because they ignore the lateral diffusion of electrons. The Monte Carlo method for the broad field three-dimensional situation in treatment planning is impractical because of the enormous computer time required. The pencil beam technique may represent a suitable compromise. The behavior of a pencil beam may be described by the multiple scattering theory or, alternatively, generated using the Monte Carlo method. Although nearly two orders of magnitude slower than the equivalent path length technique, the pencil beam method improves accuracy sufficiently to justify its use. It applies very well when accounting for the effect of surface irregularities; the formulation for handling inhomogeneous internal structure is yet to be developed.

REFERENCES

1. Ayyangar, K., Ting, J. Y., and Suntharalingam, N. (1978): Surface contour and inhomogeneity corrections in electron beam treatment planning. AAPM presentation.
2. Brahme, A., Lax, I., and Andreo, P. (1982): Electron beam dose planning using discrete gaussian beams: Mathematical background. *In press.*
3. Hogstrom, K. R., Mills, M. M., and Almond, P. R. (1981): Electron beam dose calculations. *Phys. Med. Biol.*, 26:445–459.
4. Holt, J. G., Mohan, R., Caley, R., Buffa, A., Reid, A., Simpson, L., and Laughlin, J. S. (1978): Memorial electron beam AET treatment planning system. In: *Practical Aspects of Electron Beam Treatment Planning, Medical Physics Monograph No. 2*, edited by C. G. Orton and F. Bagne, pp. 70–79. *American Institute of Physics*, New York.
5. Hsi, S. C., Laughlin, J. S., Miller, D. W., Masterson, M. E., Simpson, L., and Pentlow, K. (1978): An experimentally based computation approach for the relationship between CT number and electron density for radiation therapy treatment planning: works in progress. AAPM, Chicago.
6. Kawachi, K. (1975): Calculation of electron dose distribution for radiotherapy treatment planning. *Phys. Med. Biol.*, 20:571–577.
7. Laughlin, J. S. (1975): High energy electron treatment planning for inhomogeneities. *Br. J. Radiol.*, 38:143–147.
8. Masterson, M. E., Thomason, C. L., McGary, R., Hunt, M. A., Simpson, L., Miller, D. W., and Laughlin, J. S. (1981): Dependence of the CT number-electron density relationship of patient size and x-ray beam filtration for fan beam CT scanners. In: *SPIE Technical Program Committee Proceedings*, San Francisco (*in press*).
9. Mohan, R., Bading, J., Caley, R., Reid, A., Ding, J., and Laughlin, J. S. (1979): Computerized electron beam dosimetry. In: *Proceedings of the Symposium on Electron Beam Therapy*, pp. 75–81.
10. Perry, D., and Holt, J. G. (1980): A model for calculating the effects of small inhomogeneities on electron beam dose distributions. *Med. Phys.*, 7:207–215.
11. Riley, R., Mohan, R., Laughlin, J. S., Goodman, M., Karpovsky, A., and Gabriel, A. (1981): Use of Monte Carlo generated pencil beam data in electron beam dosimetry. AAPM presentation.
12. Steben, J. D., Ayyangar, K., and Suntharalingham, N. (1979): Betatron electron beam characterization for dosimetry calculations. *Phys. Med. Biol.*, 24:299–309.
13. Werner, B. L., Khan, F., and Deibel, F. C. (1981): The spreading of electron beams. *In press.*

Computed Tomography in Radiation Therapy,
edited by C. C. Ling, C. C. Rogers, and
R. J. Morton. Raven Press, New York © 1983

Use of CT in Electron Beam Treatment Planning: Current and Future Development

Kenneth R. Hogstrom and Robert S. Fields

*Department of Physics and Radiotherapy, The University of Texas System Cancer Center,
M.D. Anderson Hospital and Tumor Institute, Houston, Texas 77030*

Prior to the availability of computed tomographic (CT) scanning for routine use in electron beam radiation therapy, it was often difficult to appreciate completely the distribution of dose with respect to the target volume and surrounding anatomy. This was due to a lack of both accuracy in defining target volume depth and ability to calculate the perturbation of dose due to tissue heterogeneities. Typically, electron beam energy for treatment has been based on distal tumor depth. Methods of determining tumor depth ranged from the use of standard treatment depths to transverse axial tomography. CT has not necessarily replaced those other clinical methods, but it has supplemented them and provides an anatomic map suitable to the task of treatment planning in all parts of the body.

CT provides an accurate way to identify the tumor and those tissues and structures at risk. This permits the therapist to visualize quantitatively the target volume on an individual basis. By determining the maximum depth in the target volume, the optimal beam energy may be selected for treatment. This is particularly important in treatments having critical structures distal to the target volume. The depth of the critical structures also can be assessed from CT scans, which allows a determination of dose to these structures. With knowledge of these depths, the treatment plan can be optimized, but caution is advised if the planning is done using only central axis depth dose because there may be dose perturbations due to changes in electron beam penetration and lack of scatter equilibrium. The former is due to tissue heterogeneities, and the latter is due to irregular skin contours, tissue heterogeneities, and collimation effects.

CT provides an excellent means for measuring skin contour, especially in the head and neck, where manual measurement methods may be difficult. In addition, there is no substitute for the use of CT in characterizing those tissue heterogeneities required for accurate electron beam planning. Therefore CT has opened the door for significant improvement in our electron beam treatment planning methods. Success in this area depends on both development of more accurate algorithms for dose calculation and more sophistication in our treatment techniques.

DOSE CALCULATION ALGORITHMS

Numerous papers dealing with electron beam dose calculations have appeared since the onset of electron beam therapy, and reviews of these works exist (9,11). Many of the algorithms are either completely empirical or modifications of previous algorithms developed for photon beams. Corrections for tissue heterogeneities often involve simple methods using tables of correction factors. The weakness of many of these methods is that they do not model the physics of electon beams per se, nor are they flexible enough to account for the complex patient anatomy revealed by CT scanning.

Recently the trend (1,6,10,13) has been to develop the pencil beam or strip beam algorithm, as it offers the advantage of simultaneously correcting for changes in electron beam penetration and side scatter nonequilibrium. Based on the physical laws of electron multiple coulomb scattering, the method is not only an improvement over earlier methods but lends itself to future modifications as we learn more about electron beam dosimetry. The algorithm by Hogstrom et al. (6) deals specifically with calculations using CT data on a pixel-by-pixel basis, and as it is currently being investigated clinically we limit our discussion to that work.

The pencil beam algorithm calculates dose at a point by summing the contribution of dose from each pencil beam that passes through the aperture-defining collimator. A pencil beam is defined as those electrons passing through a small, imaginary rectangle lying with the collimator plane. The dose distribution of each pencil beam is calculated by assuming that the heterogeneities underlying the central ray of each pencil beam extend laterally well outside the collimator boundaries.

The pencil beam dose distribution is characterized by a central and off-axis profile. The off-axis profile of a pencil beam is gaussian, with a σ that can be calculated using Fermi-Eyges theory (4) and is given by

$$\sigma_x^2 = (Z + L_0 + L_{air})^2 \sigma_{air}^2 + \frac{1}{2} \int_0^Z [(d\sigma^2/dZ)/(d\sigma^2/dZ)_{H_2O}] \tag{1}$$

$$\times (d\sigma^2/dZ)_{H_2O}(Z - Z')^2 dZ'$$

where Z is the depth below the skin surface; L_0 is the air gap from the collimator to the skin-surface distance (SSD); L_{air} is the air gap from the SSD to the skin surface; σ_{air} is a constant that is machine- and energy-dependent and is equal to the ratio of the 90% to 10% penumbra of a broad-field profile in air at the SSD to 2.56 times L_0; $(d\sigma^2/dZ)_{H_2O}$ is the linear angular scattering power in water at the energy E_Z corresponding to the mean electron energy at Z; and $(d\sigma^2/dZ)/(d\sigma^2/dZ)_{H_2O}$ is the energy-independent ratio of the linear angular scattering power of the tissue at Z relative to that of water. The linear scattering power ratio is determined from the CT number H using the calibration curve shown in Fig. 1.

The central axis depth dose of the pencil beam is calculated from the central axis depth dose (D_0) for the rectangular field size at the SSD (*WX* by *WY*), which is

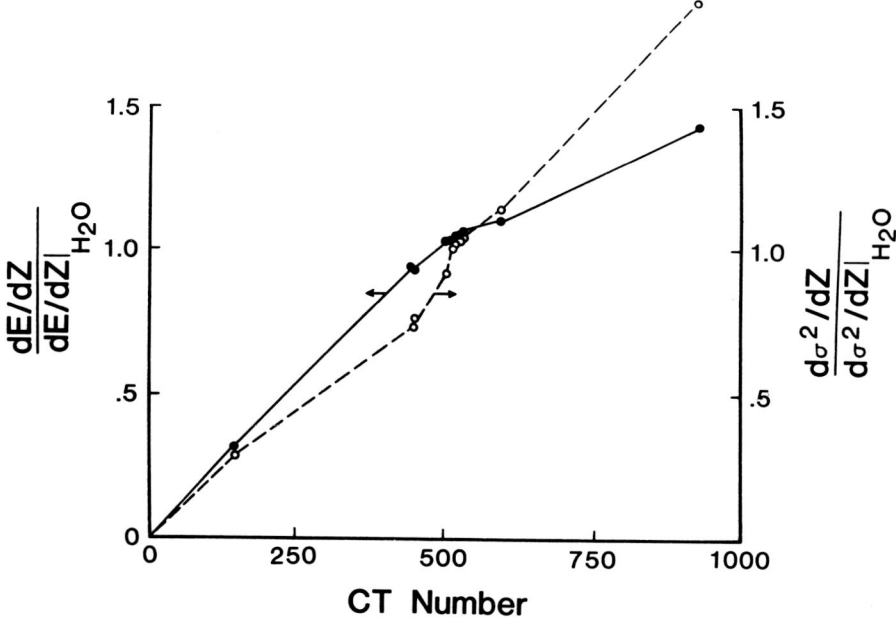

FIG. 1. Plot of linear stopping power relative to that of water versus CT number H (0 = air, 500 = water), and plot of linear scattering power relative to that of water versus CT number for electrons in human tissues, which are, in order of increasing CT number, lung, fat, adipose, red marrow, brain, kidney, muscle, liver, inner bone, compact bone.

inscribed by the actual collimator. It also depends on the effective depth (Z_{eff}) and the air gap, being given by

$$d_{pencil}(Z) = \frac{1}{2\pi\sigma_x^2}$$
$$\times \left\{ D_0(Z_{eff}) \left[erf\left(\frac{WXZ}{2\sqrt{2}\sigma_0}\right) erf\left(\frac{WYZ}{2\sqrt{2}\sigma_0}\right) \right]^{-1} \left(\frac{SSD + Z_{eff}}{SSD}\right)^2 \right\}$$
$$\times \left(\frac{SSD}{SSD + Z + L_{air}}\right)^2 \tag{2}$$

where erf is the standard error function, *WYZ* by *WYZ* is the field size projected to Z, and σ_0 is the σ_x for the geometry under which D_0 was measured. The first term in Eq. 2 is due to the variation of central axis scatter equilibrium with depth; the second term is the depth dose for an infinite field size, infinite SSD calculated from measured data; and the final term is the inverse square dependence. Critical to the evaluation is the effective depth, which is calculated by

$$Z_{\text{eff}}(Z) = \int_0^Z \left[\frac{(dE/dZ)}{(dE/dZ)_{\text{H}_2\text{O}}} \right] dZ' \tag{3}$$

where $(dE/dZ)/(dE/dZ)_{\text{H}_2\text{O}}$ is the energy-independent ratio of linear stopping power of the tissue at Z' relative to that of water. Again, the linear stopping power ratio is determined from the CT number H using the calibration curve shown in Fig. 1.

The calibration curves for the linear stopping power ratio and the linear scattering power ratio have been determined in the following manner. Lung, fat, muscle, inner bone, hard bone, etc. tissue substitutes of known composition and density are prepared (3) as inserts into a CT phantom. The phantom is scanned and the CT number H is determined. Then the effective x-ray energy that most accurately predicts H is determined. If one then calculates the linear stopping and scattering power ratios at 10 MeV and the CT numbers at the effective x-ray energy for actual tissues, the calibration curves of Fig. 1 can be constructed.

This algorithm uses measured data, corrects for variable air gap, makes an effective depth correction due to tissue heterogeneities, and makes a scatter correction due to both irregular skin surface and tissue heterogeneities. Furthermore, corrections for patient anatomy can be made using CT data on a pixel-by-pixel basis. Disadvantages of the algorithm are that computation time presently constrains us to assume that anatomic features adjacent to the slice of calculation do not vary significantly in size or shape.

Recently a study using TLD in tissue substitute phantoms of the head has been performed to assess the accuracy of the algorithm in its present form (7). These results show that the algorithm is good to approximately $\pm 4\%$ in the target volume or ± 4 mm in regions of sharp dose gradients (i.e., penumbra, distal edge) in most circumstances, but that greater errors occur in cases where air cavities lie deep beneath the skin and where air cavities are narrow and parallel to the incident beams. In addition, the single-slice calculation can lead to greater errors in regions where the anatomic features change significantly from slice to slice, as is the case in the area of the nose. Nevertheless, the algorithm is an improvement to previous clinical dosimetry and can give valuable information with respect to tumor dose, hot or cold spots, and coverage of the isodose line selected for treatment.

PATIENT CASES

In the two cases presented, the patients were scanned on the General Electric (GE) 8800 CT scanner in the treatment position. The scans were then transferred via magnetic tape to the GE RT/Plan therapy planning system for hardcopy printout. The scans were then input as contours into a separate computer for electron beam dose calculations. Therefore the present isodose distributions have been calculated by characterizing the anatomy according to average CT number within any contours rather than on a pixel-by-pixel basis. Selecting the shape and average CT number within any contour is a very subjective process and confirms our belief that planning on a pixel-by-pixel basis is desirable.

Case I

A patient presented with a recurrent soft tissue sarcoma to the posterior medial thoracic wall. The patient was CT scanned to determine the depth to the spinal cord and the thickness of the thoracic wall, necessary for electron beam energy selection for a posterior field. The scout view of the CT scan is shown in Fig. 2 and the central CT scan slice in Fig. 3. Three CT scan slices were obtained at the center and just inside the inferior and superior field borders to determine tumor

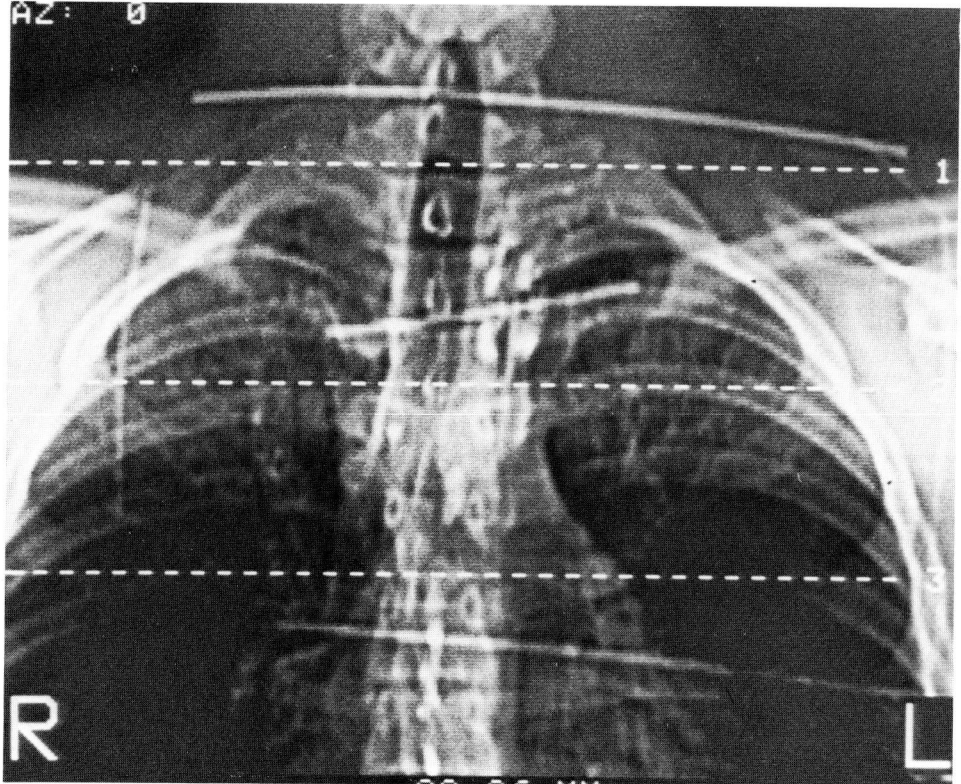

FIG. 2. Scout view of CT scan of patient with a recurrent soft tissue sarcoma to the posterior medial thoracic wall. Radiopaque catheters delineate the treatment portal. The dashed lines indicate the levels of the limited CT scan.

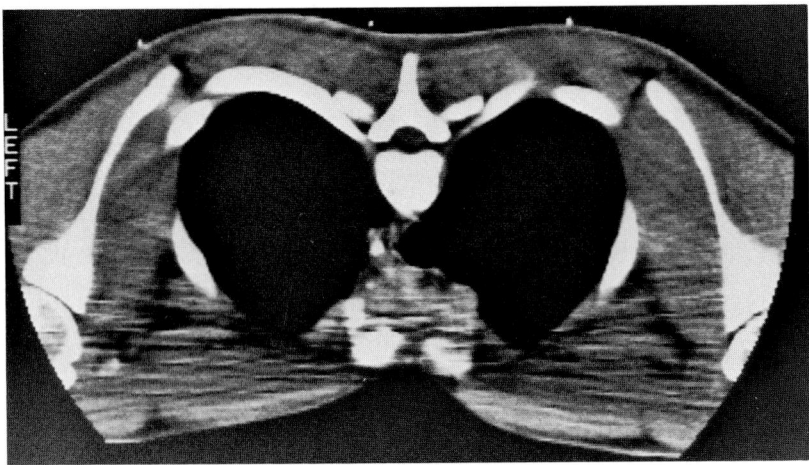

FIG. 3. CT scan slice 2 of Fig. 2 passing through the center of the field. The depth of the spinal cord and lung localization are easily obtained.

coverage and minimum spinal cord depth. The end slices were without evidence of disease, thus confirming adequate coverage, and the minimum cord depth was found to be 4.1 cm in the central slice, compared with 3.2 cm in the inferior slice. A 13-MeV electron beam was being considered for treatment, and the dose distribution has been plotted in Fig. 4 for the central CT slice. The cord receives a considerable dose, especially at the inferior border of the field where the cord depth is less (Fig. 4). When calculating the cord dose, one should be aware that the spinous process does not completely shield the cord, and that this could cause a distal (anterior) shift of the isodose lines by approximately 2 mm at some locations. The amount of irradiated lung is easily seen. A 9-MeV electron beam dose distribution also was calculated, showing essentially no lung or cord dose but a 1.5 cm proximal shift of the 90% isodose line. Based on this information, the therapist selected an 11-MeV electron beam with a reduction to 9 MeV at midtreatment. The last four fractions were given with 6 MeV to boost the scar tissue. The resulting depth dose of the mixed beams is plotted in Fig. 5 using the mixing program developed by Fields et al. (5). It shows a skin dose of 5,677 rads, a cord dose of 4,735 rads at 3.2 cm, and a dose of 5,525 rads at a depth of 2.7 cm, the depth of prescription by the therapist.

Because the anatomic features slowly vary in adjacent CT slices, a great deal of confidence is placed in the calculated dose distributions. This, coupled with the ease of obtaining tumor, cord, and lung localization from limited CT scans, has made scanning routine for this type of patient.

Case II

A patient presented with recurrent chronic parotiditis. Typically, patients with tumor in this area receive a mixture of 17 MeV electrons and 18 MV photons, as

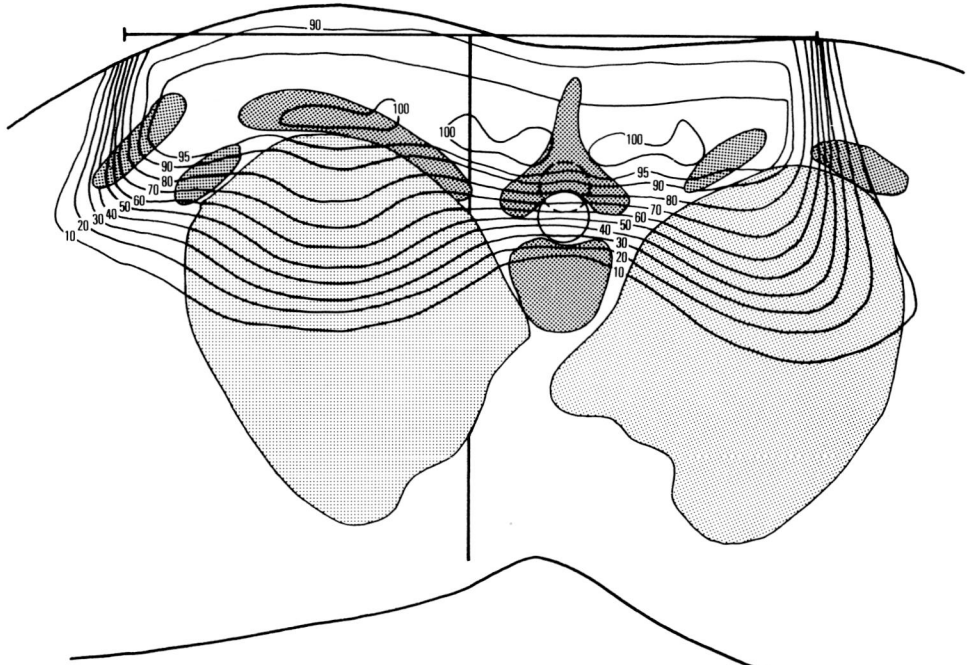

FIG. 4. Dose distribution in the central CT scan plane (Fig. 3) from a 13-MeV electron beam. The dashed circle is the location of the spinal cord relative to the skin surface on the inferior CT slice, where cord depth is at a minimum.

discussed by Tapley (12). Electrons are used to spare the contralateral side, and photons are mixed so as to provide skin sparing and a more uniform dose distribution across the target volume. A procedure for optimizing the mixture has been developed by Fields et al. (5). However, the treatment aim in this case was to deliver 2,000 rads in 10 fractions to decrease the activity and inflammation of the parotid gland. With treatment of benign disease, sparing of normal tissue is requisite. Also, because the dose to the treatment volume is relatively low compared to that for treatment of malignant disease, the high surface dose with the electron beam is of less importance. Therefore electron beam radiation only is desired to minimize the contralateral dose.

The patient was CT scanned for localization of the parotid gland and to determine maximum depth of the target volume for use in treatment planning. Figure 6 shows the scout view, and Fig. 7 shows the CT scan passing through the primary area of interest. The maximum depth of the parotid gland was determined to be 3.2 cm on the CT scan, and it was then decided to treat to 90% at 4 cm. When calculating the electron beam dose distribution, the CT scan was useful in that it indicated the location of the mandible and the skin surface, the latter being difficult to determine by manual methods due to the irregular shape of the ear. Both 13- and 17-MeV electron beam dose distributions were provided to the therapist for evaluation, and

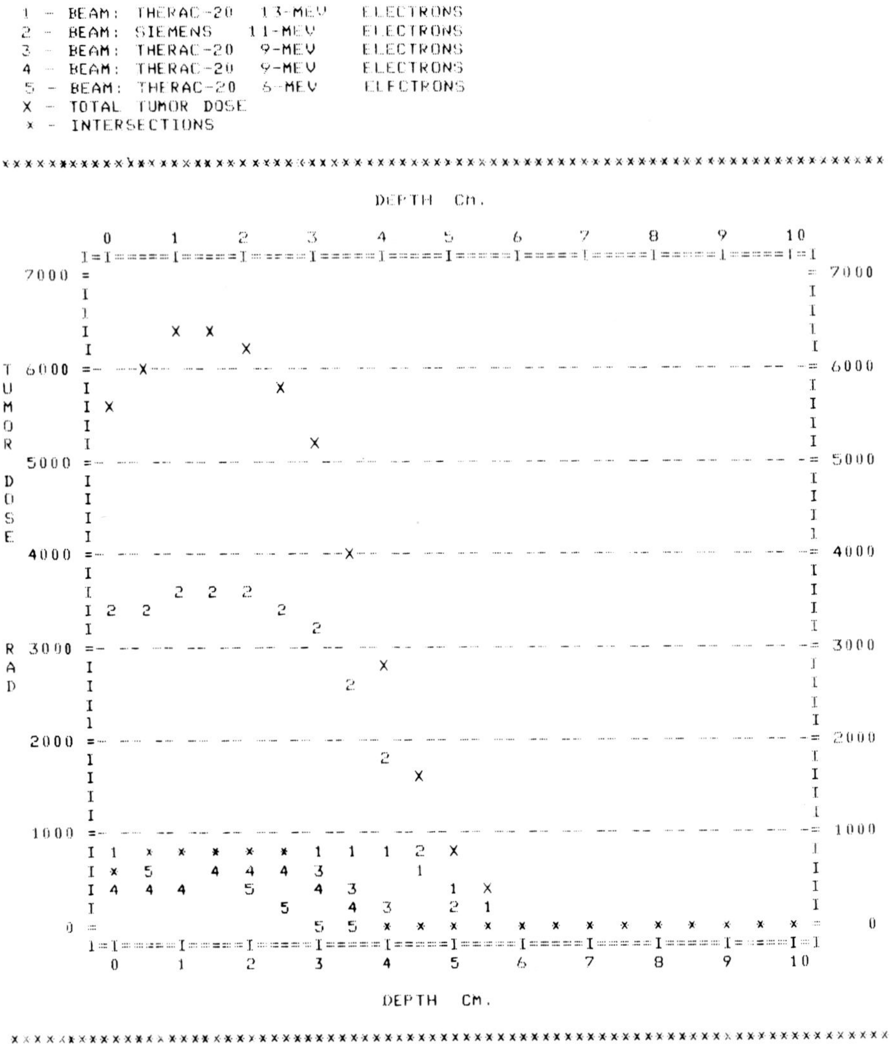
1 – BEAM: THERAC-20 13-MEV ELECTRONS
2 – BEAM: SIEMENS 11-MEV ELECTRONS
3 – BEAM: THERAC-20 9-MEV ELECTRONS
4 – BEAM: THERAC-20 9-MEV ELECTRONS
5 – BEAM: THERAC-20 6-MEV ELECTRONS
X – TOTAL TUMOR DOSE
x – INTERSECTIONS
DEPTH CM.
TUMOR DOSE RAD
0
1000
2000
3000
4000
5000
6000
7000
0 1 2 3 4 5 6 7 8 9 10
DEPTH CM.

FIG. 5. Central axis depth dose calculated by EMIX of 13, 11, 9, and 6 MeV electrons mixed in the completed treatment of case I.

the latter is shown in Fig. 8. Note the 10% hot spot in dose due to scatter off the ear. No significant hot or cold spots are generated distal to the edges of the mandible, in agreement with previous calculations and measurements that typically show a hot spot of approximately 5%. The shifting of the isodose curves due to the mandible is seen in the 95% isodose line. Note, however, that this shift decreases and spreads laterally with depth due to side scatter. The 13-MeV distribution reduced the 90% depth from approximately 5.1 cm to 3.6 cm at the posterior border of the mandible. Based on this information, it was decided to treat the patient with a 3:2 mixture of

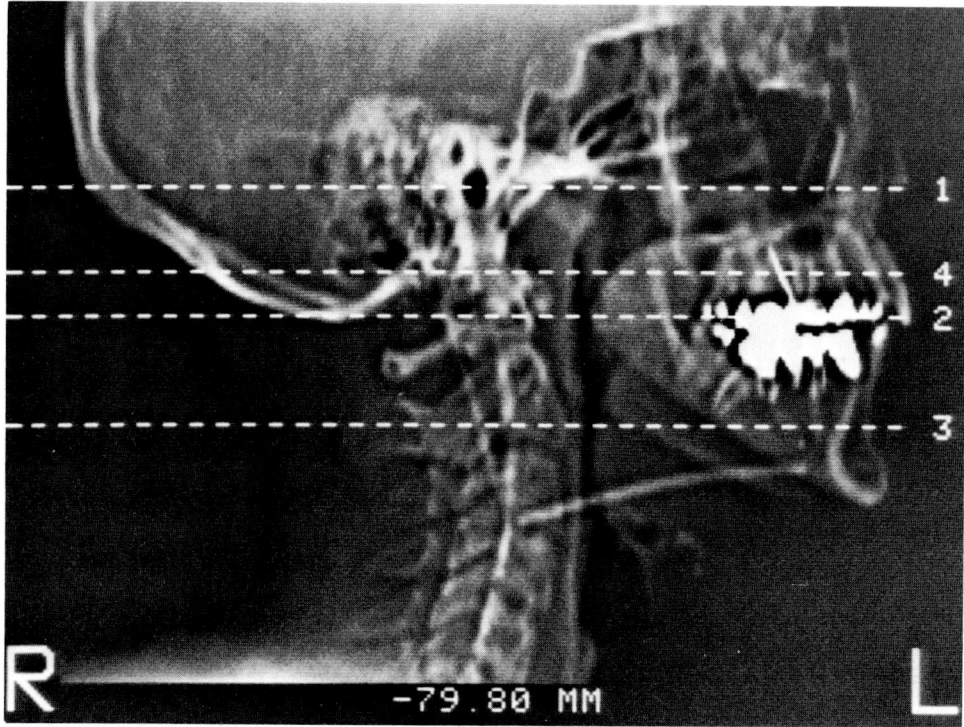

FIG. 6. Scout view of CT scan of a patient with parotiditis. Radiopaque catheters delineate the treatment portal. The dashed lines indicate the levels of the limited CT scan.

17-MeV/13-MeV electrons, which resulted in a 4.2-cm penetration to the 90% isodose line.

FUTURE OF CT IN ELECTRON BEAM THERAPY

The future of CT in electron beam therapy lies in our ability to: (a) implement in routine clinical use those techniques currently available; (b) improve the speed, sophistication, and ease of calculating dose distributions for routine clinical setups; and (c) develop new techniques whose potential now exists with CT scanning.

As discussed earlier, we can use CT scans to assess maximum target volume depth and depth to critical structures for selection of beam energy and determination of dose to critical structures. Dose distributions superimposed on the anatomy are particularly rich in such assessment. When calculating dose we should realize that corrections for effective depth are required in regions containing heterogeneities. We have seen the influence of lung and mandible in the cases described. In regions of irregular skin surface and heterogeneities, it is beneficial to have dose calculations that correct for side scatter nonequilibrium. This is particularly true when treating tumors of the nose with posterior extension. Calculations show hot spots (approx-

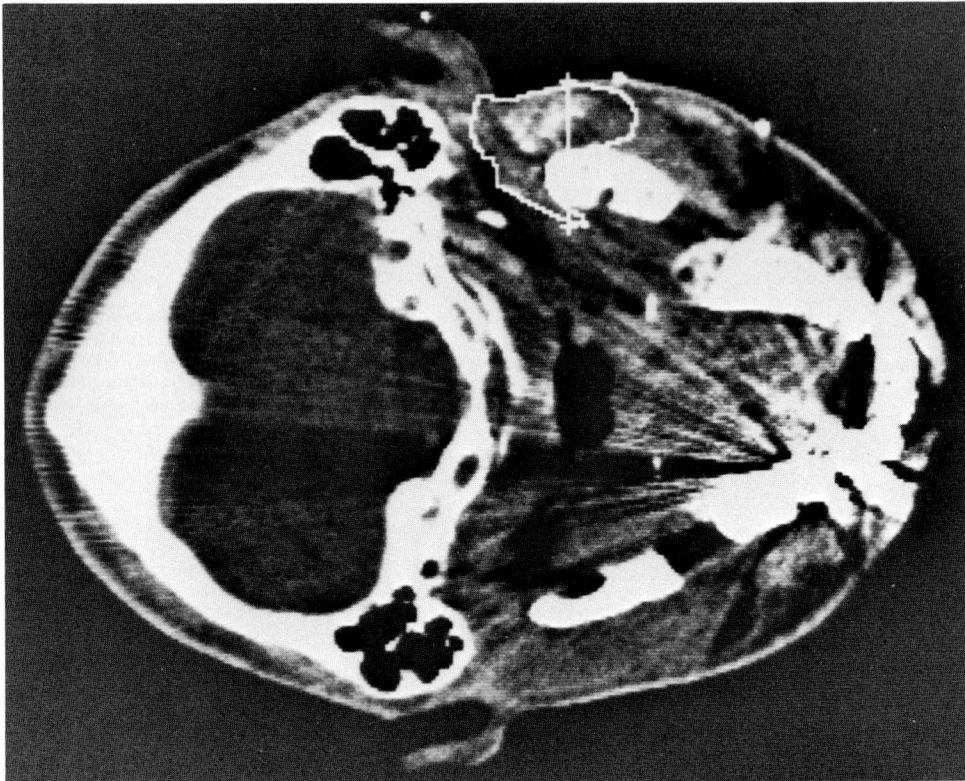

FIG. 7. CT scan slice 4 of Fig. 5 passing through the deepest extension of the parotid. Calcification is seen in the gland, and the dashed line generously outlines its extension. The line segment indicates a maximum depth of 3.2 cm through soft tissue and mandible.

imately 20% increase in dose) beneath the lateral borders of the nose caused by the irregular skin surface and cold spots (approximately 25% decrease in dose) in the septum due to both the irregular skin surface and the nasal air cavities (7). Reevaluation of our current treatment techniques using CT anatomy and sophisticated dose-calculation algorithms could lead to modification of some of our treatment plans.

Because CT now provides accurate anatomic maps useful for treatment planning, it is now the task of the medical physicist to provide more sophisticated dose calculations so that the therapist can have greater confidence in the dose distributions. Although the pencil beam algorithms are a step in the right direction, they require more computation time than we normally expect. Furthermore, we must extend the algorithm's capability to calculate using anatomy in adjacent CT slices. Measurements in a Rando phantom at the level of the base of the nose by Hogstrom et al. (7) have shown this to be desirable at this anatomic location. As irregular fields are commonplace using electrons, the algorithms should have that capability. Presently, the main weakness of pencil beam algorithms is their ability to account

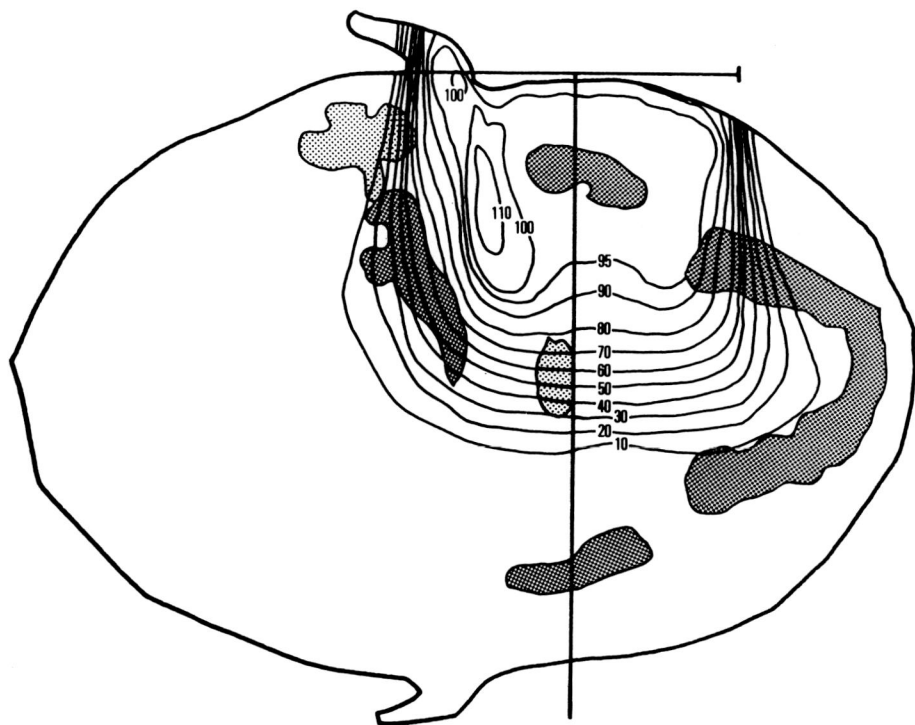

FIG. 8. Dose distribution in CT slice 4 (Fig. 7) through the parotid gland from a 17-MeV electron beam. Note the hot spot of 110% due to ear scattering and the mandible influencing isodose lines in its shadow. (7.6 × 6.0 cm; 100 cm SSD.)

accurately for heterogeneities either long and parallel to the incident beam or distal to the skin surface. Improvements in speed, sophistication, and ease of clinical use will not come easy and will require coordinated research.

A sounder knowledge of the use of CT in electron beam treatment planning should lead to the development of more sophisticated treatment techniques. The influence of heterogeneities may modify the dose distribution from what is expected, and as a result an increase in mixing with photon beams may be advantageous. This influence is a factor to be considered, in addition to those discussed by Fields et al. (5), for determining an electron-photon mix. We may see more tailoring of electron beams in individual treatments based on CT anatomy. For example, determination of chest wall thickness should allow pseudo arc therapy, in which energy is varied as the arc is rotated (8). Finally, the use of compensating bolus for tailoring the beam penetration versus transverse position is particularly attractive (2). This technology is routinely used in heavy charged particle therapy but requires software and technological capabilities.

In conclusion, we should look at CT scanning as potentially beginning a new era in electron beam treatment planning. Some techniques can readily be implemented in the clinic, but we have yet to realize the potential which exists.

ACKNOWLEDGMENTS

This work was supported in part by research grant CA-06294 from the National Cancer Institute.

REFERENCES

1. Ayyangar, K., Leonard, C., and Sunthralingam, N. (1980): Computerization of electron beams for treatment planning. *Med. Phys.*, 7:440.
2. Chu, F. C. H. (1981): Electron beam therapy of breast cancer. In: *Proceedings of the Symposium on Electron Beam Therapy*, edited by F. C. H. Chu and J. S. Laughlin, pp. 83–88. Memorial Sloan-Kettering Cancer Center, New York.
3. Constantinou, C. (1978): Tissue substitutes for particulate radiations and their use in radiation dosimetry and radiotherapy. Ph.D. thesis, University of London.
4. Eyges, L. (1948): Multiple scattering with energy loss. *Phys. Rev.*, 74:1534–1535.
5. Fields, R. S., Spanos, W. J., Tapley, N., duV., Cundiff, J. H., and Sampiere, V. A. (1980): Computer optimization for combining electron and photon beams. *Int. J. Radiat. Oncol. Biol. Phys.*, 6:144.
6. Hogstrom, K. R., Mills, M. D., and Almond, P. R. (1981): Electron beam dose calculations. *Phys. Med. Biol.*, 26:445–459.
7. Hogstrom, K. R., Mills, M. D., Cundiff, J. H., Almond, P. R., Fields, R., and McNeese, M. D. (1981): Clinical evaluation of an electron beam algorithm. *Med. Phys.*, 8:577.
8. Mok, E. C., Boyer, A. L., and Fullerton, G. D. (1981): Computer based dosimetry for multi-energy electron, pseudo-arc technique. *Med. Phys.*, 8:575.
9. Nusslin, F. (1979): Computerized treatment planning in therapy with fast electrons: a review of procedures for calculating dose distribution. *Medicamundi*, 24:112–118.
10. Perry, D. J., and Holt, J. G. (1980): A model for calcuating the effects of small inhomogeneities on electron beam dose distributions. *Med. Phys.*, 7:207–215.
11. Sternick, E. S. (1978): Algorithms for computerized treatment planning. In: *Practical Aspects of Electron Beam Treatment Planning, Medical Physics Monograph No. 2*, edited by C. G. Ortin and F. Bagne, pp. 52–69. American Institute of Physics, New York.
12. Tapley, N.duV. (ed.) (1976): *Clinical Applications of the Electron Beam.* Wiley, New York.
13. Werner, B. L., Khan, F. M., and Deibel, F. C. (1982): The spreading of electron beams. *Med. Phys.*, 9:180–187.

Computed Tomography in Radiation Therapy,
edited by C. C. Ling, C. C. Rogers, and
R. J. Morton. Raven Press, New York © 1983

Clinical Perspective

R. J. Berry

Department of Oncology, The Middlesex Hospital Medical School, London, England

The success of this volume must be credited to the organizers for structuring the presentation of the material so well. This is reflected in the way the individual presentations fit together. Moreover, the organizers made sure that the clinicians and the physicists both presented their approaches. I would like to try to put the various problems in perspective.

TYPES OF LESIONS

Among our 6 million population in south London, 25,000 new cancer cases present for treatment per year; roughly that is 4,000 new cancer cases per million population per year. This is also a good general figure for the Western world. On the average in the United Kingdom, one-third of the cases are treated by radiotherapy as part of their primary management (Table 1).

One in five new cancers is a carcinoma of the lung, and at the moment one-third of these undergo radiotherapy. There are two quite different groups here, however. On the one hand, there is a selected group of patients with non-oat-cell carcinoma

TABLE 1. *New patients with cancer[a]*

Site	% Of all new cancers	% Treated by radiotherapy
Lung	19	33
Colon/rectum	12	5
Breast	11	47
Skin	11	51
Gynecologic region	8	46
Stomach/esophagus	8	8
Bladder	5	36
Leukemia/lymphoma	5	24
Prostate	4	14
Pancreas	3	3
Head and neck	3	78
Brain	1	36

[a]From South Thames Cancer Registry, 1975: Evidence to London Health Planning Consortium. Report of the Study Group on Radiotherapy and Oncology, November 1979.

of the bronchus. All of our diagnostic skills must be put to use for these patients to exclude disseminated disease, and all of our therapeutic skills, both in terms of tumor localization with CT and treatment planning to spare normal tissue structures must be used. Despite this admonition, however, the evidence is still conflicting about this lesion, although there are a number of reports from groups who treat selected cases with high doses of radiation and who have long-term survivors.

These patients must be carefully distinguished from the vast majority of patients who should receive palliative treatment only. The latter patients should have the simplest management that keeps the length of hospitalization and the cost at a minimum.

Colorectal cancer, the next most common malignancy, is a lesion for which, at the moment, radiotherapists do nothing. Occasionally some of the recurrences are irradiated for palliative treatment, but basically we are not involved. Yet there is an argument which says that this is an anatomic area where cure could be effected by the combined treatment of irradiation and surgery. This is a new area for study, where treatment planning may be vitally important because if the colorectal tumor can be treated, it is in a structure which is itself highly radiosensitive.

Treatment of carcinoma of the breast exemplifies a changing technology. About 50% of these lesions are now treated with radiotherapy. There is currently tremendous pressure on the physician to preserve the breast by more limited surgery, and so a higher proportion of patients will be treated by irradiation with the breast intact. Hence radiotherapeutic techniques will demand greater consideration about the effect on normal tissues. This is an area where much needs to be done: maximizing the treatment to the organ of interest while minimizing scattered and unwanted radiation to normal tissue.

The treatment of skin tumors will remain very much as it is now. They require no imaging. The treatment of gynecological tumors is also probably not going to change very much.

Carcinomas of the stomach and esophagus comprise less than 10% of all new malignancies. However, CT imaging has allowed, for the first time, the exact localization of these lesions.

Carcinoma of the bladder, of particular interest to my department, is a lesion on which we believe CT has had a major impact. We will only know in a few years' time whether, with selection of cases for radiotherapy solely by CT-aided assessment of tumor response, we are doing as well as with the more brutal approach of preoperative radiotherapy and cystectomy.

Leukemia is a systemic disease, and, except for the lymphomas, sophisticated treatment planning is already required.

Localized carcinoma of the prostate is now curable, and more of these lesions will present for treatment by radiotherapy. Surgical treatment in this disease is becoming rare.

Carcinoma of the pancreas is another lesion not treated by irradiation, although CT imaging has allowed us to determine the location of the tumor. Moreover, a number of American studies involving small numbers of cases of inoperable carcinoma of the pancreas have reported early results that indicate tumor local control by irradiation, or at least long-term palliation. These findings could increase population of patients presenting to our radiotherapy departments.

Little change is likely in the treatment of head, neck, and brain tumors. However, it is clear that the techology discussed in this volume may itself change radiotherapy practice.

WHO SHOULD HAVE A CT SCANNER?

There is a very different organization of radiotherapy practice in the United States than that in England. Suntharalingam noted that more than half the total departments surveyed in the United States treated less than 300 new patients per year. A center that size makes it difficult to justify dedicated machinery, or even major-use machinery, compared to an organization such as ours where the individual cancer-treatment centers tend to be much larger. The different geographies contribute to the differences in our systems as well—none of our patients has to travel more than 50 miles for treatment.

TECHNICAL ASPECTS

Tremendous strides have been made in display graphics. This is an area where the ability of the physician to think pictorially is important. One of the problems here lies in training the young physician to relate these pictures to what they actually see and feel on the patient. We do not teach the relation to surface anatomy anymore, and so it will be important to educate the new physicains in this area.

Another problem that must be faced with this new technology is that once an image is seen on a display screen or is reinforced by hard copy, one tends to implicitly believe both the pictures and the numbers. It must be kept in mind that we still lack total confirmation that the abnormalities we see even in diagnostic CT scans are histopathologically accurate.

The quantitative information we obtain in terms of tissue densities must be considered in terms of the limitations on the interpretation of those numbers from CT numbers. The dose distributions from our present relatively simplified algorithms include approximations whose limits may not be appreciated by those who are using them, especially not by the physcians. The current algorithms need strict testing by measurements of dose on complex phantoms. We must take a close look at the errors which exist in some of the commercial systems, because in some cases these systems are being used beyond the limits for which they were intended.

MISCELLANEOUS CONSIDERATIONS

A major point made by Lichter about volume localization being more important than tumor localization emphasizes the need for the physician to detail what a given gross tumor volume means in terms of the risk of spread of disease. It is still necessary for physicians to know basic anatomy and physiology, which regrettably is being less well taught in medical schools today.

Lichter also distinguished between the diagnostic approach being qualitative and the radiotherapeutic approach to CT information being quantitative. I take issue with that. The diagnostician also quantitates, but visually in terms of gray scales or color—pattern recognition is basically quantitative.

Goodenough introduced a very useful concept, the voxel. Too often we think about the cross-sectional pictures obtained by CT scan as a single slice that is infinitely thin, and that the pixel represents the entire picture. This is a volume element, however, and it is comprised of many half-volume effects which are important. The quantitative measurement depends on what is actually included in the slice. That is one problem we must give more consideration to, in terms of both qualitative imaging and in what use we make quantitatively of the CT numbers.

Another problem is the difference between computed and measured data. We must be able to believe the numbers the machines provide us. Yet even some of the good commercial treatment planning systems still produce data with errors that are of a magnitude which is unacceptable. This is a particular problem for small centers where the personnel simply do not have the experience to know the limitations of their systems. It boils down to an ethical problem for the commercial enterprise that wants to sell its system but is constrained to describe its limitations.

One of the important changes occurring in the United Kingdom and which will hopefully take place in the United States as well is that we are breaking down the traditional radiologic and nuclear medicine departments. In their place, we are creating central imaging departments, with the radiologist being recognized as an imaging consultant to whom the clinician turns to say: "Which of the technologies available is the best one to deal with the clinical problem that I have?"

Roughly one-third of all cancer deaths occur in patients in whom treatment of the primary disease has failed. However, even if patients are to die eventually of metastatic disease, they need not always go through the misery of primary recurrence. This, then, is an area to work on.

A number of contributors to this volume implied that CT will replace the simulator. A healthy approach to diagnosis and therapy is to say: "Let us look at the whole patient. Let us reconstruct in three dimensions what is going on inside the patient and aim the radiation beams at it." Furthermore, the pseudosurgical approach of peering down the beam using a simulator leaves something to be desired. This method can produce a distorted picture, particularly in the breast, if the examiner is inexperienced. Moreover, simulators have often been an excuse for radiotherapists to take poor x-ray pictures. Hence replacement of the simulator by real three-dimensional reconstruction is a good move.

Another point to be considered is how to structure the liaison with one's diagnostic colleagues in centers where the patient numbers are not large enough to justify a dedicated scanner. We need some positive dialogue along these lines—how one can make use, in a positive interactive way, of somebody else's scanner.

A very important point was made by Henkleman. He said that we should aim for a precision no greater than about twice that which a clinician can attain. That is probably a good goal at which to aim. There is no point looking for the 1% error in dose that is impossible to detect. Even under the best radiobiological conditions, we can detect only about a 7% difference in dose (the best percentage ever claimed). Ten percent differences are probably more realistic for most situations. Thus looking for errors of 5% that can be corrected is probably a reasonable goal.

FINAL COMMENT

The field of CT in radiotherapy is maturing quite nicely, the initial ferment having calmed down. Like the maturing of good wine, the maturing of radiotherapy contains the proper elements for quality, both in terms of the pictorial display of information needed to localize a tumor and in terms of the information required for optimizing the distribution of radiation dose. Given the right conditions, our field will reach its maturity, and its fruits will improve with time.

Computed Tomography in Radiation Therapy,
edited by C. C. Ling, C. C. Rogers, and
R. J. Morton. Raven Press, New York © 1983

Physics and Engineering Perspective

J. R. Cunningham

The Ontario Cancer Institute, Toronto, Ontario, Canada

It is clear that computed tomography (CT) has provided an impetus for various new developments, from the clinical point of view as well as in terms of computer hardware and software, and ideas about how to display images and data. The chapters in this volume have presented, for example, interesting examples of imaginative displays, and there has been much discussion about the handling of photon beams and more recently electron beams for treatment planning.

Early in this volume there was a comparison of the uses of CT for diagnostic and therapy purposes, and it was pointed out that the requirements for these two areas are different: The diagnostic use is qualitative, and radiotherapy use is quantitative. These two biases formed the basis for different approaches and different sets of specifications, different needs for the quality of images, and the way those images are handled. It was also pointed out that CT images are perhaps not as quantitative as radiotherapists would like them to be.

Certain specifications were recommended for CT in radiotherapy, including those related to the hardware: a large opening; rapid scans, which have implications for the engineering of cooling targets and moving pieces of machinery on the scanners; the need for thin slices; and the need for many slices. There were also some software-related requirements: the need for scout views and for sagittal, coronal, and even oblique views to be readily available.

According to the literature and contributions to this volume, treatment plans are changed as a result of using CT. Some report that as many as 50% are altered for this reason.

The possibility, and perhaps the inevitability, of the CT scanner performing at least some of the functions now carried out on the simulator was discussed. It was pointed out that the simulator performed two functions distinctly different from those of the CT scanner. One was the "simulating" or "mimicking" of actual treatments once decisions had been made. The other concerned the procedures that are part of the decision-making process itself—part of the treatment planning. It is the latter function that the CT scanner can assume, which might have implications as to the design of future simulators.

The accuracy and stability of scanners and the numbers they produce were discussed, and it was noted that the CT numbers are not a clean function of the densities of tissues. There are artifacts that affect these numbers as well as instabilities in the system itself.

There was some discussion about the problem of scanners being dedicated to radiotherapy. This is an issue that arises often and is not likely to be solved in the immediate future.

There was some discussion about patient position and that it must be the same for the diagnostic CT as it is for radiotherapy. These problems include the effects of position, the difficulty of getting the patient into position because of the size of the opening, and the fact that patients cannot always hold their position. It would be advantageous if the openings were large enough to allow patients to have their arms in treatment position or to allow the proper placement of alignment devices. The problem of positioning the patient for CT is not different in principle from the problem of positioning for radiotherapy itself. As such, it is not a new problem.

There were a number of additional recommendations. We should unequivocally record the locations of scans already taken. There are two resolution requirements: high spatial resolution for diagnostic scanning and high contrast resolution for radiotherapy.

The problem of data transfer from the scanner to the treatment-planning computer was discussed. Magnetic tape is not well liked, although it is, in fact, probably the most universally used medium. Hence in spite of complaints—from the point of view of transferring images from one device to another (from the scanner to the treatment planning computer or from one system to another)—one may always have to deal with the magnetic tape.

Some new developments are called for. These include placing error bars on the output in some way and displaying other types of information, e.g., LET. Of course, this is particularly relevant for heavy-particle irradiation.

When we use the term "optimization," we are manipulating not just doses but also biological responses. Thus sooner or later our treatment planning and processing of the scans must give us some information on biological parameters, e.g., dose responses.

There is the question of accuracy versus precision, with proponents of each. Some deem accuracy to be more important, particularly from the point of view of establishing dose-response curves. I would like to underscore that view. In the long term, the acquisition of further information may be one of the most important contributions the scanner makes in radiotherapy; that is, for the first time, we may be able sometime in the future to generate good response-versus-dose data. At present we draw sigmoid-shaped curves and draw conclusions from them, but we really do not know exactly what those curves look like.

The availability of hard copy that the radiotherapist can carry away and mark is an important advance. One should not be forced to make a decision about a patient at a time when one is under pressure, viewing a terminal with people milling around. There is a great danger of operating in a "no-think mode" under these circumstances.

There are problems in carrying out inhomogeneity corrections. It may be that this should be viewed as a pertubation problem and that the procedure should be to make a good dose calculation for the unperturbed reference (the water-equivalent situation) and deal with inhomogeneities as a correction or an adjustment to that.

Standard methods have been developed for purposes of manual calculations and are indeed still applied in many cases to our computer procedures. Understanding them is indeed still relevant.

Three-dimensional calculations are desirable to some, and some investigators are concerned about the number of slices necessary and how close together slices should be. Another question concerns the resolution that should be required for some of this work. Some strive for an accuracy of about ±5% in the overall dose; this is probably a reasonable figure, but it includes all variations in the chain of events in dosimetry. The implication is that our inhomogeneity corrections should be accurate to approximately the 3% level. That result comes directly from the procedure of adding errors in quadrature.

The discussion on inhomogeneities in the volume dealt only with photon beams, although there was some suggestion that these processes should be examined for electron beams as well.

Monte Carlo calculations received somewhat of a "bad press" at one stage. Whatever the future of this type of calculation, it is certainly true that Monte Carlo calculations are a valid and useful alternative to experiments. They allow one to carry out calculations which can be used as references to which other methods can be compared.

Subject Index

Subject Index

A

Abdominal lymphoma, 50–51
Abdominal region radiotherapy, 37–53
Absorbed dose calculation, 187–196
Absorption coefficient method, 193
Absorption equivalent thickness (AET),
 193, 229–230
Accuracy versus precision, 260
ADAC systems, 183
AET (absorption equivalent thickness),
 193, 229–230
Afterloading technique, 109
Age diffusion equation method, 194
Age diffusion pencil beam, 232
Air, bowel, 49–50
Alignment lights, 151
Alignment marks, 150–151
Aluminum discs, CT value of, 133–135
Anatomy, internal
 involuntary patient motion on, 46–48
 patient position effect on, 42–46
Antrum, carcinoma of, 91, 92, 94–96,
 98
Artifacts, CT, 127–128
Artronix PC-12 system, 189
Astrocytomas, low-grade (LGA),
 85–86
Attenuation coefficient
 effective, 210–211
 mass, 123–124
 total, 124
Attenuation method, effective, 190
Attenuation profiles, X-ray, 122

B

Back-projection, 122
Batho method, 212–214
Beam
 electron, *see* Electron beam *entries*
 photon, *see* Photon beam, external
Bladder area, average, 56

Bladder carcinoma, 57–63
Blur size, 128
Bolus material, 152
Bone, primary sarcomas of, 78
Bowel air, 49–50
Brachytherapy, CT in, 109–118
Brachytherapy dose calculations, 19,
 194–195
Brain, dose response for tumor and,
 84–86
Brain tumors, dose optimization and,
 81–87
Breast, opposite, dose to, 106
Breast cancer
 field configurations in, 102–105
 primary, 99–107
Breast carcinoma, 110, 112–114
Breathing, effect of, 47, 151–152
Bronchogenic carcinoma, 31–33
 staging, 27–31

C

C (correction factor), 209
Calibration, CT, 223–226
Cancer, *see also* Carcinoma; Tumors
 breast, *see* Breast cancer
 colon, 52
 pancreatic, 51–52
Carcinoma, *see also* Cancer; Tumors
 of antrum, 91, 92, 94–96, 98
 bladder, 57–63
 breast, 110, 112–114
 bronchogenic, *see* Bronchogenic
  carcinoma
 esophageal, 33–34
 of larynx, 90, 91
 lung, 155–164
 pancreatic, 43
 prostatic, 64–71, 112, 114–115
 rectal, recurrent, 70–73